Periodontitis: Diagnosis and Treatment

Periodontitis: Diagnosis and Treatment

Editor: Joel Turner

AMERICAN
MEDICAL PUBLISHERS
www.americanmedicalpublishers.com

AMERICAN
MEDICAL PUBLISHERS
www.americanmedicalpublishers.com

Cataloging-in-Publication Data

Periodontitis : diagnosis and treatment / edited by Joel Turner.
p. cm.
Includes bibliographical references and index.
ISBN 978-1-63927-780-3
1. Periodontitis. 2. Periodontal disease. 3. Periodontal disease--Diagnosis.
4. Periodontal disease--Treatment. 5. Dental therapeutics. I. Turner, Joel.
RK450.P4 P47 2023
617.601--dc23

American Medical Publishers,
41 Flatbush Avenue,
1st Floor, New York,
NY 11217, USA

ISBN 978-1-63927-780-3 (Hardback)

Contents

Preface

Periodontitis is an inflammatory condition impacting the tissues adjoining the teeth. In the earlier stages, the gums become red and swollen and it can also result in bleeding. In its severe form, periodontitis can cause bone loss, and teeth might come loose or can fall out. It usually occurs because of the bacteria present in the mouth contaminating the surrounding tissue and teeth. Diagnosis is done by visual examination of the gum tissue surrounding the teeth. The examination can also be done through X-rays searching for loss of bone around the teeth. Its treatment can involve professional cleaning of teeth regularly and practicing good oral hygiene, such as brushing and flossing the teeth. In some of the cases, the treatment can require antibiotics and dental surgery. This book elucidates the concepts and innovative models around prospective developments with respect to the diagnosis and treatment of periodontitis. Those in search of information to further their knowledge will be greatly assisted by it.

The researches compiled throughout the book are authentic and of high quality, combining several disciplines and from very diverse regions from around the world. Drawing on the contributions of many researchers from diverse countries, the book's objective is to provide the readers with the latest achievements in the area of research. This book will surely be a source of knowledge to all interested and researching the field.

In the end, I would like to express my deep sense of gratitude to all the authors for meeting the set deadlines in completing and submitting their research chapters. I would also like to thank the publisher for the support offered to us throughout the course of the book. Finally, I extend my sincere thanks to my family for being a constant source of inspiration and encouragement.

Editor

1

Association of Insufficient or Excess Sleep with Type 2 Diabetes Mellitus in the Presence of Periodontitis

Se-Yeon Kim [1], Ji-Soo Kim [1], Min-Ji Byon [1,2], Hyun Kyung Kang [3] and Jin-Bom Kim [1,2,*]

1 Department of Preventive and Community Dentistry, School of Dentistry, Pusan National University, 49 Busandaehak-ro, Yangsan 50612, Korea; secan00@naver.com (S.-Y.K.); psily1@naver.com (J.-S.K.); kyura2@naver.com (M.-J.B.)
2 BK21 FOUR Project, School of Dentistry, Pusan National University, Yangsan 50612, Korea
3 Department of Dental Hygiene, Silla University, Baekyang-daero, 700, Sasang-gu, Busan 46958, Korea; kanghk75@gmail.com
* Correspondence: jbomkim@pusan.ac.kr

Abstract: We aimed to investigate the effects of sleep duration on impaired fasting glucose and diabetes in Korean adults with periodontal disease. This cross-sectional study was performed using data for 10,465 subjects aged >19 years who completed the periodontal examination and questionnaires in the Sixth Korea National Health and Nutrition Examination Survey (2013–2015). The effect of sleep was confirmed by a complex-sample multinomial logistic regression analysis. Confounding variables were age, sex, household income, education level, smoking status, and sleep duration. Of all participants, 25.7% had periodontitis, of which 28.6% had fasting serum glucose disorder and 14.2% had diabetes. Among participants with periodontitis, the prevalence of diabetes was 1.49 times higher in participants with an average sleep duration of ≥8 h than those with an average sleep duration of 6–7 h. The prevalence of diabetes among participants without periodontitis was 1.49 times and 1.57 times higher in participants with an average sleep duration of ≤5 and ≥8 h, respectively, than those with an average sleep duration of 6–7 h. We found that altered sleep duration may be a risk factor for diabetes and that proper sleep duration is important to control diabetes incidence.

Keywords: sleep; inadequate sleep; excessive sleep; impaired fasting glucose; type 2 diabetes mellitus; periodontitis

1. Introduction

Stress, increasing activity time, and advancements in electronic devices have resulted in major sleep deficits in modern society [1]. People sleep one-third of their lifetime. According to a simple behavioral definition, sleep is a reversible behavioral state of perceptual disengagement from and unresponsiveness to the environment [2]. The circadian sleep rhythm is considered to influence sleep habits [3]. An adequate amount of good-quality sleep affects immune system response and body functioning, so high-quality sleep duration is a very important parameter for health enhancement and maintenance [4]. Moreover, lack of sleep can result in physical and psychological disorders [5].

Inappropriate sleep duration and poor sleep quality have been recently reported to be risk factors for diabetes mellitus (DM) [6,7]. Too much or too little sleep disrupts glycemic control in both prediabetes and type 2 diabetic patients. In addition, inadequate sleep duration increases the risk of obesity and metabolic syndrome and can increase mortality rates [8].

Sleep duration has also been associated with the prevalence of dyslipidemia [9]. Sleep durations above or below the median of 7 to <8 h per night are associated with an increased prevalence of hypertension. Circadian misalignments such as shift work are also associated with an increased risk of developing type 2 diabetes [10]. Korean adults have an average sleep duration of 6.8 h, which is less than the sleep duration in OECD (Organization for Economic Cooperation and Development) countries [11].

Diabetes is a group of chronic metabolic diseases characterized by hyperglycemia resulting from defects in insulin secretion, insulin action, or both. Periodontal disease is known as the sixth most common complication of DM [12,13]. Diabetic patients have been shown to present with a higher prevalence and severity of periodontal disease than non-diabetic patients [14].

The most evident change in patients with diabetes is the decrease in external defense mechanisms and the resultant increased susceptibility to infections. The major signs in the oral cavity are changes in periodontal tissues; gingival enlargement; gingival polyps; formation of abscess; gingival bleeding; periodontal disease; tooth mobility [15]. The prevalence of periodontitis in patients whose serum glucose level was not regulated was higher than that in individuals with regulated glucose levels and patients without glycemic control showed increased severity of periodontal disease [16]. Regardless of the type of diabetes, diabetic patients experience a significant increase in periodontal tissue destruction. Mattout et al. reported that compared to non-diabetic patients, diabetic patients showed greater destruction of periodontal tissues such as gingivitis and clinical attachment loss (CAL) [17].

The risk of diabetes has also been shown to increase with chronic periodontal disease [18]. The pathophysiologic mechanism of the association between periodontal disease and diabetes is likely to be complex and bidirectional [19]. The purpose of this study was to investigate the effects of sleep duration on impaired fasting glucose and diabetes in participants with periodontal disease.

2. Materials and Methods

2.1. Data Sources

This study was based on data obtained from the Sixth Korea National Health and Nutrition Examination Survey (KNHANES-VI), which was conducted from 2013 to 2015 by the Korea Centers for Disease Control and Prevention. KNHANES is conducted annually using a rolling sampling design, which involves a complex, stratified, multistage probability-cluster survey of a large representative sample of the non-institutionalized civilian population in South Korea. The purpose of this survey was to gather national data about the health status and behaviors as well as the nutritional intake of the Korean population. KNHANES-VI included highly structured health-related questionnaires, a nutrition survey, and an oral health examination conducted by trained dentists.

This cross-sectional analysis was restricted to adult participants aged >19 years, among all 15,099 participants in KNHANES-VI, who had undergone the oral health examination and completed the health-related questionnaires (20,219,595 weighted samples). Participants with one or more missing answers in the questionnaires and participants without oral health examination data were excluded from the analysis. We eventually included 10,465 individuals who had undergone clinical oral health examinations and completed the questionnaires, which included data for demographic socioeconomic variables, sleep duration, diabetic status, and prevalence of periodontal disease from KNHANES-VI (Figure 1).

All participants gave their informed consent for inclusion before their participation in the study. The study was conducted in accordance with the Declaration of Helsinki, and the protocol was approved by the Ethics Committee of Institutional Review Board of KCDC (2013-07CON-03-4C, 2013-12EXP-03-5C). Since 2015, the KNHANES has been exempted from review following the Bioethics and Safety Act.

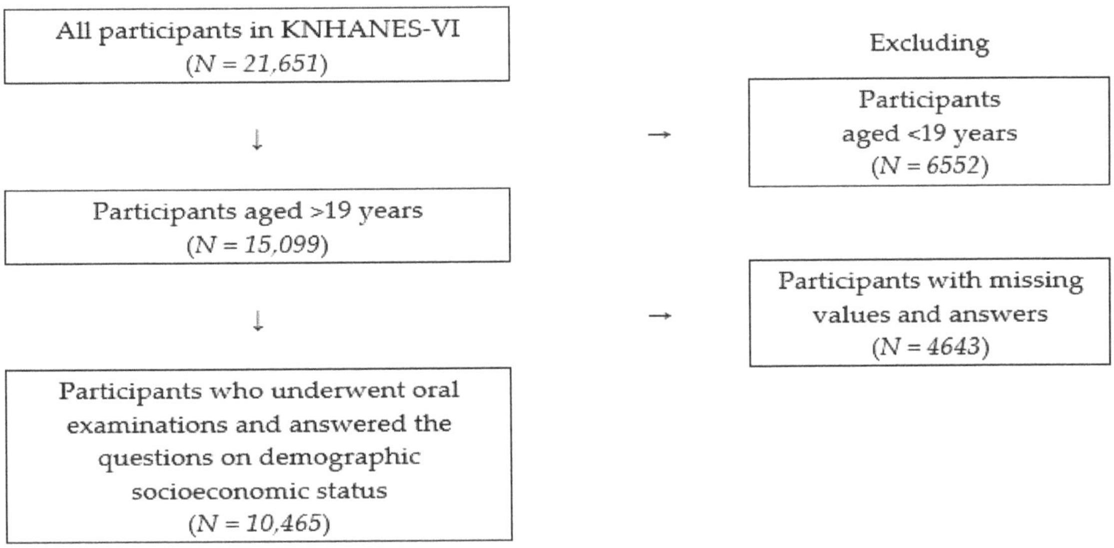

Figure 1. Flowchart for sampling of study participants (KNHANES-VI: Sixth Korea National Health and Nutrition Examination Survey).

2.2. *Variables*

Household income level was determined as the gross household income, divided by the square root of the number of household members and categorized as low, low-middle, middle-high, or high for family size. Educational level was categorized as junior high school, high school, or college and more.

Among the lifestyle variables, smoking status was classified as current smoker, past smoker, and non-smoker. Sleep duration was classified into three groups based on an average sleep time of 6.8 h in this study: inadequate sleep (less than 5 h); normal sleep duration (6 to 7 h); excessive sleep (more than 8 h).

The community periodontal index (CPI) was used to measure periodontitis in the KNHANES, and the oral cavity was divided into the following sextants: #18–14, #13–23, #24–28, #34–38, #33–43, and #44–48. CPI was selected as a tool for evaluating the periodontal health status of population by the World Health Organization (WHO) [20]. The CPI was rated on the following scale from 0 to 4: 0 = normal, 1 = gingivitis with bleeding on probing, 2 = presence of calculus, 3 = probing depth (PD) of 4–5 mm, 4 = PD of 6 mm or more. CPI grades 1 to 2 were defined as absence of periodontitis and CPI grades 3 to 4 were defined as periodontitis. If CPI grades 3 or 4 were present in at least one of the sextants examined for periodontal health, the participant was regarded as a patient with periodontitis. Periodontal assessment was conducted by calibration-trained dentists using a CPI probe (WHO CPI probe, Osung, Korea). Measurements of CAL, pocket depth, and periodontal treatment status were not performed in the KNHANES (2013–2015).

Dependent variables were classified as non-diabetic (fasting serum glucose: FSG < 100 mg/dL), fasting serum glucose disorder ($100 \leq$ FSG ≤ 125 mg/dL), and diabetic (FSG ≥ 126 mg/dL or taking hypoglycemic agent or insulin injection). In this study fasting serum glucose disorder means only impaired glucose not diagnosed with diabetes, and it means prediabetes.

2.3. *Statistical Analysis*

Statistical analyses were performed with the Statistical Package for the Social Sciences (SPSS), version 25 (IBM SPSS Statistics for Windows, Armonk, NY, USA). A plan file was produced by calculating stratified variables with a layer for dispersion estimation, clustered enumeration districts, and weighted samples with an integral weight of 3 years of existing examination survey–nutrition relation weight. Participants were divided into three groups on the basis of the presence or absence of DM and prediabetes. Each group was then divided into a non-periodontitis group and a periodontitis group, according to the CPI value. The chi-squared test was used for assessing the periodontitis status of participants and demographic socioeconomic variables. Statistically significant variables were analyzed by complex-sample multinomial logistic regression analysis to evaluate the odds ratio (OR) and 95% confidence interval (CI). Complex-samples multinomial logistic regression analysis was performed to assess the association between sleep duration and prediabetes and diabetes in participants with periodontal disease. Sex, age, education level, household income level, smoking status, and average sleep duration were used as confounding variables.

3. Results

Of the participants, 25.7% had periodontitis. The prevalence of periodontitis by sex was 58.9% in male and 41.1% in female. The proportion of participants with periodontitis increased with age. Higher education and income levels were associated with a low prevalence of periodontitis. Average sleep duration was 6.8 h in Korean adults. The prevalence of periodontitis for those with ≤5 and ≥8 h of sleep was 16.2% and 17.8%, respectively. In assessments based on smoking status, 23.5% of participants with periodontitis were past smokers and 30.9% were current smokers. Among the participants with periodontitis, 28.6% had prediabetes and 14.2% had diabetes. Among those without periodontal disease, 17.4% had prediabetes and 4.5% had diabetes (Table 1).

Table 1. The prevalence of periodontitis by demographic and socioeconomic parameters, smoking status, and sleeping duration.

	Total (%)			**No Periodontitis (%)**			**Periodontitis (%)**			***p*-Value**
Variable	**DM**	**IFG**	**NDM**	**DM**	**IFG**	**NDM**	**DM**	**IFG**	**NDM**	
Sex										<0.001
Male	8.4	24.4	67.2	5.3	21.5	73.3	15.6	31.2	53.3	
Female	5.7	16.2	78.2	3.9	13.9	82.2	12.3	24.9	62.9	
Age group (years)										<0.001
19–34	1.1	9.1	89.8	0.9	9.0	90.1	3.5	10.2	86.3	
35–44	4.5	20.7	74.8	3.6	18.6	77.7	7.3	28.1	64.5	
45–54	8.3	26.8	64.8	5.8	24.4	69.8	12.6	31.0	56.4	
55–64	16.0	31.8	52.2	12.0	30.8	57.2	20.9	33.0	46.2	
>65	21.2	28.3	50.5	19.6	28.6	51.8	22.8	28.1	49.2	
Education level										<0.001
≤Junior high school	16.2	28.9	55.0	13.4	26.0	60.5	19.4	32.2	48.5	
High school	5.5	20.0	74.5	3.2	17.3	79.5	12.9	28.6	58.5	
≥College	4.6	16.8	78.6	3.2	15.0	81.8	10.4	24.7	64.9	
Household income level										<0.001
Low	13.3	22.2	64.5	7.7	19.2	73.1	22.8	27.2	50.1	
Low-Middle	8.4	19.6	72.0	5.6	17.3	77.1	15.9	25.6	58.4	
Middle-High	5.4	20.2	74.5	3.8	16.7	79.5	10.5	31.1	58.4	
High	5.6	20.3	74.1	3.8	17.7	78.6	12.1	29.3	58.6	
Smoking status										<0.001
Current smoker	7.7	24.1	68.2	4.2	21.0	74.8	14.3	29.8	55.9	
Past smoker	9.7	25.4	64.9	6.1	23.0	70.9	17.5	30.7	51.7	
Non-smoker	5.9	17.1	77.0	4.2	14.7	81.1	12.5	26.6	60.9	
Estimate sleeping duration										<0.001
≤5 h	9.3	23.2	67.5	6.3	20.3	73.4	16.2	30.0	53.8	
6–7 h	6.2	20.3	73.5	4.4	17.3	78.3	11.9	29.4	58.7	
≥8 h	7.5	18.8	73.6	4.1	16.4	79.5	17.8	26.0	56.1	

DM: diabetes mellitus; IFG: impaired fasting glucose; NDM: no diabetes mellitus.

Among participants with periodontitis, in comparison with those with a normal sleep duration of 6–7 h, participants with an average sleep duration of less than 5 h showed a 1.49-fold higher prevalence of diabetes while those with an average sleep duration of ≥8 h showed a 1.57-fold higher prevalence of diabetes. Among participants without periodontitis, in comparison with participants with normal sleep duration, those with an average sleep duration of <5 h showed 1.25-fold and 1.53-fold higher prevalence of prediabetes and diabetes, respectively (Tables 2 and 3). The confounding variables were not controlled in Tables 2 and 3.

Table 2. The prevalence of fasting serum glucose disorder and diabetes without periodontitis.

Variables	IFG	DM
	Crude OR (95% CI)	Crude OR (95% CI)
Sex		
Male	**1.74 (1.53–1.99)**	**1.51 (1.21–1.90)**
Female	1.00	1.00
Age	**0.61 (0.58–0.65)**	**0.41 (0.38–0.45)**
Education level		
≤Junior high school	**2.35 (1.97–2.81)**	**5.66 (4.27–7.51)**
High school	**1.19 (1.03–1.39)**	1.03 (0.77–1.37)
≥College	1.00	1.00
Household income level		
Low	1.17 (0.92–1.47)	**2.20 (1.55–3.11)**
Low-Middle	1.00 (0.83–1.19)	**1.51 (1.12–2.03)**
Middle-High	0.93 (0.79–1.10)	0.99 (0.73–1.36)
High	1.00	1.00
Smoking status		
Current smoker	**1.55 (1.30–1.84)**	1.07 (0.78–1.47)
Past smoker	**1.79 (1.50–2.13)**	**1.66 (1.24–2.23)**
Non-smoker	1.00	1.00
Estimate sleeping duration		
≤5 h	**1.25 (1.03–1.52)**	**1.53 (1.14–2.07)**
≥8 h	0.94 (0.80–1.10)	0.91 (0.70–1.20)
6–7 h	1.00	1.00

IFG: impaired fasting glucose; DM: diabetes mellitus; independent variable: diabetes mellitus (ref. non-diabetic patient); cOR: crude odds ratio; 95% CI: 95% confidence interval; crude odds ratios and 95% confidence interval were estimated by complex-samples multinomial logistic regression analysis; Bold letters indicate statistically significant differences.

To investigate the effect of sleep duration on the prevalence of diabetic participants with periodontitis, a complex-samples multinomial logistic regression analysis was performed after adjusting the findings for sex, age, socioeconomic variables, and smoking (Table 4). Periodontitis increased the prevalence of prediabetes and DM in total. The prevalence of prediabetes and DM adjusted for sleep duration was 1.28-fold higher and 1.86-fold higher in participants with periodontitis. The prevalence of diabetes was 1.49-fold higher in periodontitis participants with an average sleep duration of >8 h. However, in participants without periodontitis with a sleep duration of ≥8 h, the prevalence of diabetes was 1.57-fold higher than that in participants with a normal sleep duration of 6–7 h. Moreover, the diabetes incidence was 1.49-fold higher in participants without periodontitis with sleep duration of ≤5 h compared to that in participants with normal sleep duration of 6–7 h.

Table 3. The prevalence of fasting serum glucose disorder and diabetes with periodontitis.

Variables	IFG	DM
	Crude OR (95% CI)	Crude OR (95% CI)
Sex		
Male	**1.48 (1.22–1.79)**	**1.50 (1.18–1.90)**
Female	1.00	1.00
Age	**0.76 (0.70–0.82)**	**0.56 (0.51–0.63)**
Education level		
≤Junior high school	**1.74 (1.37–2.22)**	**2.48 (1.82–3.38)**
High school	**1.28 (1.01–1.64)**	1.37 (0.98–1.91)
≥College	1.00	1.00
Household income level		
Low	1.08 (0.81–1.45)	**2.21 (1.56–3.12)**
Low-Middle	0.88 (0.68–1.14)	1.32 (0.96–1.83)
Middle-High	1.06 (0.83–1.36)	0.87 (0.61–1.23)
High	1.00	1.00
Smoking status		
Current smoker	1.22 (0.97–1.53)	1.24 (0.93–1.67)
Past smoker	1.36 (1.07–1.72)	**1.65 (1.25–2.19)**
Non-smoker	1.00	1.00
Estimate sleeping duration		
≤5 h	1.11 (0.85–1.46)	**1.49 (1.09–2.04)**
≥8 h	0.93 (0.74–1.16)	**1.57 (1.19–2.07)**
6–7 h	1.00	1.00

IFG: impaired fasting glucose; DM: diabetes mellitus; independent variable: diabetes mellitus (ref. non-diabetic patient); crude OR: crude odds ratio; 95% CI: 95% confidence interval; crude odds ratios and 95% confidence interval were estimated by complex-samples multinomial logistic regression analysis; bold letters indicate statistically significant differences.

Table 4. Effect of sleep duration on fasting serum glucose and diabetes with periodontitis and non-periodontitis.

Variables			IFG	DM
			Adjusted OR (95% CI)	Adjusted OR (95% CI)
Total	Periodontitis	Yes	**1.28 (1.13–1.46)**	**1.86 (1.55–2.23)**
		No	1.00	1.00
	Sleep duration	≤5 h	1.09 (0.92–1.30)	1.17 (0.93–1.48)
		≥8 h	1.03 (0.90–1.18)	**1.29 (1.05–1.57)**
		6–7 h	1.00	1.00
Non-Periodontitis	Sleep duration	≤5 h	1.12 (0.91–1.38)	**1.49 (1.09–2.04)**
		≥8 h	1.13 (0.95–1.34)	**1.57 (1.19–2.07)**
		6–7 h	1.00	1.00
Periodontitis	Sleep duration	≤5 h	1.06 (0.80–1.41)	1.24 (0.89–1.73)
		≥8 h	0.90 (0.72–1.14)	**1.49 (1.12–1.98)**
		6–7 h	1.00	1.00

IFG: impaired fasting glucose; DM: diabetes mellitus; independent variable: diabetes mellitus (ref. non-diabetic participants); adjusted for sex, age, educational level, income level, smoking status; adjusted OR: adjusted odds ratio; 95% CI: 95% confidence interval. Adjusted odds ratios and 95% confidence intervals were estimated by complex-samples multinomial logistic regression analysis; Bold letters indicate statistically significant differences.

4. Discussion

The pathophysiologic mechanism underlying the association between sleep and DM is likely to be complex and bidirectional. Epidemiological evidence on this link, however, is not yet conclusively established. Therefore, we investigated the effects of sleep duration on impaired fasting glucose levels and diabetes in participants with periodontal disease by using data from the Sixth KNHANES

(2013–2015). We found that altered sleep duration could be a risk factor for an increased incidence of diabetes regardless of periodontitis, and that proper sleep duration is important for diabetes.

The sleep–wake cycle is a complex phenomenon that encompasses several physiological and behavioral oscillations [21]. Sleep is a biological process that is essential for all human beings and is the most basic requirement for a healthy daily life. Insufficient sleep duration increases the risk of premature death [22]. In the normal sleep–wake cycle, immune system indicators like the number of undifferentiated naïve T cells and the production of pro-inflammatory cytokines exhibit peaks during early nocturnal sleep, whereas circulating numbers of immune cells with immediate effects or functions, like cytotoxic natural killer cells, as well as anti-inflammatory cytokine activity peak during daytime wakefulness [4]. Thus, sleep health may be promoted for therapeutic control of chronic infections and inflammatory and neuropsychiatric diseases [23].

In addition, short sleep duration could be a significant risk factor for diabetes [6]. Sleep deprivation has become a global phenomenon, and short sleep duration adversely affects human physical health [24]. Adequate amount and quality of sleep are important for metabolic control in patients with type 2 diabetes. Too short or too long sleep durations disrupt glycemic control in both prediabetic and type 2 diabetic patients. The development of impaired glucose tolerance is associated with periodontitis. Periodontitis is more common in diabetes patients and worsens with this condition. In particular, duration of diabetes, fasting serum glucose, glycated hemoglobin (HbA1c) levels, and compliance to self-management of diabetes were significantly correlated with periodontal health among individuals with type 2 diabetes [25].

Periodontal disease is a chronic inflammatory disease characterized by the destruction of the tooth-supporting connective tissues in response to subgingival infection with various periodontal pathogens [14]. The risk of periodontitis has been reported to be 1.34 times higher in subjects with a sleep duration of less than 7 h per day on average [26]. In this study, however, the prevalence of diabetes associated with periodontal disease was observed in participants with sleep durations <5 h or with more >8 h than in participants with normal sleep duration. The prevalence of diabetes was 1.49-fold higher in periodontitis participants with an average sleep duration of <5 h compared to that in participants with a sleep duration of 6–7 h, while the prevalence was 1.57-fold higher in those with a typical average sleep duration of ≥8 h. In the case of fasting serum glucose, the prediabetes stage, the incidence of prediabetes without periodontal disease was higher with longer sleep duration than in participants with proper sleep duration. Sleep problems were associated with disturbances in cortisol responses to stress, as well as changes diurnal cortisol output in people with DM [27]. The increasing level of cortisol make it difficult to control fasting serum glucose in DM. Therefore, sleep quality deteriorated due to more than usual or insufficient sleep can lead to an increase in prediabetes and DM. The results of this study were similar to previous result of another study outlining the relationship between sleep duration and periodontitis in Korean adult women [28].

Nakada et al. reported that fatigue worsened systemic health in rats and increased gingival inflammation and alveolar bone loss in experimental periodontitis [29]. In our study, the prevalence of diabetes was 1.49-fold higher in periodontitis participants with an average sleep duration of ≥8 h than that in participants with normal sleep duration. However, corresponding prevalence in participants without periodontitis who slept for ≥8 h was 1.57-fold higher compared to that in participants with a normal sleep duration. Moreover, the diabetes incidence was 1.49-fold higher in participants without periodontitis and sleep duration ≤5 h compared to that in participants with normal sleep duration. Dumitrescu et al. reported that the disturbed sleep index was associated with oral health status and behavior [30]. This study had some limitations as it was a cross-sectional analysis and based solely on information gained from KNHANES-VI. Although we analyzed the prevalence of prediabetes and DM in participants without periodontitis and with periodontitis, more various variables should be considered to establish the accurate relationship as type 2 diabetes is a multifactorial disease. Furthermore, it is necessary to study variables that may be associated with hormones as well as prediabetes and DM.

5. Conclusions

Our findings suggested that periodontitis can increase the risk of prediabetes and DM. We also investigated the effects of sleep duration on prediabetes and DM in participants with periodontitis and non-periodontitis. We found that longer/shorter sleep duration may be a risk factor for diabetes and that the proper sleep duration could be good for prevention of diabetes. It is necessary to develop a comprehensive health promotion program that can improve the sleeping habits of adults and to combine oral health programs to prevent periodontitis and diabetes.

Author Contributions: All authors contributed extensively to the work presented in this paper. S.-Y.K. wrote the entire manuscript. J.-B.K. provided the idea for the study. M.-J.B. performed the statistical analyses. J.-S.K. and H.K.K. performed the literature review. J.-B.K. conceived the study and coordinated and helped with the drafting of the manuscript. All authors have read and agreed to the published version of the manuscript.

References

1. Akerstedt, T.; Knutsson, A.; Westerholm, P.; Theorell, T.; Alfredsson, L.; Kecklund, G. Sleep Disturbances, Work Stress and Work Hours: A Cross-Sectional Study. *J. Psychosom. Res.* **2002**, *53*, 741–748. [CrossRef]
2. Carskadon, M.A.; Dement, W.C. *Normal Human Sleep: An Overview Principles and Practice of Sleep Medicine*, 5th ed.; Elsevier Saunders: St. Louis, MO, USA, 2005; pp. 13–23.
3. Liu, X.; Uchiyama, M.; Shibui, K.; Kim, K.; Kudo, Y.; Tagaya, H.; Suzuki, H.; Okawa, M. Diurnal preference, sleep habits, circadian sleep propensity and melatonin rhythm in healthy human subjects. *Neurosci. Lett.* **2000**, *280*, 199–202. [CrossRef]
4. Besedovsky, L.; Lange, T.; Born, J. Sleep and immune function. *Pflugers Arch.* **2012**, *463*, 121–137. [CrossRef] [PubMed]
5. Cauter, E.V.; Spiegel, K.; Tasali, E.; Leproult, R. Metabolic consequences of sleep and sleep loss. *Sleep Med.* **2008**, *9*, S23–S28. [CrossRef]
6. Gangwisch, J.E.; Heymsfield, S.B.; Boden-Albala, B.; Buijs, R.M.; Kreier, F.; Pickering, T.G.; Rundle, A.G.; Zammit, G.K.; Malaspina, D. Sleep duration as a risk factor for diabetes incidence in a large US sample. *Sleep* **2007**, *30*, 1667–1673. [CrossRef]
7. Knutson, K.L.; Ryden, A.M.; Mander, B.A.; Cauter, E.V. Role of sleep duration and quality in the risk and severity of type 2 diabetes mellitus. *Arch. Intern. Med.* **2006**, *166*, 1768–1774. [CrossRef]
8. Knutson, K.L. Sleep Duration and Cardiometabolic Risk: A Review of the Epidemiologic Evidence. *Best Pract. Res. Clin. Endocrinol. Metab.* **2010**, *24*, 731–743. [CrossRef]
9. Lee, H.J.; Jeong, Y.W.; Kim, H.J.; Jeong, R.H. Association between Sleep Duration and Prevalence of Dyslipidemia in Korean Adults: The Sixth Korean National Health and Nutrition Examination Survey. *Korean J. Family Pract.* **2019**, *9*, 485–491. [CrossRef]
10. Knutsson, A.; Kempe, A. Shift work and diabetes—A systematic review. *Chronobiol. Int.* **2014**, *31*, 1146–1151. [CrossRef]
11. OECD iLibrary. OECD Social Indicators. Available online: https://doi.org/10.1787/19991290 (accessed on 1 June 2020).
12. Löe, H. Periodontal disease: The sixth complication of diabetes mellitus. *Diabetes Care* **1993**, *16*, 329–334. [CrossRef]
13. Saini, R.; Saini, S.; Sugandha, R. Periodontal disease: The sixth complication of diabetes. *J. Family Community Med.* **2011**, *18*, 31. [CrossRef] [PubMed]
14. Pihlstrom, B.L.; Michalowicz, B.S.; Johnson, N.W. Periodontal diseases. *Lancet* **2005**, *366*, 1809–1820. [CrossRef]
15. Casanova, L.; Hughes, F.J.; Preshaw, P.M. Diabetes and periodontal disease: A two-way relationship. *Br. Dent. J.* **2014**, *217*, 433–437. [CrossRef] [PubMed]
16. Tsai, C.; Hayes, C.; Taylor, G.W. Glycemic control of type 2 diabetes and severe periodontal disease in the US adult population. *Community Dent. Oral Epidemiol.* **2002**, *30*, 182–192. [CrossRef] [PubMed]
17. Mattout, C.; Bourgeois, D.; Bouchard, P. Type 2 diabetes and periodontal indicators: Epidemiology in France 2002–2003. *J. Periodontal Res.* **2006**, *41*, 253–258. [CrossRef]
18. Gurav, A.; Jadhav, V. Periodontitis and risk of diabetes mellitus. *J. Diabetes* **2011**, *3*, 21–28. [CrossRef] [PubMed]

19. Ship, J.A. Diabetes and oral health: An overview. *J. Am. Dent. Assoc.* **2003**, *134*, 4S–10S. [CrossRef] [PubMed]
20. Ainamo, J.; Barmes, D.; Beagrie, G.; Cutress, T.; Martin, J.; Sardo-Infirri, J. Development of the World Health Organization (WHO) community periodontal index of treatment needs (CPITN). *Int. Dent. J.* **1982**, *32*, 281–291.
21. Brown, R.E.; Basheer, R.; McKenna, J.T.; Strecker, R.E.; McCarley, R.W. Control of sleep and wakefulness. *Physiol. Rev.* **2012**, *92*, 1087–1187. [CrossRef]
22. Kim, Y.; Wilkens, L.R.; Schembre, S.M.; Henderson, B.E.; Kolonel, L.N.; Goodman, M.T. Insufficient and excessive amounts of sleep increase the risk of premature death from cardiovascular and other diseases: The Multiethnic Cohort Study. *Prev. Med.* **2013**, *57*, 377–385. [CrossRef]
23. Irwin, M.R. Why sleep is important for health: A psychoneuroimmunology perspective. *Annu. Rev. Psychol.* **2015**, *66*, 143–172. [CrossRef]
24. Grover, V.; Malhotra, R.; Kaur, H. Exploring association between sleep deprivation and chronic periodontitis: A pilot study. *J. Indian Soc. Periodontol.* **2015**, *19*, 304–307. [CrossRef]
25. Kim, E.-K.; Lee, S.G.; Choi, Y.H.; Won, K.C.; Moon, J.S.; Merchant, A.T.; Lee, H.-K. Association between diabetes-related factors and clinical periodontal parameters in type-2 diabetes mellitus. *BMC Oral Health* **2013**, *13*, 64. [CrossRef]
26. Wiener, R.C. Relationship of routine inadequate sleep duration and periodontitis in a nationally representative sample. *Sleep Disord.* **2016**, *2016*, 9158195. [CrossRef] [PubMed]
27. Hackett, R.A.; Dal, Z.; Steptoe, A. The relationship between sleep problems and cortisol in people with type 2 diabetes. *Psychoneuroendocrinology* **2020**, *117*, 104688. [CrossRef] [PubMed]
28. Do, K.-Y.; Lee, E.-S. Relationship between Sleep Duration and Periodontitis in Korean Adult Women: Data from Korea National Health and Nutrition Examination Survey 2014. *J. Dent. Hyg. Sci.* **2017**, *17*, 298–305. [CrossRef]
29. Nakada, T.; Kato, T.; Numabe, Y. Effects of fatigue from sleep deprivation on experimental periodontitis in rats. *Comp. Study* **2015**, *50*, 131–137. [CrossRef] [PubMed]
30. Dumitrescu, A.L.; Toma, C.; Lascu, V. Associations among sleep disturbance, vitality, fatigue and oral health. *Oral Health Prev. Dent.* **2010**, *8*, 323–330.

2

German Dentists' Preferences for the Treatment of Apical Periodontitis

Jonas Conrad [1], Jan Retelsdorf [2], Sameh Attia [3], Christof Dörfer [1] and Mohamed Mekhemar [1,*]

1 Clinic for Conservative Dentistry and Periodontology, School of Dental Medicine, Christian-Albrecht's University, 24105 Kiel, Germany; conrad@konspar.uni-kiel.de (J.C.); doerfer@konspar.uni-kiel.de (C.D.)
2 Department of General, Faculty of Education, Intercultural and International Comparative Education University of Hamburg, 20146 Hamburg, Germany; jan.retelsdorf@uni-hamburg.de
3 Department of Cranio Maxillofacial Surgery, Justus-Liebig University, 35392 Giessen, Germany; sameh.attia@dentist.med.uni-giessen.de
* Correspondence: mekhemar@konspar.uni-kiel.de

Abstract: Currently, there is no standard treatment protocol for apical periodontitis (AP). Thus, restorable teeth might get extracted and replaced prosthetically. This study evaluated German dentists' preferred AP treatment decisions and the influencing factors for selecting tooth retention by initial/repeated surgical/non-surgical root-canal treatment (RCT) or extraction with/without prosthetic replacement. Through an online-survey, participants ($n = 260$) rated different treatment options for four case scenarios with AP in anterior/posterior teeth without/with previous RCT. Statistical analysis included the Friedman test for intra-case comparisons and Chi-squared test for factor-associations ($p \leq 0.05$). Tooth retention using initial/repeated RCT was ranked first in all scenarios and rated as (very) appropriate by most participants, while implant-supported crowns (ISC) and apicoectomy had the second ratings. ISC were preferred more on posterior teeth or previous root-canal-treated teeth. Rating levels of treatment options displayed significant differences for all case scenarios. Posterior tooth retention by RCT demonstrated a significant association with work experience. Tooth retention with previous RCT displayed a significant correlation with dentists' privately insured patients. Most dentists preferred tooth preserving with initial/repeated RCT, while others selected non-evidence-based choices. This reflects a lack of consensus of AP treatment decisions in Germany. Fixed treatment guidelines and further evaluation of treatment–decision-correlated factors are recommended for correct treatment planning.

Keywords: Root canal treatment; endodontic treatment; apical periodontitis; oral disease; health-related quality of life; German dentists; treatment decision

1. Introduction

Helping patients to keep a healthy and functional dentition is an ultimate aim of dentistry and public oral health. Besides being a marker of functional aging, patients' loss of dentition has been linked with a higher occurrence of dementia, psychological distress, and a poor health related quality of life [1,2]. An important dilemma often discussed by clinicians is when teeth should be extracted and restored instead [3]. This problem should be increasingly recognized by the dental society as making treatment decisions that do not consider the patients' preferences or quality of life can affect the public health severely.

Apical periodontitis (AP), a highly prevalent dental disease resulting from an endodontic infection of the root canal system, is one of the main reasons for tooth extraction [4]. The prevalence of AP increases during life and by the age of 50 years one in two individuals is affected by this disease [4]. Treatment options of AP include mainly root-canal treatment (RCT) or the extraction of the affected tooth [5]. In case of tooth extraction, the edentulous area can be restored by fixed or removable dental prostheses (FDP and RDP, respectively), implant supported crowns (ISC), or remains edentulous. Another possible treatment modality includes apicoectomy after an unsuccessful RCT [6].

Previous studies present different perspectives among dentists on the correct treatment plan for AP [4,7–12]. Besides several disagreements about radiographic analyses and radiographic based treatment decisions, dentists also display no agreement on treatment choices in different clinical circumstances. Furthermore, the investigations display that clinical decision-making may be reliant on the dentist's clinical experience and education, as well as the working environment and oral health systems in the involved countries [4,7,8,13,14]. By identifying and addressing this gap among clinicians' treatment decisions, an academic society can provide predictive guidelines and an effective development of skills and knowledge to the dentists (as required) to preserve and improve the oral public health and quality of life of the patients.

Earlier investigations have compared clinical decisions for the treatment of AP among dentists in different countries using survey models [4,7–10,12]. Several surveys involved investigations of patients' periapical radiographs under a specified clinical scenario, after which the dentists chose the preferred treatment plan. Other surveys sent diverse clinical scenarios to different dentist groups and revealed that clinical backgrounds and experiences, as well as factors related to the region of dental education and practice can affect the chosen treatment plan for AP. To the best of our knowledge, there is no definite treatment protocol for teeth with AP, raising the concerns that some affected but restorable teeth might get extracted and affect the oral health-related quality of life of patients negatively [5,15,16].

In Germany, all residents are required by law to have a health insurance. Nearly 90% of the inhabitants have statutory health insurance and about 10% are privately insured. Statutory insurers basically offer the same standard medical treatments, prescription drugs, and health care services. The standard benefits likewise include dental check-ups, dental and gingival treatment, as well as orthodontic procedures. When it comes to dental implants and prosthetics, statutory health insurers recompense a fixed amount. Before starting any prosthetic or implant-associated dental work, the dentist provides a treatment and cost plan that must be submitted to the insurer. The insurer afterwards decides the costs covered and how much the patient has to pay by himself. Private health insurers may cover special services as treatment by a senior consultant or head of department, having a private hospital room, as well as special dental treatments including prostheses and dental implants. The included private insurance benefits are specified in the individual policy [17].

Thus, the aim of the current survey was to evaluate German dentists' preferences for the treatment of teeth with AP in northern Germany via four different case scenarios including the selection of tooth retention using RCT compared to tooth extraction followed by replacement with ISC/FDP/RDP or no replacement. Furthermore, this survey intended to investigate whether various influencing factors are associated to the first-ranked treatment option selected for each of the different case scenarios presented in the survey.

2. Materials and Methods

2.1. Study Population and Methodology

In the current study, data on dentists' treatment selection preferences was collected using an online survey as previously described [10] with slight modifications in the available clinical scenarios to adapt to the German oral healthcare system. The questionnaire was translated into the German language by an authorized translation expert and was pilot tested by a focus group of ten dentists from northern Germany. The focus group represented dentists from private practices and university clinics. It included variations of gender, age, as well as in work and educational experience. Furthermore, the survey was validated [18] by five experts in the fields of dentistry, psychology, and web-based surveys at the University of Kiel and transformed into an online survey using a web-based survey tool (Unipark, QuestBack GmbH, Cologne, Germany). After the approval by the University of Kiel Ethics Board (D499/16) the survey link was sent by email to all registered dentists at the state dental council (Zahnärztekammer Schleswig-Holstein, Kiel, Germany) in the northern state of Schleswig-Holstein, Germany ($N = 2270$). The introductory text in the email briefly explained the research project and assured anonymity and voluntary participation to the dentists. No financial incentives or gifts were promised to the participants and no exclusion criteria were defined (e.g., age, gender, or nationality).

In the first part of the questionnaire participants' sociodemographic data such as gender, work experience, current employment situation, specialty education, location of their practice/workplace, performed treatment spectrum, and the percentage of privately insured patients in their dental practice/workplace was gathered.

In the second part participants were provided with four written, clinical scenarios of a 50-year-old patient suffering from an AP on a permanent tooth:

Case Scenario 1 (CS1)—AP on a permanent, anterior tooth with no root canal filling;
Case Scenario 2 (CS2)—AP on a permanent, posterior tooth with no root canal filling;
Case Scenario 3 (CS3)—AP on a permanent, anterior tooth with root canal filling;
Case Scenario 4 (CS4)—AP on a permanent, posterior tooth with root canal filling.

For CS1 and CS2, participants were asked to assess the following treatment options according to their preferences:

1. Tooth retention using RCT followed by a coronal restoration;
2. Tooth retention using apicoectomy followed by a coronal restoration;
3. Tooth extraction followed by replacement with ISC;
4. Tooth extraction followed by replacement with FDP;
5. Tooth extraction followed by replacement with RDP;
6. Tooth extraction followed by no replacement.

For CS3 and CS4, participants were asked to assess the following treatment options according to their preferences:

1. Tooth retention using non-surgical endodontic retreatment followed by a coronal restoration;
2. Tooth retention using apicoectomy followed by a coronal restoration;
3. Tooth extraction followed by replacement with ISC;
4. Tooth extraction followed by replacement with FDP;
5. Tooth extraction followed by replacement with RDP;
6. Tooth extraction followed by no replacement.

All fictive patients presented in the case scenarios had private health insurance and no medical records or underlying diseases to eliminate bias in decision-making caused by financial or systemic health situations of the patients. The response scale for each treatment option displayed three choices: 'very appropriate', 'appropriate', and 'not appropriate'.

2.2. Sample Size Calculation

To determine the number of responding dentists needed for a significant database, the following conditions were defined for the sample size calculation:

1. Number of sent emails to registered dentists in the northern state of Schleswig-Holstein, Germany ($N = 2270$);
2. A confidence level of 95%;
3. A margin of error of 6%.

Based on these conditions it was determined that within Schleswig-Holstein in northern Germany at least 239 dentists were needed for a statistically significant sample size.

2.3. Statistical Analysis

Data from the online questionnaire was digitally recorded by the web-based survey tool and analyzed using PASW (Predictive Analysis Software) Statistics for Windows software (SPSS Inc., Version 18.0.0, Chicago, Ill., USA). The Shapiro–Wilk-Test was performed to test for normality of the data. Data was not normally distributed. Statistical comparisons of the different ratings of treatment choices by the participants within each case scenario were performed using the non-parametric Friedman test. The mean rating value points of each treatment option was evaluated by giving value points (VP) to each answer of the participants ("very appropriate" = 1VP; "appropriate" = 2VP and "not appropriate" = 3VP). Chi-square tests for independence were used for association analysis between participant-related factors (gender, work experience, location of practice, treatment spectrum in the dental practice and percentage of privately insured patients) and the most preferred treatment options (smallest mean rating value points) stated in each case scenario of the survey. Statistical significance was set at $p < 0.05$.

3. Results

3.1. Participation and Sociodemographic Data

A total of 366 dentists participated in the survey with 260 completed questionnaires resulting in a statistically significant sample. Participants included female and male dentists with different years of work experience. The majority of respondents (71.5%) were self-employed in their practice. Most of the participants were general practitioners with few specialized dentists mainly in the fields of implantology, endodontics, and periodontology.

The locations of the respondents' workplaces were evenly distributed with the smallest group located in the suburban area (18.5%).

Slightly more than one third (34.6%) of the respondents stated a proportion of 20–40% of privately insured patients, while the majority of participants indicated to have a smaller percentage of statutory insured patients (Table 1)

Table 1. Sociodemographic and professional data of the survey participants.

Sociodemographic and Professional Characteristics	Distribution (n = 260)
Sex	
Male	149 (57.3%)
Female	111 (42.7%)
Work experience	
0–9 years	70 (26.9%)
10–19 years	56 (21.5%)
>19 years	134 (51.5%)
Employment status [1]	
Currently practicing in own practice	186 (71.5%)
Employed dentist in (panel/private) practice	36 (13.8%)
Employed dentist during assistantship in (panel/private) practice	17 (6.5%)
Director/head of a university clinic	0 (0%)
Senior dentist at a university clinic	2 (0.8%)
Assistant dentist at a university clinic	12 (4.6%)
Medical officer (military)	3 (1.2%)
Not practicing/retired	5 (1.9)

Table 1. *Cont.*

Sociodemographic and Professional Characteristics	Distribution (n = 260)
Dental specialization [1]	
No specialization/GP	250 (96.2%)
Orthodontist	0 (0%)
Oral surgery	6 (2.3%)
Periodontology	2 (0.8%)
Public health	0 (0%)
Maxillofacial surgery	2 (0.8%)
Certified focus of treatment [1]	
Geriatric dentistry	4 (1.5%)
Endodontology	29 (11.2%)
Functional analysis/therapy	4 (1.5%)
Implantology	39 (15.0%)
Aesthetic dentistry	4 (1.5%)
Pediatric dentistry	8 (3.1%)
Laser dentistry	0 (0%)
Periodontology	21 (8.1%)
Prosthodontics	10 (3.8%)
Restorative dentistry	4 (1.5%)
Other dental specialization or focus of treatment	8 (3.1%)
Location of practice	
Inner city/commercial subcenter	61 (23.5%)
Urban area	75 (28.8%)
Suburban area	48 (18.5%)
Rural area	76 (29.2%)
Provided treatment services [1]	
Root canal treatment	255 (98.1%)
Tooth extraction	249 (95.8%)
Implantology (with/without restoration)	131 (50.4%)
Non-surgical endodontic retreatment	214 (82.3%)
Endodontic microsurgery (e.g., apicoectomy)	86 (33.1%)
FDP	251 (96.5%)
RDP	243 (93.5%)
Privately insured patients	
0–20%	150 (57.7%)
20–40%	90 (34.6%)
40–60%	17 (6.5%)
60–80%	3 (1.2%)
80–100%	0 (0%)

[1] The sum of this group may be more than n = 260 (100%) because multiple answers were possible. GP: General practitioner; FDP: Fixed dental prostheses; RDP: Removable dental prostheses.

Statements about the provided treatment services showed varying distributions of treatment spectra (TS1–TS4) performed in the dentists' workplaces (Table 2).

Table 2. Proportions of the four subgroups based on categories of treatment spectrum performed in the dental practice.

Subgroup	Distribution (n = 260)
TS1: practicing endodontics but not implants	129 (49.6%)
TS2: practicing implants but not endodontics	5 (1.9%)
TS3: practicing both	126 (48.5%)
TS4: practicing neither	0 (0%)

3.2. Rating of the Case Scenarios

Tooth retention using RCT followed by a coronal restoration was the first-ranked treatment option in CS1 (Table 3) and CS2 (Table 4), while tooth retention using non-surgical endodontic retreatment followed by a coronal restoration was the first-ranked treatment option in CS3 (Table 5) and CS4 (Table 6). Second choice treatment preferences in all case scenarios were either tooth retention using apicoectomy followed by a coronal restoration or tooth extraction followed by replacement with ISC (Tables 3–6)

Table 3. Preferences of survey participants regarding case scenario 1 in %, mean rating value and results of the Friedman test comparing all treatment choices.

Case Scenario 1: AP on a Permanent, Anterior Tooth with no Root Canal Filling					
Treatment Choices	Very appropriate (1 value point)	Appropriate (2 value points)	Not appropriate (3 value points)	Mean rating value	Friedman test
Tooth retention using RCT followed by a coronal restoration	84.6	15.0	0.4	1.2	$p < 0.001$
Tooth retention using apicoectomy followed by a coronal restoration	9.2	42.7	48.1	2.4	
Tooth extraction followed by replacement with ISC	6.2	50.4	43.5	2.4	
Tooth extraction followed by replacement with FDP	1.9	36.9	61.2	2.6	
Tooth extraction followed by replacement with RDP	0.0	7.3	92.7	2.9	
Tooth extraction followed by no replacement	0.0	2.3	97.7	3.0	

AP: Apical periodontitis. RCT: Root canal treatment. ISC: Implant supported crown. FDP: Fixed dental prostheses. RDP: Removable dental prostheses.

Table 4. Pre-preferences of survey participants regarding case scenario 2 in %, mean rating value and results of the Friedman test comparing all treatment choices.

Case Scenario 2: AP on a Permanent, Posterior Tooth with no Root Canal Filling					
Treatment Choices	Very appropriate (1 value point)	Appropriate (2 value points)	Not appropriate (3 value points)	Mean rating value	Friedman test
Tooth retention using RCT followed by a coronal restoration	77.3	21.5	1.2	1.2	$p < 0.001$
Tooth extraction followed by replacement with ISC	12.7	54.2	33.1	2.2	
Tooth retention using apicoectomy followed by a coronal restoration	6.9	44.6	48.5	2.4	
Tooth extraction followed by replacement with FDP	4.6	44.2	51.2	2.5	
Tooth extraction followed by no replacement	0.4	26.2	73.5	2.7	
Tooth extraction followed by replacement with RDP	0.4	16.2	83.5	2.8	

Table 5. Preferences of survey participants regarding case scenario 3 in %, mean rating value and results of the Friedman test comparing all treatment choices.

Case Scenario 3: AP on a Permanent, Anterior Tooth with Root Canal Filling					
Treatment Choices	very appropriate (1 value point)	Appropriate (2 value points)	not appropriate (3 value points)	MEAN rating value	Friedman test
Tooth retention using non-surgical endodontic retreatment followed by a coronal restoration	76.5	23.1	0.4	1.2	$p < 0.001$
Tooth retention using apicoectomy followed by a coronal restoration	16.9	43.1	40.0	2.2	
Tooth extraction followed by replacement with ISC	7.7	56.2	36.2	2.3	
Tooth extraction followed by replacement with FDP	2.3	42.7	55.0	2.5	
Tooth extraction followed by replacement with RDP	0.0	13.1	86.9	2.9	
Tooth extraction followed by no replacement	0.0	3.1	96.9	3.0	

Table 6. Preferences of survey participants regarding case scenario 4 in %, mean rating value and results of the Friedman test comparing all treatment choices.

Case Scenario 4: AP on a Permanent, Posterior Tooth with Root Canal Filling					
Treatment Choices	Very appropriate (1 value point)	Appropriate (2 value points)	Not appropriate (3 value points)	Mean rating value	Friedman test
Tooth retention using non-surgical endodontic retreatment followed by a coronal restoration	63.5	35.4	1.2	1.4	$p < 0.001$
Tooth extraction followed by replacement with ISC	14.2	56.5	29.2	2.2	
Tooth retention using apicoectomy followed by a coronal restoration	12.7	45.4	41.9	2.3	
Tooth extraction followed by replacement with FDP	4.6	43.5	51.9	2.5	
Tooth extraction followed by no replacement	0.8	26.5	72.7	2.7	
Tooth extraction followed by replacement with RDP	0.4	17.7	81.9	2.8	

Statistical analysis displayed statistically significant differences ($p < 0.05$) between all four case scenarios' mean rating values of the different treatment options (Tables 3–6).

For CS2, the factors' analysis showed a significant positive correlation ($p < 0.05$) between the first-ranked treatment option (tooth retention after RCT/retreatment) and increasing work experience of the dentists. Significantly more female dentists (83%) also decided to preserve the tooth in CS2 by endodontic treatment, compared to the male counterpart (72.5%). For CS3 and CS4, a significant positive correlation was observed between the first-ranked treatment option (tooth retention by non-surgical endodontic retreatment) and higher numbers of privately insured patients at the dental practice (Table 7).

Table 7. *p*-value of statistical association analysis by Chi-squared tests between the first-ranked treatment option of the four different case scenarios and different factors.

Case Scenarios	Gender	Work Experience	Location of the Practice	Category of Performed Treatment Spectrum	Percentage of Privately Insured Patients
Case scenario 1	0.29	0.11	0.32	0.52	0.42
Case scenario 2	0.05	0.01	0.94	0.80	0.92
Case scenario 3	0.09	0.07	0.34	0.15	<0.001
Case scenario 4	0.23	0.04	0.62	0.52	<0.001

The background color marks the significance.

4. Discussion

Recently, there has been rising attention describing the consequences of disease or medical decisions by measuring its effect on patients' daily living and quality of life [5]. Numerous efforts have been employed to evaluate the relationship between quality of life and health related factors, leading to the widely spread term health-related quality of life. Evaluations of health-related quality of life have been widespread in medical areas as well as within fields of dentistry and oral health. Oral health is an essential part of general health, therefore it contributes extensively to health-related quality of life at biological, psychological, as well as social levels. Several studies previously reported the negative effect of tooth loss on the quality of life of dental patients [19]. Treatment of AP, a very prevalent dental condition, is a complex process in which dentists are regularly confronted with the difficult question of whether to save the affected teeth or to extract them [4,20]. It has been described as the first stage of all other developments of periapical endodontic lesions, either in an acute or chronic direction and its treatment modalities have been thoroughly discussed in various studies [21]. Nevertheless, up to the present time there is no definite treatment protocol or recommendation for teeth with AP. Thus, this survey aimed to evaluate for the first time German dentists' preferences in northern Germany for the treatment of teeth with AP.

In this survey 2270 dentists from the state of Schleswig-Holstein in northern Germany were invited to participate via the dental regulatory body's email register and a statistically significant sample size of 260 dentists completed the online questionnaire, displaying a similar response rate (11.4%) among the dental community reported in other studies in northern Germany [22,23]. Most of the non-responders did not contribute for no explicit reason or due to the absence of a reward, as observed in similar studies [4]. Sociodemographic data of the participants showed a similar gender distribution compared to the dental population in Germany and Europe (Table 1) [24,25]. The majority of the survey participants were dentists with no specialization (general practitioners), currently practicing in their own practice with a work experience of more than 20 years (Table 1). This corresponds to the reported average age and equivalent professional characteristics among dentists in Schleswig-Holstein, Germany [22,23]. Almost all participants of the study performed RCT in their workplace but only half of them performed implant treatments and one third of them performed endodontic microsurgeries (Table 1). This can be explained as RCT are commonly performed by general practitioners and are considered one of the basic dental treatments in Germany. Implantology and endodontic microsurgery, however, are more specialized treatment options that require further education, practical experience, and patients who are able to afford these procedures financially [26]. These results revealed that for most sociodemographic data that could be compared, variances between the relatively small study sample and its counterpart of dentists in northern Germany were rather non-significant, suggesting a minimal response bias. Consequently, the study participants can be considered as an acceptable and representative sample of Schleswig-Holstein's dentists.

Making treatment decisions is considered one of the most difficult aspects challenging any healthcare professional [27]. It shows a high level of complexity due to the expectations of the patient, and the contemplations the health care professional must make in selecting a treatment that is not only effective, but additionally maximizes benefits and health-related quality of life of the patient while minimizing risks. Often the construction of a decision selecting a definite treatment option may be linked to empirical principles or experiences of the dentist, which explains why dental education or training affects the treatment choices of oral healthcare professionals [28]. This effect may arise from differences in the diagnosis or identification of certain conditions [29], the preferred decisions to treat these conditions according to the dentist's awareness of the risks and progression of the disease, as well as the most appropriate procedure applied for treatment [30]. Furthermore, the practice of dentistry imitates market principles in which the patients' or clinicians' sensitivity to financial burdens, costs, and health insurance coverage of different treatments besides the patients' cooperation might influence the treatment decision by dentists and their patients [31,32]. Treatment recommendations or decisions might also be affected by the medical and dental history of the patient [33], as well as the specific tooth or surface to be treated [34], in which the dental community also tends to disagree. Indeed, all factors affecting the treatment decisions by oral healthcare professionals can be divided into patient-related (PRF), practice/education-related (ERF), and tooth-related factors (TRF), providing the base for dentists in their judgements and treatment planning [35,36]. In the current survey the practice/education- and tooth-related levels were addressed, while patient-related factors were excluded as explained above to eliminate predisposition in decision-making produced by financial or systemic health circumstances of the fictive patients.

From among the treatment options study participants could select, tooth retention using RCT or non-surgical endodontic retreatment followed by a coronal restoration was noticeably the first-ranked treatment option for all four case scenarios (Tables 3–6). This expresses a strong tendency towards tooth preservation when considering the treatment options for AP among dentists in Schleswig-Holstein addressing the contemporary dilemma facing dentists worldwide, whether to treat the teeth endodontically or extract them for a prosthetic procedure. This result can be expected due to the priority given by the German oral health system in the last decade to preventive and conservative dental care instead of prosthetic treatment, supported by financial incentives for tooth preserving measures and introduction of preventive and conservative dentistry principles in the dental curricula and education (ERF) [37]. Similar results were described previously in Canada [10], as well as South Korea [4]. Nevertheless, these surveys additionally reported a correlation between treatment preferences and the dental specialization. Since in Germany, as observed in this survey, the number of dental specialists is considered lower than of North American and other international dental societies and there are fewer state-recognized, post-graduate specialization programs, a differentiation of this kind was not feasible in the current investigation [26,38]. Unlike the first-ranked treatment preference, the second-rated treatment option in all case scenarios showed varying answers of the participating dentists. However, these choices seem to be affected mainly by the tooth location and difficulty of the treatment (TRF). For anterior teeth (CS1 and CS3), the second-rated preference was tooth retention using apicoectomy followed by a coronal restoration, while for posterior teeth (CS2 and CS4), the treatment option was tooth extraction followed by replacement with ISC (Tables 3–6). This finding concurs with previously published results and can be explained by the fact that apicoectomy on a posterior tooth is technically challenging (especially on the palatal root apex) and displays lower success rates than the anterior region due to access difficulties and complicated anatomical properties of the posterior teeth [10,39,40]. Further association analysis of the first-ranked treatment options revealed significant positive correlations between the treatments of choice in CS2 and CS4 (Table 7) and higher work experience. More years of work experience can be associated with advanced practical skills [41]. This could explain the enhanced preference for root canal (re)treatment on posterior teeth which often present a more challenging root canal system than anterior teeth [40]. Another observed significance correlated the preferred treatment in CS3 and CS4 positively (Table 7) to the higher percentage of privately insured patients in the dentist's practice. Dental practices with a higher percentage of privately insured patients might have more specialized technical equipment as endodontic microscopes, as well as higher skills using them to perform root canal retreatment [42,43]. This may be attributed to the fact that privately insured patients find it easier to finance this complex and cost-intensive treatment option which is often not covered by statutory insurance. Both observed associations can correspondingly be ascribed to all three mentioned levels of factors affecting the treatment decisions in dental practice (PRF, ERF, and TRF). Female participants also presented a significantly higher tendency to preserve posterior teeth by RCT in CS2 only when compared to male dentists (Table 7). This corresponds to previous findings describing gender as one of the potential dentist-related associated factors connected with the decision to retain compromised teeth and showing a higher inclination of female clinicians towards tooth preservation [35,44]. Nevertheless, gender as an influencing factor on clinical treatment decisions seems to be less important than the other factors being only significant in one CS in the current study and similarly observed and explained in previous investigations [10,12].

As clinical dentistry is becoming progressively complex and patients more educated, evidence-based dental care is nowadays looked upon as the "gold standard" of dental treatment worldwide [30]. This entitles the patients to receive correct information about state-of-the-art treatment techniques and possibilities from their dentist, as clinician's opinions can affect the final decision of their patient [45,46]. Although many participants of this study displayed an obvious tendency following evidence-based treatment of AP and tooth preservation, the results indicated some obsolete or non-evidence-based treatment recommendations. For example, almost half of the respondents in CS1 and CS2 (Tables 3 and 4) have surprisingly ranked the treatment option "tooth retention using apicoectomy followed by a coronal restauration" as "(very) appropriate" although this option is not indicated scientifically until primary RCT has failed [47]. Such lack of consensus has already been reported for teeth with AP and previous RCT and endorses the described claims of subjective and inconsistent treatment recommendations [48,49]. Previously reported factors disturbing the adoption of modern and evidence-based dental technology and science in decision making, such as psychosocial and behavioral factors, as well as a complex interplay of perceived benefits might provide an explanation of this observation [50,51]. The outcomes of this survey reflect the current clinical situation of the dental society in Germany and worldwide, where, even though dentists are capable of saving a tooth with AP through endodontic treatment, some clinicians are more likely to extract the tooth for implantation or recommend other non-evidence-based treatment options. Despite academic and dental associations' efforts to increase clinical agreement concerning the treatment of AP, a consensus has still not been reached and many dentists continue to depend only on their clinical experience and other personalized factors. Patients generally prefer to save their restorable teeth over tooth extraction [52]. Providing the best care and treatment to patients according to their preferences within the evidence-based scope of treatment is the chief duty of every clinician. Consequently, continuous and proper education and dental training should be offered to the dental society. This could be fulfilled by reviewing and re-evaluating the endodontic education programs on under- and postgraduate levels, as well as targeting the diagnostic and clinical skills of the dentists and also improving their self-efficacy and self-perceived competence [53]. Equally important, advanced diagnostic methods, such as artificial intelligence-guided techniques, should be introduced to support the clinical decision-making process based on scientific evidence and train the dentists to correctly interpret and diagnose the conditions [54]. In addition, further evaluation and consideration of the factors affecting the treatment decisions of AP (ERF, PRF, and TRF) should be performed to establish scientifically-based treatment guidelines for AP and guarantee a dental health system allowing the correct treatment of the patients.

Limitations of the Study

The following limitations have to be acknowledged. One main disadvantage of this cross-sectional study is that the data analyzed are restricted to the available information. On the other hand, misdiagnoses and misinterpretations in this type of study are also known to be equally distributed. In this investigation the observed treatment decisions of German dentists cannot be attributed completely to the analyzed factors and socioenvironmental data. Examining further co-variables and conditions such as additional clinical case scenarios (including different teeth as premolars) and further sociodemographic observations (including age, financial challenges, and place of initial training) could play a key role influencing the outcomes of the survey. Moreover, the present investigation examined a relatively small sample of dentists in the state of Schleswig-Holstein in northern Germany. The results obtained may not be representative for other German states or generalizable on all dentists in Germany. However, it could serve as an indicator of German dentists' main preferences due to the equality of dental education and training in Germany as explained in previous studies [24]. Furthermore, it may be important to add radiographic diagnosis and patient symptoms to the clinical case scenarios as they could be crucial to make the correct treatment decisions [4]. Yet, because of considerable inter- and intra-observer variability and radiographic interpretation divergences as previously reported in comparable studies related to endodontic treatment [10,55], radiographic images were intentionally left out in the case scenarios to avoid similar complications. Another significant limitation of this investigation is the potential presence of social desirability bias when answering the questions of the survey. Respondents may tend to deliver responses based on textbook recommendations, which might not necessarily reflect their actual clinical performs. This bias might also continue in spite of the confidentiality promised to participating dentists. Furthermore, the lack of knowledge about time from endodontic treatment to the present could also be considered a limiting factor of this investigation. It is also not known whether the apical status has improved or not after RCT. However, these conditions are also unknown among comparable studies, and the results from the current investigation are largely harmonious with other studies in the literature.

5. Conclusions

This survey investigated for the first time preferences of dentists in the state of Schleswig-Holstein in northern Germany for the treatment of AP and the factors affecting their decisions. The majority of dentists preferred tooth retention using RCT or non-surgical endodontic retreatment followed by a coronal restoration, while the less preferred option was tooth extraction and replacement with an ISC or apicoectomy followed by a coronal restoration. The observed results reflected a significant positive association between retention of posterior teeth using RCT or non-surgical endodontic retreatment and the work experience of the dentists, as well as the preference for retention of previously root canal filled teeth and the higher percentage of privately insured patients in the dentist's practice.

The results reveal a lack of consensus regarding the indication of different treatment options for AP among the dentists in Germany and indicates a personalized, non-evidence-based decision making by some clinicians. To ensure correct evidence-based patient guidance throughout the treatment process, an establishment of definite treatment protocols for AP besides continuous advanced endodontic education and clinical training for general practitioners are recommended. Furthermore, other external factors affecting the treatment decisions on financial and insurance-related levels should be considered and re-evaluated to prevent any interference with the guidelines.

Author Contributions: Conceptualization, M.M., J.C., J.R., S.A., and C.D.; data curation, J.C.; investigation, M.M. and J.C.; methodology, M.M., J.C., J.R., and S.A.; project administration, J.R. and C.D.; software, J.C.; supervision, C.D. and M.M.; validation, M.M. and S.A.; writing—original draft, J.C. and M.M.; writing—review and editing, J.R., C.D., and S.A. All authors have read and agreed to the published version of the manuscript.

Acknowledgments: The authors would like to thank every dentist who participated in this study and the state dental council (Zahnärztekammer Schleswig-Holstein) that helped to distribute the survey-link among its members. The authors would also like to thank the University of Kiel and the state of Schleswig-Holstein, Germany, for the financial support through the Open Access Funds.

References

1. Chen, J.; Ren, C.J.; Wu, L.; Xia, L.Y.; Shao, J.; Leng, W.D.; Zeng, X.T. Tooth loss is associated with increased risk of dementia and with a dose-response relationship. *Front. Aging Neurosci.* **2018**, *10*, 415. [CrossRef] [PubMed]

2. Kaur, P.; Singh, S.; Mathur, A.; Makkar, D.K.; Aggarwal, V.P.; Batra, M.; Sharma, A.; Goyal, N. Impact of dental disorders and its influence on self esteem levels among adolescents. *J. Clin. Diagn. Res.* **2017**, *11*, ZC05–ZC08. [CrossRef] [PubMed]
3. Setzer, F.C.; Kim, S. Comparison of long-term survival of implants and endodontically treated teeth. *J. Dent. Res.* **2014**, *93*, 19–26. [CrossRef] [PubMed]
4. Lee, J.; Kang, S.; Jung, H.I.; Kim, S.; Karabucak, B.; Kim, E. Dentists' clinical decision-making about teeth with apical periodontitis using a variable-controlled survey model in South Korea. *BMC Oral Health* **2020**, *20*, 23. [CrossRef] [PubMed]
5. Wigsten, E.; Kvist, T.; Jonasson, P.; EndoReCo; Davidson, T. Comparing quality of life of patients undergoing root canal treatment or tooth extraction. *J. Endod.* **2020**, *46*, 19–28. [CrossRef]
6. Kui, A.I.; Labuneţ, A.J.; Popescu, C.; Popa, D.; Lascu, L. Dentists' perspectives on the choice of treatment of teeth with apical periodontitis. *Clujul Med.* **2018**, *91*, 98–103. [CrossRef] [PubMed]
7. McCaul, L.K.; McHugh, S.; Saunders, W.P. The influence of specialty training and experience on decision making in endodontic diagnosis and treatment planning. *Int. Endod. J.* **2001**, *34*, 594–606. [CrossRef] [PubMed]
8. Dechouniotis, G.; Petridis, X.M.; Georgopoulou, M.K. Influence of specialty training and experience on endodontic decision making. *J. Endod.* **2010**, *36*, 1130–1134. [CrossRef]
9. Bigras, B.R.; Johnson, B.R.; BeGole, E.A.; Wenckus, C.S. Differences in clinical decision making: A comparison between specialists and general dentists. *Oral Surg. Oral Med. Oral Pathol. Oral Radiol. Endodontol.* **2008**, *106*, 139–144. [CrossRef]
10. Azarpazhooh, A.; Dao, T.; Figueiredo, R.; Krahn, M.; Friedman, S. A survey of dentists' preferences for the treatment of teeth with apical periodontitis. *J. Endod.* **2013**, *39*, 1226–1233. [CrossRef]
11. von Arx, T.; Roux, E.; Burgin, W. Treatment decisions in 330 cases referred for apical surgery. *J. Endod.* **2014**, *40*, 187–191. [CrossRef] [PubMed]
12. Taha, N.A.; Albashaireh, Z.S.; Alfied, R.G. Endodontic decision making for asymptomatic root-filled teeth with apical periodontitis—A radiographic survey. *Aust. Endod. J.* **2019**, *45*, 40–45. [CrossRef] [PubMed]
13. Su, H.; Liao, H.F.; Fiorellini, J.P.; Kim, S.; Korostoff, J. Factors affecting treatment planning decisions for compromised anterior teeth. *Int. J. Periodontics Restor. Dent.* **2014**, *34*, 389–398. [CrossRef]
14. Parirokh, M.; Zarifian, A.; Ghoddusi, J. choice of treatment plan based on root canal therapy versus extraction and implant placement: A mini review. *Iran. Endod. J.* **2015**, *10*, 152–155. [CrossRef] [PubMed]
15. Chercoles-Ruiz, A.; Sanchez-Torres, A.; Gay-Escoda, C. endodontics, endodontic retreatment, and apical surgery versus tooth extraction and implant placement: A systematic review. *J. Endod.* **2017**, *43*, 679–686. [CrossRef] [PubMed]
16. Brignardello-Petersen, R. Evidence about success of endodontic treatment or retreatment versus tooth extraction and implant placement is not sufficient for making clinical decisions. *J. Am. Dent. Assoc.* **2017**, *148*, e110. [CrossRef]
17. InformedHealth.org. Available online: https://www.ncbi.nlm.nih.gov/books/NBK65083 (accessed on 12 October 2020).
18. Tsang, S.; Royse, C.F.; Terkawi, A.S. Guidelines for developing, translating, and validating a questionnaire in perioperative and pain medicine. *Saudi J. Anaesth.* **2017**, *11*, S80–S89. [CrossRef]
19. Haag, D.G.; Peres, K.G.; Balasubramanian, M.; Brennan, D.S. Oral conditions and health-related quality of life: A systematic review. *J. Dent. Res.* **2017**, *96*, 864–874. [CrossRef]
20. Berlinck, T.; Tinoco, J.M.; Carvalho, F.L.; Sassone, L.M.; Tinoco, E.M. Epidemiological evaluation of apical periodontitis prevalence in an urban Brazilian population. *Braz. Oral Res.* **2015**, *29*, 51. [CrossRef]
21. Juerchott, A.; Pfefferle, T.; Flechtenmacher, C.; Mente, J.; Bendszus, M.; Heiland, S.; Hilgenfeld, T. Differentiation of periapical granulomas and cysts by using dental MRI: A pilot study. *Int. J. Oral Sci.* **2018**, *10*, 17. [CrossRef]
22. Hertrampf, K.; Wenz, H.J.; Koller, M.; Wiltfang, J. Comparing dentists' and the public's awareness about oral cancer in a community-based study in Northern Germany. *J. Cranio-Maxillofac. Surg.* **2012**, *40*, 28–32. [CrossRef] [PubMed]
23. Hertrampf, K.; Wenz, H.J.; Koller, M.; Grund, S.; Wiltfang, J. The oral cancer knowledge of dentists in Northern Germany after educational intervention. *Eur. J. Cancer Prev.* **2011**, *20*, 431–437. [CrossRef] [PubMed]

24. Mekhemar, M.; Conrad, J.; Attia, S.; Dorfer, C. Oral health attitudes among preclinical and clinical dental students in Germany. *Int. J. Environ. Res. Public Health* **2020**, *17*, 4253. [CrossRef] [PubMed]
25. Eaton, K.A.; Ramsdale, M.; Leggett, H.; Csikar, J.; Vinall, K.; Whelton, H.; Douglas, G. Variations in the provision and cost of oral healthcare in 11 European countries: A case study. *Int. Dent. J.* **2019**, *69*, 130–140. [CrossRef]
26. Ziller, S.; Eaton, K.E.; Widstrom, E. The healthcare system and the provision of oral healthcare in European Union member states. Part 1: Germany. *Br. Dent. J.* **2015**, *218*, 239–244. [CrossRef]
27. Malykh, V.L.; Rudetskiy, S.V. Approaches to medical decision-making based on big clinical data. *J. Health Eng.* **2018**, *2018*, 3917659. [CrossRef]
28. Nalliah, R.P. Clinical decision making—choosing between intuition, experience and scientific evidence. *Br. Dent. J.* **2016**, *221*, 752–754. [CrossRef]
29. Chipchase, S.Y.; Chapman, H.R.; Bretherton, R. A study to explore if dentists' anxiety affects their clinical decision-making. *Br. Dent. J.* **2017**, *222*, 277–290. [CrossRef]
30. Kishore, M.; Panat, S.R.; Aggarwal, A.; Agarwal, N.; Upadhyay, N.; Alok, A. Evidence based dental care: Integrating clinical expertise with systematic research. *J. Clin. Diagn. Res.* **2014**, *8*, 259–262. [CrossRef]
31. Vernazza, C.R.; Rousseau, N.; Steele, J.G.; Ellis, J.S.; Thomason, J.M.; Eastham, J.; Exley, C. Introducing high-cost health care to patients: Dentists' accounts of offering dental implant treatment. *Community Dent. Oral Epidemiol.* **2015**, *43*, 75–85. [CrossRef]
32. Shrirao, N.D.; Deshmukh, S.P.; Pande, N.A.; Radke, U.M. An evaluation of patient's decisions regarding dental prosthetic treatment. *J. Indian Prosthodontic Soc.* **2016**, *16*, 366–371. [CrossRef]
33. Sivakumar, A.; Thangaswamy, V.; Ravi, V. Treatment planning in conservative dentistry. *J. Pharm. Bioallied. Sci.* **2012**, *4*, S406–S409. [CrossRef] [PubMed]
34. Uhlen, M.M.; Valen, H.; Karlsen, L.S.; Skaare, A.B.; Bletsa, A.; Ansteinsson, V.; Mulic, A. Treatment decisions regarding caries and dental developmental defects in children-a questionnaire-based study among Norwegian dentists. *BMC Oral Health* **2019**, *19*, 80. [CrossRef] [PubMed]
35. Lang-Hua, B.H.; McGrath, C.P.; Lo, E.C.; Lang, N.P. Factors influencing treatment decision-making for maintaining or extracting compromised teeth. *Clin. Oral Implant. Res.* **2014**, *25*, 59–66. [CrossRef] [PubMed]
36. Bader, J.D.; Shugars, D.A. Variation, treatment outcomes, and practice guidelines in dental practice. *J. Dent. Educ.* **1995**, *59*, 61–95. [CrossRef]
37. Saekel, R. China's oral care system in transition: Lessons to be learned from Germany. *Int. J. Oral Sci.* **2010**, *2*, 158–176. [CrossRef]
38. Schleyer, T.; Eaton, K.A.; Mock, D.; Barac'h, V. Comparison of dental licensure, specialization and continuing education in five countries. *Eur. J. Dent. Educ.* **2002**, *6*, 153–161. [CrossRef]
39. Dagli, R.J.; Tadakamadla, S.; Dhanni, C.; Duraiswamy, P.; Kulkarni, S. Self reported dental health attitude and behavior of dental students in India. *J. Oral Sci.* **2008**, *50*, 267–272. [CrossRef]
40. Öğütlü, F.; Karaca, İ. Clinical and radiographic outcomes of apical surgery: A clinical study. *J. Maxillofac. Oral Surg.* **2018**, *17*, 75–83. [CrossRef]
41. Iqbal, A. The factors responsible for endodontic treatment failure in the permanent dentitions of the patients reported to the college of dentistry, the university of aljouf, kingdom of Saudi Arabia. *J. Clin. Diagn. Res.* **2016**, *10*, Zc146–Zc148. [CrossRef]
42. Wenteler, G.L.; Sathorn, C.; Parashos, P. Factors influencing root canal retreatment strategies by general practitioners and specialists in Australia. *Int. Endod. J.* **2015**, *48*, 417–427. [CrossRef] [PubMed]
43. Low, J.F.; Dom, T.N.M.; Baharin, S.A. Magnification in endodontics: A review of its application and acceptance among dental practitioners. *Eur. J. Dent.* **2018**, *12*, 610–616. [CrossRef] [PubMed]
44. Ghasemi, H.; Murtomaa, H.; Torabzadeh, H.; Vehkalahti, M.M. knowledge of and attitudes towards preventive dental care among Iranian dentists. *Eur. J. Dent.* **2007**, *1*, 222–229. [CrossRef] [PubMed]
45. Foster, K.H.; Harrison, E. Effect of presentation bias on selection of treatment option for failed endodontic therapy. *Oral Surg. Oral Med. Oral Pathol. Oral Radiol. Endodontol.* **2008**, *106*, e36–e39. [CrossRef]
46. Taibah, S.M. Dental professionalism and influencing factors: Patients' perception. *Patient Prefer. Adherence* **2018**, *12*, 1649–1658. [CrossRef]
47. Del Fabbro, M.; Corbella, S.; Sequeira-Byron, P.; Tsesis, I.; Rosen, E.; Lolato, A.; Taschieri, S. Endodontic procedures for retreatment of periapical lesions. *Cochrane Database Syst. Rev.* **2016**, *10*, Cd005511. [CrossRef]

48. Jang, J.H.; Lee, J.M. Surgical endodontic management of infected lateral canals of maxillary incisors. *Restor. Dent. Endod.* **2015**, *40*, 79–84. [CrossRef]
49. Karamifar, K.; Tondari, A.; Saghiri, M.A. Endodontic periapical lesion: An overview on the etiology, diagnosis and current treatment Modalities. *Eur. Endod. J.* **2020**, *5*, 54–67. [CrossRef]
50. Ghoneim, A.; Yu, B.; Lawrence, H.; Glogauer, M.; Shankardass, K.; Quiñonez, C. What influences the clinical decision-making of dentists? A cross-sectional study. *PLoS ONE* **2020**, *15*, e0233652. [CrossRef]
51. Parashos, P.; Messer, H.H. The diffusion of innovation in dentistry: A review using rotary nickel-titanium technology as an example. *Oral Surg. Oral Med. Oral Pathol. Oral Radiol. Endodontol.* **2006**, *101*, 395–401. [CrossRef]
52. Azarpazhooh, A.; Dao, T.; Figueiredo, R.; Krahn, M.; Friedman, S. A survey of patients' preferences for the treatment of teeth with apical periodontitis. *J. Endod.* **2013**, *39*, 1534–1541. [CrossRef]
53. Baaij, A.; Özok, A.R. Influence of method of teaching endodontics on the self-efficacy and self-perceived competence of undergraduate dental students. *Eur. Endod. J.* **2018**, *3*, 31–37. [CrossRef] [PubMed]
54. Endres, M.G.; Hillen, F.; Salloumis, M.; Sedaghat, A.R.; Niehues, S.M.; Quatela, O.; Hanken, H.; Smeets, R.; Beck-Broichsitter, B.; Rendenbach, C.; et al. Development of a deep learning algorithm for periapical disease detection in dental radiographs. *Diagnostics* **2020**, *10*, 430. [CrossRef]
55. Sherwood, I.A. Pre-operative diagnostic radiograph interpretation by general dental practitioners for root canal treatment. *Dentomaxillofac. Radiol.* **2012**, *41*, 43–54. [CrossRef] [PubMed]

Mechanical Debridement with Antibiotics in the Treatment of Chronic Periodontitis: Effect on Systemic Biomarkers

Sudhir L. Munasur [1], Eunice B. Turawa [1], Usuf M.E. Chikte [2] and Alfred Musekiwa [1,]*

[1] Division of Epidemiology and Biostatistics, Department of Global Health, Faculty of Medicine and Health Sciences, Stellenbosch University, Cape Town 7530, South Africa; munasurs@gmail.com (S.L.M.); Eunice.Turawa@mrc.ac.za (E.B.T.)

[2] Division of Health Systems and Public Health, Department of Global Health, Faculty of Medicine and Health Sciences, Stellenbosch University, Cape Town 7530, South Africa; umec@sun.ac.za

* Correspondence: alfred.musekiwa@gmail.com

Abstract: In this systematic review, we assessed the effectiveness of systemic antibiotics as an adjunctive therapy to mechanical debridement in improving inflammatory systemic biomarkers, as compared to mechanical debridement alone, among adults with chronic periodontitis. We searched relevant electronic databases for eligible randomized controlled trials. Two review authors independently screened, extracted data, and assessed risk of bias. We conducted meta-analysis, assessed heterogeneity, and assessed certainty of evidence using GRADEPro software. We included 19 studies (n = 1350 participants), representing 18 randomized controlled trials and found very little or no impact of antibiotics on inflammatory biomarkers. A meta-analysis of eight studies demonstrated a mean reduction of 0.26 mm in the periodontal pockets at three months (mean difference [MD] −0.26, 95%CI: −0.36 to −0.17, n = 372 participants, moderate certainty of evidence) in favor of the antibiotics. However, results from five studies reporting clinical attachment level (mm) yielded little or no difference at three months (MD −0.16, 95% CI: −0.35 to 0.03, n = 217 participants) between antibiotic and placebo groups. There is little or no evidence that adjunctive systemic antibiotics therapy improves inflammatory systemic biomarkers, compared to mechanical debridement alone, among adults with chronic periodontitis.

Keywords: chronic periodontitis; mechanical debridement; antibiotics; systemic biomarkers

1. Background

According to the World Health Organization (WHO), oral diseases are the most common non-communicable diseases with severe periodontal disease being the 11th most prevalent disease worldwide [1]. Periodontal disease is a chronic inflammatory disease of the periodontium and the most prevalent infectious oral condition [2]. Although the disease can be treated and prevented, it is the most frequent cause of tooth loss in adults. The signs and symptoms of periodontitis include persistent halitosis, red or swollen gingiva, tender or bleeding gingiva, painful mastication, loose teeth, and gingival recession. A new identification and classification system of periodontitis was developed in 2017 whereby the 1999 classification of chronic periodontitis is incorporated under the category of periodontitis (previously considered as either chronic or aggressive) [3]. The prevalence of periodontitis ranges 5–15% in most populations [4]. Globally, periodontal disease had an estimated prevalence of 750,847,000, incidence of 89,840,000, and 4,898,000 years lived with disability (YLD), in 2016 [5].

The diagnosis of periodontal disease is based on clinical measures such as bleeding on probing, pocket probing depth, and attachment loss, as well as radiological evidence of bone destruction [6]. Periodontal treatment entails the elimination of biofilm and microbial deposits from the root surfaces, thus reducing the inflammatory host response and tissue destruction [7,8]. Although there are several treatment approaches for periodontitis, conservative mechanical debridement (scaling and root planing [SRP]) has been the most common therapy [9]. Depending on the severity of inflammation, mechanical debridement combined with systemic antibiotic use has been advocated as a treatment possibility. However, there is currently insufficient scientific evidence to support or refute whether systemic antibiotics effectively enhances a positive outcome in chronic periodontal disease [10–15].

Therefore, this systematic review assessed the effectiveness of systemic antibiotics as an adjunctive therapy to mechanical debridement in the improvement of inflammatory systemic biomarkers, as compared to mechanical debridement alone, among adults with chronic periodontitis, using evidence from published randomized controlled trials.

2. Methods

This systematic review followed the preferred reporting items for systematic reviews and meta-analyses (PRISMA) statement for reporting systematic reviews and meta-analyses of studies that evaluate healthcare interventions [16]. The protocol for study was registered with the International Prospective Register of Systematic Reviews (PROSPERO), (registration number: RD42017059053).

2.1. *Criteria for Considering Studies for This Review*

2.1.1. Types of Studies

We included all randomized controlled trials (RCTs), published between January 2000 and October 2019, evaluating systemic antibiotics combined with mechanical debridement versus mechanical debridement alone or with placebo. Quasi-randomized controlled trials were also eligible, as well as studies in abstract only, with relevant results. Non-randomized trials and observational studies met the exclusion criteria.

2.1.2. Types of Participants

We included adults, aged 18 years and older, diagnosed with periodontal disease with or without co-morbidities such as diabetes mellitus, cardiovascular diseases, chronic obstructive pulmonary disease, and chronic kidney disease.

2.1.3. Types of Interventions

Experimental

All interventions that included mechanical debridement combined with adjunctive systemic antibiotics for the treatment of chronic periodontitis.

Control

The trials compared antibiotics versus placebo or no antibiotic, with mechanical debridement in either arm of the intervention.

2.1.4. Types of Outcome Measures

Primary Outcomes

The primary outcomes were changes in blood levels of inflammatory biomarkers such as Matrix Metalloproteinases (MMPs), Tissue Inhibitors of MMPs (TIMPs), Cytokines/Interleukins (IL-1β, IL-6 and IL-8), C-Reactive Protein (CRP), Glycosylated Hemoglobin (HbA1c), and Tumor Necrosis Factor alpha (TNF-α).

Secondary Outcomes

The secondary outcomes were periodontal parameters including pocket depth and clinical attachment level (CAL).

2.2. Search Methods for Identification of Studies

We adopted the following search terms and strategy: "anti-bacterial agents" [medical subject headings (MeSH)] OR "anti-infective" OR "systemic antibiotics" OR "antibiotic OR "antibiotic therapy") AND (periodontitis OR "chronic periodontitis" OR "periodontal diseases" [MeSH] OR "periodontitis" [MeSH].

We used the search strategy to identify relevant trials in MEDLINE database, and adapted the same strategy for other relevant electronic databases that we searched. We considered relevant RCTs published from January 2000 to October 2019 for inclusion. We did not apply any language restrictions.

2.2.1. Electronic Searches

We searched the following databases to identify relevant trials: Cochrane Oral Health Group's Trials Register, CENTRAL—Cochrane Register of Controlled Trials (of the Cochrane Library—current issue), MEDLINE (1966 to present), EMBASE (1982 to present), CINAHL (1990 -present), and Google scholar (1990–present).

2.2.2. Ongoing Trials Databases

We searched the following on-going trials registers (31 October 2019) to identify relevant trials: The meta-Register of Controlled Trials (www.controlled-trials.com), the US National Institutes of Health On-going Trials Register (www.clinicaltrials.gov), the World Health Organization International Clinical Trials Registry platform (www.who.int/trialsearch).

2.2.3. Grey Literature

We also searched the reference lists of included trials (31 October 2019) for relevant trials. We also emailed the authors of included trials and experts in the field of oral health care to identify any additional published or unpublished trials (31 October 2019). We searched the ProQuest database, Stellenbosch University database, and Google scholar (31 October 2019) and hand searched for trials not indexed in databases.

2.3. Data Collection and Analysis

2.3.1. Selection of Studies

Two review authors (SM and ET) independently screened the titles and abstracts of the search output to select potentially eligible trials using pre-specified eligibility criteria. After removing duplicates and ineligible trials, we retrieved the full-text articles of potentially relevant trials. Any disagreements were resolved through discussion or the third and fourth review authors (UMEC and AM) would add their input to enable a consensus.

2.3.2. Data Extraction and Management

Two review authors (SM and ET) also independently extracted data from each included trial using a pre-piloted data extraction form specifically designed for this review. The extracted data included study characteristics (authors, year, country and setting, and funding) and participant characteristics (study population, age, gender, periodontal disease diagnosis and severity, number of participants recruited and number of participants completing the trial, withdrawals and the reasons thereof, and overall sample size). Three review authors (SM, ET, and AM) extracted data for primary and secondary outcomes. For continuous outcomes that could be assumed normally distributed, such as pocket depth (in mm), we extracted the mean and standard deviation. For other continuous outcomes containing outliers, such as IL-1β, IL-6, IL-8, CRP, and CAL, we extracted the medians and their corresponding inter-quartile ranges (IQR). Otherwise, we extracted any other relevant data such as median ratios, 95% confidence intervals (CI), and p-values, as reported by study authors.

2.3.3. Assessment of Risk of Bias of Included Studies

Two review authors (SM and ET) independently assessed the risk of bias assessment for each of the included studies, in accordance with the guidelines in the Cochrane Handbook for Systematic Reviews of Interventions and levels of attrition were noted [17]. Each domain of risk of bias (generation of allocation sequence, allocation concealment, blinding of participants and personnel, blinding of outcome assessors, incomplete outcome data, selective outcome reporting, and other bias) were judged as either low risk, high risk, or unclear. Disagreements were resolved by discussion or by consulting AM.

2.3.4. Measures of Treatment Effect

We calculated the mean difference (MD), with its corresponding 95%CI, for continuous data with the same scale (for instance, pocket depth (mm)). Where continuous data could not be assumed to be normally distributed and study authors reported medians and ranges (for instance, CRP), we reported the median (IQR) together with any reported p-values for group comparisons, as given by study authors. For binary data, the reported odds ratios (OR) and corresponding 95% CI's and p-values were reported.

2.3.5. Unit of Analysis Issues

We performed analyses at the participant level to avoid unit of analysis errors. We did not include any crossover or cluster-randomized trials. For trials that had multiple intervention groups, we combined relevant groups to create single pairwise comparison. For one three-arm trial, we selected one pair of interventions and excluded one arm that was not relevant for this review.

2.3.6. Dealing with Missing Data

We contacted study authors to request information regarding missing data on either outcomes or risk of bias; however, we did not receive any responses. For each outcome in each trial, the denominator was the number of randomized subjects excluding any participants whose outcomes were missing. We therefore used the available case analysis and did not perform any data imputation.

2.3.7. Data Synthesis

We performed inverse variance random effects meta-analysis using RevMan statistical software version 5.3 (The Nordic Cochrane Centre, Copenhagen, Denmark) for some continuous secondary outcomes such as pocket depth (mm). To assess the extent and significance of heterogeneity, we used the I^2 test statistic and the Chi^2 test ($p < 0.1$ indicated statistical significance). Due to insufficient data, we could not pool results of many outcomes in a meta-analysis, and we reported the results separately for each study. We used GRADE Profiler (GRADEpro, version 3.6) software to assess the quality of evidence on the four main outcomes (HbA1c, MMP-8, CRP, and probing depth at 3 months) by rating the quality of evidence as either high, moderate, low, and very low certainty of evidence and summarized the results in the Summary of Findings table. Grading of the evidence considers factors such as study limitation (risk of bias), imprecision, inconsistency, indirectness of results, and publication bias [18].

3. Results

3.1. Results of the Search

The search yielded a total of 1730 titles and abstracts (1717 from electronic searches and 13 from hand searches). We excluded 1128 duplicates and remained with 602 records. We screened these 602 titles and abstracts and retained 58 records for further assessment. We also identified two additional articles from an updated search. We then retrieved full-text articles of these 60 studies and re-screened them for eligibility, from which we excluded 41 studies with reasons, thus retaining with 19 studies that we included in this review [13,15,19–35]. We report on 18 randomized controlled trials considering that two studies [26,31] were from the same trial. One trial [35] was published in French and we obtained an English translation. (Figure 1).

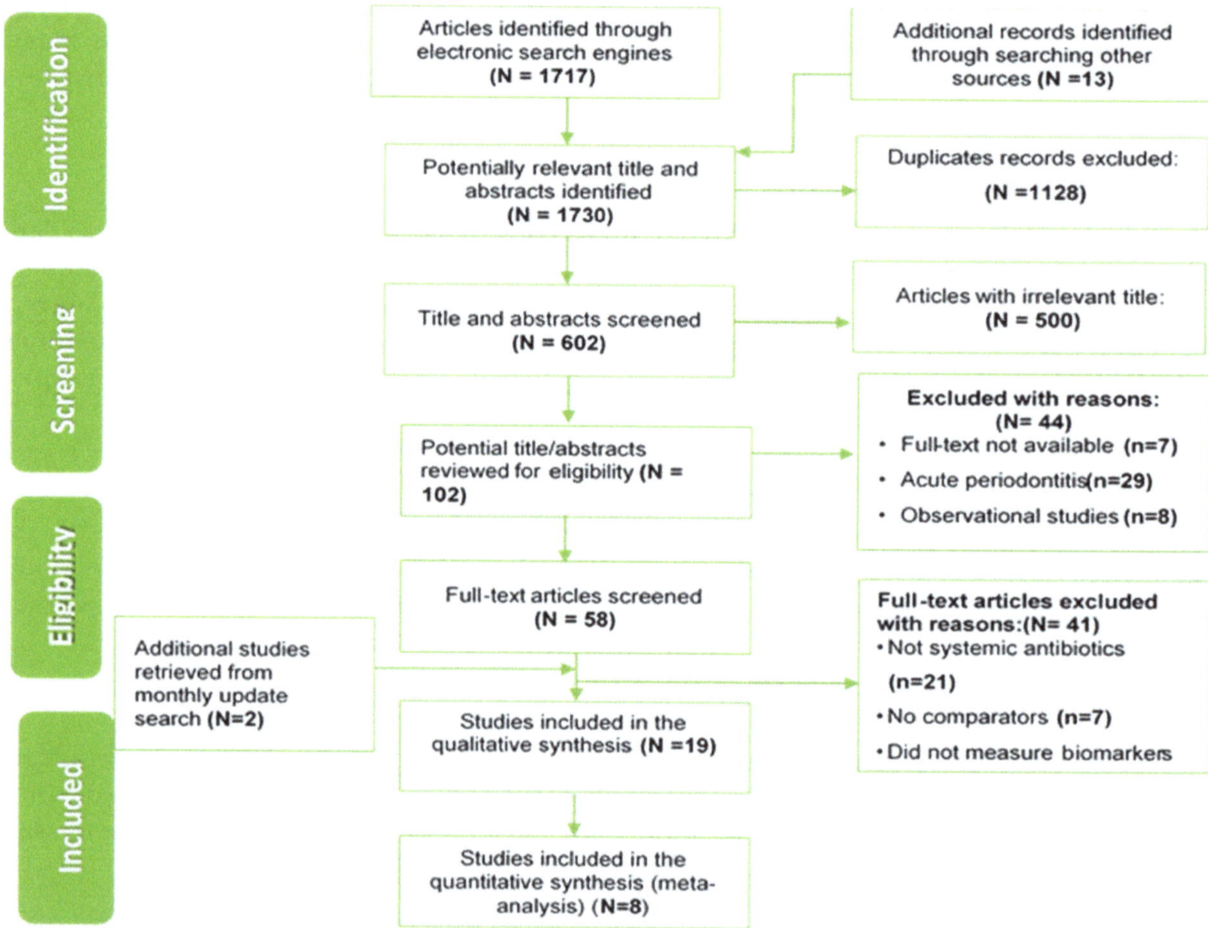

Figure 1. Search results for studies on the effect of antibiotics in addition to mechanical debridement among adults with chronic periodontitis

3.2. Settings, Participants, and Interventions

The characteristics of included studies are summarized in Table 1.

Table 1. Characteristics of included studies on the effect of antibiotics in addition to mechanical debridement among adults with chronic periodontitis.

Study ID	Country and Setting	Patients	Trial Duration	Intervention	Control
Almaghlouth 2014 [19]	School of Dental Medicine of the University of Geneva, Switzerland	40 patients with moderate-to-advanced periodontitis, aged 25–70 years	3 months	500 mg Metronidazole+ 375 mg Amoxicillin three times a day for 7 days	No placebo
Botero 2013 [20]	San Vicente de Paul Hospital Medellin, Colombia, South America	105 adults diagnosed with moderate periodontitis and diabetes	18 months	Azithromycin tablet 500 mg daily for 3 days (Group 1: Az+Scaling, Group 2: Az+Prophylaxis)	Placebo
Cionca 2009 [21]	School of Dental Medicine, University of Geneva, Switzerland	51 adult patients with moderate to advanced periodontitis, between ages of 25–70 years	1 year	500 mg Metronidazole & 375 mg Amoxicillin t.i.d × 7 days	Placebo capsules of 500 mg and 375 mg t.i.d. × 7 days
Engebretson 2011 [22]	Naomi Berrie Centre and Department of Periodontics, Columbia University Medical Centre, USA	45 Type 2 diabetes patients with chronic periodontitis, aged 50–56 years.	3 months	Group 1: 20 mg Sub-antimicrobial dose doxycycline (SDD) b.i.d × 3 months Group 2: 100 mg ADD daily × 3 months	Placebo daily × 3 months
Gaikwad 2013 [23]	Department of Periodontics, Tatyasaheb Kore Dental College, India	50 diabetes patients with chronic generalised periodontitis aged 30–70 years.	3 months	100 mg Doxycycline once daily for 15 days	No placebo
Gilowski 2012 [24]	Medical University of Silesia, Katowice, Poland	34 type 2 diabetes patients with chronic periodontitis, aged 36–68 years	3 months	20 mg doxycycline hydrochloride three times a day for 3 months	No placebo
Golub 2008 [26] and Payne 2011 [31]	University of Nebraska Medical Centre College of Dentistry and the School of Dental Medicine at Stonybrook University, Stoney Brook, USA	128 Osteopenic post-menopausal women with moderate to advanced periodontitis between the ages of 45–70 years	2 years	20 mg Sub-antimicrobial dose doxycycline (SDD) × 3 times a day for 2 years	20 mg Placebo × 3 times a day for 2 years
Golub 2001 [25]	Department of Oral Biology & Pathology, School of Dental Medicine, State University of New York at Stony Brook, USA	174 adult patients with chronic periodontitis aged 18–75 years	9 months	Group 1–4 Doxycycline 20 mg × 12 weeks (in different combinations)	Placebo × 12 weeks
Han 2012 [27]	Department of Periodontology, School of Dentistry, Ege University, Izmir, Turkey	36 patients with severe generalised chronic periodontitis in the age range of 35–54 years	6 months	500 mg Azithromycin once daily × 3 days	500 mg Placebo once daily for 3 days
Jones 2007 [28]	All four departments of Veterans Administration facilities at Greater Boston, USA	165 diabetes patients with periodontitis, mean (SD) age of 59.1(11) years	4 months	100 mg doxycycline daily for 14 days	Usual care with no placebo
Lopez 2012 [29]	Dr. Eloisa Diaz Dental Center, San José Hospital, Santiago, Chile	165 patients with Metabolic Syndrome (MetS) having periodontitis, between the ages of 35–65 years	1 year	250 mg Metronidazole t.i.d AND 500 mg Amoxicillin t.i.d for 7 days	250 mg placebo t.i.d AND 500 mg placebo t.i.d for 7 days
Miranda 2014 [30]	Department of Periodontology, Dental Research Division, Guarulhos University, Sao Paulo, Brazil	58 Type 2 diabetes patients with generalized chronic periodontitis, aged 35 years or more.	1 year	400 mg Metronidazole+ 500 mg Amoxycillin three times a day for 14 days	Placebo

Table 1. *Cont.*

Study ID	Country and Setting	Patients	Trial Duration	Intervention	Control
O'Connell 2008 [15]	Department of Oral Surgery & Periodontology, University of São Paulo Ribeiro-Preto, Brazil	30 Type 2 diabetes patients with periodontitis, aged 46–70 years	3 months	100 mg Doxycycline once daily for 2 weeks after an initial dose of 200 mg	Placebo once daily for 2 weeks after initial dose of placebo
Rooney 2002 [32]	Department of Periodontology at Bristol Dental School and Hospital, USA	66 patients with advanced chronic periodontal disease between the ages of 20–45 years	6 months	Group 1 (AM): 250 mg Amoxycillin (capsule) and 200 mg metronidazole (tablet). Group 2 (PM): 200 mg metronidazole (tablet) and placebo (lactose capsules). Group 3 (AP): 250 mg Amoxycillin (capsule) and placebo (calcium lactate tablets).	Placebo (lactose capsules) and placebo (calcium lactate tablets).
Saleh 2016 [33]	Oral Health Centre, University of Western Australia, Australia	37 adults with generalized moderate to advanced chronic periodontitis, age of 30 years and older	3 months	Group 1: 500 mg Amoxicillin and 200 mg Metronidazole administered every 8 h for 7 days Group 2: 500 mg Azithromycin administered every 8 h for 7 days	Placebo capsules were administered every 8 h for 7 days
Soto 2016 [35]	Two university clinics in the city of Cali (Colombia), and the Universidad del Valle (university of Valle)	81 patients with moderate to severe chronic periodontitis, aged between 25 and 70 years	12 weeks	500 mg Azithromycin per day, for 5 days	Placebo
Tuter 2007 [13]	Department of periodontology of Gazi University, Ankara, Turkey	36 patients with both chronic periodontitis and coronary artery disease (CAD), and age < 70 years	6 weeks	20 mg Sub-antimicrobial dose doxycycline (SDD) three times daily for 6 weeks	20 mg Placebo, three times daily for 6 weeks
Winkel 2001 [34]	Clinic for Periodontology Amsterdam and the Clinic for Periodontology Utrecht, The Netherlands	49 patients with generalised severe periodontitis, mean age of at least 40 years	6 months	375 mg Amoxicillin in combination with 250 mg metronidazole to be taken every 8 h for next 7 days was given.	Similar placebos every 8 h for next 7 days was given

The trials were conducted in academic hospitals mainly in developed countries: Six from the USA [22,25,26,28,31,32]; five from South America (Colombia [20,35], Brazil [15,30] and Chile [29]); five from Europe (Switzerland [19,21], Poland [24], Turkey [13,27]); and one from Australia [33]. Only one study was from a developing country, India [23]. None of the included studies were conducted in Africa.

In total, 1350 participants (18 trials) were included in the analysis for this review. The age of the participants ranged from 18 to 75 years old. Participants were all diagnosed with moderate-to-advanced chronic periodontitis with or without comorbidities. Eight trials included participants with no comorbidities [19,21,25,27,32–35]. Seven trials [15,20,22–24,28,30] included participants with hyperglycemia (diabetes), one trial [13] recruited participants with coronary artery disease (CAD), another trial [29] included participants with metabolic syndrome (MetS), and the last trial reported by two studies [26,31] assessed osteopenic postmenopausal women (Table 1).

All included trials assessed the effect of antibiotics compared with placebo or no antibiotic with mechanical debridement in both groups. The duration of the trials ranged from 6 weeks to 18 months. The intervention groups had broad spectrum antibiotics as an adjunct to the non-surgical therapies received. Combination of interventions varied across included trials. Four trials [20,27,33,35] evaluated the effect of 500 mg azithromycin in the treatment group compared to placebo. Seven trials examined the effects of doxycycline against either a placebo [15,22,25,26] or no placebo [23,24,28]. Seven trials investigated the effect of a combination of metronidazole and amoxicillin, albeit utilizing different dosages, versus either placebo [21,29,30,32–34] or no placebo [19] (Table 1).

Some of the trials were multi-arm. One trial [20] randomized patients into three treatment groups: Non-surgical therapy plus azithromycin, non-surgical therapy plus placebo, and supragingival prophylaxis plus azithromycin; we analyzed the first two groups and excluded the third group since it had no SRP. The second trial [22] was also a three-arm trial with conventional subgingival debridement combined with either sub-antimicrobial-dose doxycycline (SDD), anti-microbial dose doxycycline (ADD), or placebo. The third trial [25] consisted of four groups of various 20 mg doxycycline prescriptions versus placebo. The fourth trial [32] was a four-arm trial where all patients received quadrant SRP and were then prescribed 250 mg amoxicillin and 200 mg metronidazole (AP) or lactate and metronidazole (PM) or amoxicillin and calcium lactate (AP) or lactate and calcium lactate (PP). The fifth trial [33] is a three-arm trial, the first group received 200 mg metronidazole plus 500 mg amoxicillin, the second group were given 500 mg azithromycin, and the control group received placebo. For the analysis of these multi-arm trials, we combined the antibiotic groups to create single pairwise comparison with the placebo.

3.3. *Risk of Bias of Included Studies*

The risk of bias assessments for each included study are summarized in Figure 2. We judged 12 studies at low risk of random sequence generation (selection bias) because they reported using computer generated random numbers [19–22,25–31,33]. The remaining seven studies were unclear on how they generated the random allocation sequence [13,15,23,24,32,34,35].

We judged six studies at low risk of allocation concealment (selection bias) because four reported use of opaque, sealed, and coded envelopes to conceal the assignment [19,20,29,30] and two described the assignment as being concealed and allocation visually indistinguishable [22,27]. Thirteen studies were unclear on how they concealed allocation [15,21,23–26,28,31–35].

We judged 13 studies at low risk of performance bias because they reported adequate masking of participants and personnel (dentist, dental technician, and dental assistant) [13,19–21,24–27,30–33,35]. Information provided by the authors of five studies was unclear [15,22,23,29,34]. We judged one study at high risk of performance bias because the dentist, dental technician, dental assistant, and participants, were not masked [28].

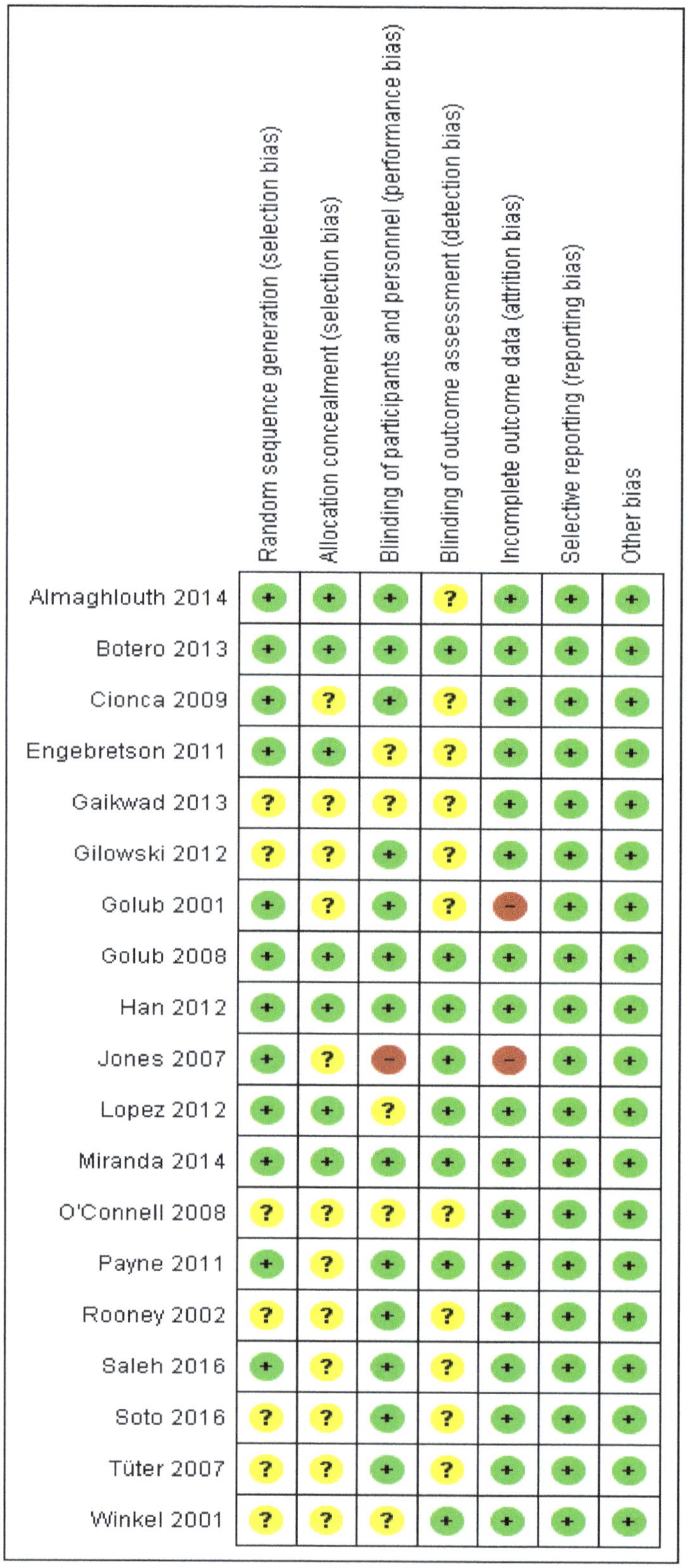

Figure 2. Risk of bias graph for studies assessing mechanical debridement with antibiotics in the treatment of periodontitis.

We judged eight studies at low risk of detection bias because they described an adequate method of blinding outcome assessors [20,26–31,34]. The remaining 11 studies were unclear of detection bias [13,15,19,21–25,32,33,35].

We judged 17 studies at low risk of attrition bias since they had low attrition [13,15,19–24,26,27,29–35]. We judged two studies at high risk of attrition bias because they had more than 15% of participants not completing the study and did not impute missing data [25,28].

We judged all the 19 included studies at low risk of reporting bias because they reported all expected outcomes as pre-specified in their methods.

We did not identify any other risk of bias in any of the 19 included studies.

3.4. Effects of Interventions

The GRADE Summary of Findings Table summarizes the results for four outcomes (Pocket depth (mm) at three months, HbA1c, MMP-8, and CRP levels) (Table 2). The detailed results for each of the primary and secondary outcomes follows.

Table 2. GRADE Summary of Findings Table for studies assessing mechanical debridement with antibiotics in the treatment of periodontitis.

Summary of Findings Table:

Antibiotic compared to placebo in the treatment of chronic periodontitis

Patient or population: Adult patients diagnosed with chronic periodontitis
Setting: Academic dentistry hospitals or clinics in developed countries
Intervention and Comparison: Antibiotic compared placebo or no antibiotic

Outcomes	Anticipated Absolute Effects * (95% CI)		Relative Effect (95% CI)	№ of Participants (studies)	Certainty of the Evidence (GRADE)	Comments
	Risk with Placebo	Risk with Antibiotic				
Pocket depth (mm) at 3 months	The mean pocket depth (mm) at 3 months was **0**	MD **0.26 lower** (0.36 lower to 0.17 lower)	-	372 (8 RCTs)	⨁⨁⨁◯ MODERATE [a]	Meta-analysis of eight studies with 372 participants show an antibiotic effect of reducing pocket depth by 0.26 mm compared to the placebo (moderate certainty of evidence). One other study found reduction in favour of the antibiotics, however results were presented as medians and ranges. Three other studies found little or no difference between the antibiotic and placebo groups.
Glycosylated Haemoglobin (HbA1c)	See comment	not pooled	-	487 (7 RCTs)	⨁◯◯◯ VERY LOW [b,c]	Six studies with 382 participants found little or no difference in the effect of antibiotics on haemoglobin levels compared to the placebo group. One study with 105 participants was unclear on the differences between the antibiotic and placebo groups.
MMP-8	See comment	not pooled	-	234 (4 RCTs)	⨁◯◯◯ VERY LOW [c,d]	Three small studies with 106 participants found little or no impact of antibiotic therapy on MMP-8 levels. One study with 128 participants found a 60% reduction in favour of antibiotics during a 2-year period.
C-Reactive Protein (CRP)	See comment	not pooled	-	504 (5 RCTs)	⨁⨁◯◯ LOW [c]	Three studies with 282 participants found little or no difference in CRP levels between the antibiotic and placebo groups. One study with 40 participants was unclear on the inter-group differences. One study with 182 participants found a small antibiotic effect of 18% decrease.

* **The risk in the intervention group** (and its 95% confidence interval) is based on the assumed risk in the comparison group and the **relative effect** of the intervention (and its 95% CI). **CI**: Confidence interval; **MD**: Mean difference

GRADE Working Group grades of evidence
High certainty: We are very confident that the true effect lies close to that of the estimate of the effect
Moderate certainty: We are moderately confident in the effect estimate: The true effect is likely to be close to the estimate of the effect, but there is a possibility that it is substantially different
Low certainty: Our confidence in the effect estimate is limited: The true effect may be substantially different from the estimate of the effect
Very low certainty: We have very little confidence in the effect estimate: The true effect is likely to be substantially different from the estimate of effect

a. Downgraded for indirectness as most studies were done in developed countries and results may not be generalizable globally; b. One study (Jones 2007) had high risk of performance and attrition bias; c. Indirectness: Outcomes were reported in different forms by studies and could not be pooled in a meta-analysis. In addition most studies were done in developed countries and results may not be generalizable globally. d. Three studies had small sample sizes of below 40.

3.5. Primary Outcomes

3.5.1. Cytokines/Interleukins

Three studies reported on IL-1β [15,19,26]. One study [19] assessed 40 participants (19 receiving antibiotic and remaining 21 placebo) and observed peak values of IL-1β in four patients at baseline (values ranging from 4.8 to 226.5 pg/mL), but no peak values were detected in any of the patients after three months. Another study [26] assessed gingival crevicular fluid (GCF) IL-1β levels in 128 postmenopausal women (64 in subantimicrobial-dose doxycycline (SDD) antibiotic group and 64 in placebo group) with chronic periodontitis, however there was no significant difference in the median GCF IL-1β levels between the two treatment groups after one-year or two-years' time-point, as reported by the study authors. The third study [15] evaluated 30 participants with type 2 diabetes and periodontitis (15 intervention and 15 placebo) but found no reduction in the concentration of IL-1β between baseline and three months (it remained at mean (standard error [SE]) of 0.3(0.3) pg/mL); however, the study authors did not give separate results for the intervention and placebo groups.

Three studies reported IL-6 [15,19,31]. One study [19] reported that a participant had a peak value of IL-6 of 216.3 pg/mL at baseline out of 40 periodontally diseased participants but there were no participants with peaked values after three months. Meanwhile, it is not clear whether the participants received antibiotic or placebo. The second study [15] reported a decrease in IL-6 in the mean (SE) of 2.1(0.3) at baseline to 1.1 (0.2) at 3 months ($p = 0.005$) for 30 participants with type 2 diabetes and periodontitis; however, the authors did not report separate values for the intervention and control groups except to say that there were no significant differences observed between treatment groups. The third study [31] found no significant difference in IL-6 level between the antibiotic group (SDD) and placebo group in 128 post-menopausal women with chronic periodontitis after two years (40% SDD versus 46% placebo; odds ratio [OR] 0.72, 95%CI: 0.30 to 1.69, $p = 0.4$).

One study [19] reported a peak value in IL-8 of 38.3 pg/mL at baseline for one participant, which rose to 39.6 after three months; but it is not clear whether the participant received antibiotic or placebo. Another study [15] reported a slight increase in IL-8 from mean (SE) of 9.0 (1.1) at baseline to 10.6 (2.5) at three months ($p = 0.621$) for 30 participants with type 2 diabetes and periodontitis; however, the study did not give separate values for intervention and placebo groups except to say there were no significant differences observed between treatment groups.

3.5.2. C-Reactive Protein (CRP)

Five studies reported on CRP [13,19,29,31,35]. From our GRADE assessments, we found little or no antibiotic effect on CRP levels (low certainty of evidence after downgrading two levels for indirectness). In one study [19], peak values of CRP were observed in four participants at baseline (values ranging from 13.4 to 52.6 μg/mL) and in three participants at three months (14.1 to 33.4 μg/mL); however, the study authors gave no indication of how many of the participants with these peak values received antibiotics. Another study [29] assessed CRP levels in participants with metabolic syndrome where 82 participants received amoxicillin and metronidazole while 83 participants received placebo. Although the mean CRP levels decreased significantly at 9 and 12 months, there were no significant differences between the two treatment groups at three months. In a third study [31], the SDD antibiotic intervention significantly reduced median hs-CRP by 18% over a period of two years compared to the placebo and the ratio of medians of SDD versus placebo (0.82, 95%CI: 0.70 to 0.97, $p = 0.02$). A fourth study [13] also assessed the effect of the SDD antibiotic on high-sensitivity CRP (hs-CRP) compared to placebo; however, although there were significant improvements between baseline and six weeks in both groups, there was no significant difference between groups at six weeks ($p = 0.628$). The fifth study [35] reported hs-CRP at baseline and 12 weeks and found that treatment with azithromycin antibiotic decreased the hs-CRP from 4.33 mg/L to 2.99 mg/L while the placebo treatment increased from 4.59 mg/L to 5.61 mg/L. Although they did not compare these intra-group changes, they found no significant differences between groups at 12 weeks (p = 0.4630); we could not calculate the 95%CI for mean difference since standard deviations were not reported.

3.5.3. MMP-8

Four studies reported MMP-8 [13,24,26,27]. From our GRADE assessments, we found little or no impact of antibiotic therapy on MMP-8 levels (very low certainty of evidence after downgrading one level for imprecision due to low sample size and two levels for indirectness). One study [24] randomized 34 participants (17 receiving SDD and 17 receiving placebo) with chronic periodontitis and type 2 diabetes; although MMP-8 decreased significantly between baseline and three months among the SDD group while an increase was observed in the placebo group, there was no significant difference between the two groups according to the study authors. In the second study [26], the SDD significantly reduced the odds of increased MMP-8 levels by 60% compared to placebo during the two-year period of study (OR 0.40, 95%CI: 0.21 to 0.77, p = 0.006) among the 128 postmenopausal women with periodontitis (64 in each group). In the third study [27], 36 participants with generalized chronic periodontitis (18 receiving azithromycin and 18 receiving placebo) showed no significant differences in GCF MMP-8 concentration between the two treatment groups from baseline to six months. The fourth study [13] demonstrated no significant differences in MMP-8 between the SDD and placebo group among the 36 participants with chronic periodontitis at pre- and post- six-week time points, according to study authors.

3.5.4. TIMP-1

One study [31] reported TIMP-1 and found no significant difference between the antibiotic group (SDD) and placebo group: TIMP-1 among the 128 postmenopausal women with chronic periodontitis after two years; ratio of medians of SDD versus placebo (0.96, 95%CI: 0.78 to 1.18, p = 0.7), according to study authors.

3.5.5. HbA1c

Seven studies reported HbA1c levels [15,20,22–24,28,30]. From our GRADE assessments, we found little or no antibiotic effect on HbA1c levels (very low certainty of evidence after downgrading one level for high risk of bias and two levels for indirectness). One study [23] found no significant difference in HbA1c levels (%) at four months of treatment between the SDD and placebo groups among the 50 participants with type 2 diabetes and chronic generalized periodontitis (Mean (SD) 7.00 (0.76) SDD versus 7.11 (0.99) Placebo; p = 0.710); however, the different sample sizes in each treatment group at four months were not given. The second study [24] also found no significant difference in HbA1c (%) at three months after treatment with SDD compared to placebo among 34 patients with type 2 diabetes and chronic periodontitis (Median (interquartile range (IQR)) 6.3 (5.5 to 7.3) SDD versus 6.7 (6.3 to 7.7) Placebo; p = 0.8). The third study [28] evaluated the effect of SDD versus placebo after four months of treatment among 165 veterans (83 receiving SDD antibiotic and 82 placebo) with periodontitis and poorly controlled diabetes; there was no significant difference in the percent achieving either HbA1c decreases of either > 0.5 or > 1.0 (55% versus 52% (p = 0.38) or 41% versus 34% (p = 0.31), respectively). In the fourth study [20], the antibiotic group had a reduction of 0.8% versus 0.3% in the placebo group at nine months; however, no comparison p-value was calculated between the two treatment groups. In the fifth study [22], the mean HbA1c after three months decreased by 0.9% (7.2% to 6.3%) in the SDD group, increased slightly by 0.3% (7.5% to 7.8%) in the ADD group, but remained the same at 8.5% in the placebo group; there were no significant differences between the antibiotic groups and the placebo, according to the study authors. The sixth study [30] assessed metronidazole plus amoxycillin versus placebo among 58 (29 per group) participants with type 2 diabetes and periodontitis but found no significant difference in HbA1c levels (%) between the two treatment groups at baseline, three months, six months, and after one year of treatment (p = 0.35, 0.55, 0.33, and 0.62, respectively). The seventh study [15] found no significant difference in HbA1c (%) improvement between the SDD group

(1.5%) and placebo group (0.9%) after three months among 30 participants with periodontitis and type 2 diabetes.

3.6. Secondary Outcomes

3.6.1. Probing Depth (PD)

(a) PD (mm)

Eight trials [15,19–21,23,30,33,34] measured PD (mm) at three months and a random effects meta-analysis of their results yielded a statistically significant antibiotic effect of reducing PD by 0.26 mm (mean difference [MD] −0.26, 95% confidence interval [CI]: −0.36 to −0.17, n = 372 participants, 8 trials, Figure 3) and there was no significant heterogeneity between trials (Chi^2 = 7.40, degrees of freedom [df] = 7, p = 0.39, I^2 = 5%). A funnel plot was constructed and it showed no evidence of publication bias (Figure 4). From our GRADE assessments, this was moderate certainty of evidence after downgrading one level for indirectness since the studies were done mainly in developed countries only.

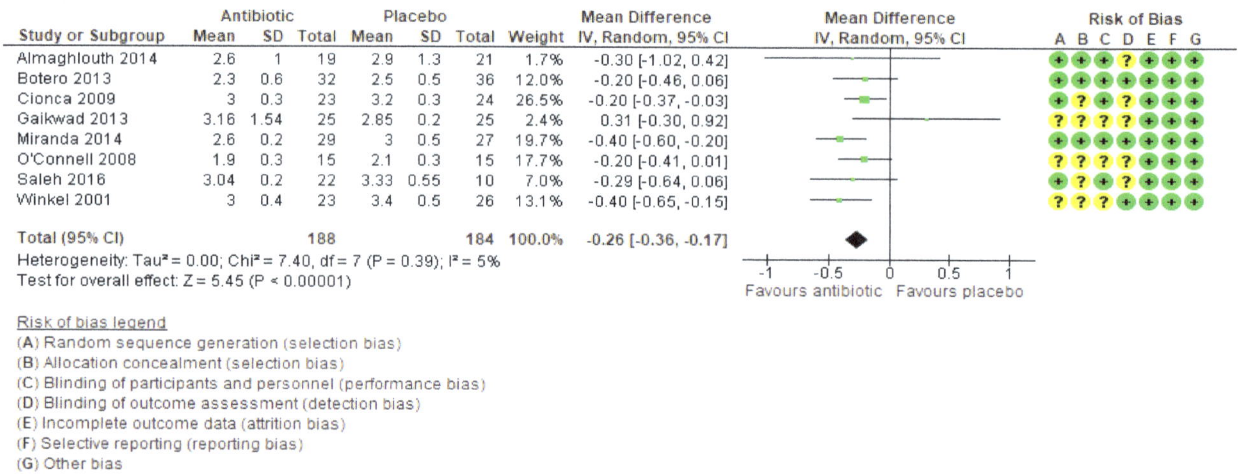

Figure 3. Meta-analysis of probing depth (in mm) after three months for studies assessing mechanical debridement with antibiotics in the treatment of periodontitis.

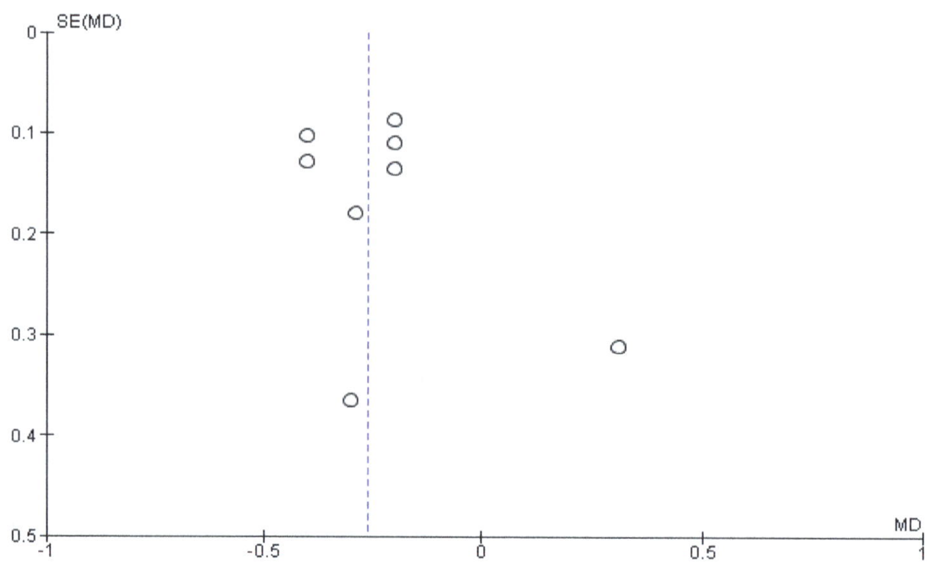

Figure 4. Funnel plot for the meta-analysis of probing depth (in mm) after three months of treatment with either antibiotics or placebo among adult chronic periodontitis patients.

One trial [24] also assessed PD (mm) at three months but there were no significant differences between treatment groups; the results are only reported in a figure (box and whisker plot) from which values for analysis cannot be accurately extracted. A second trial [27] measured PD reduction (in mm) from baseline to three months and found no significant difference between antibiotic and placebo groups (MD 0.25, 95% CI -0.05 to 0.55, n = 28 participants). A third trial [13] found statistically significant improvements in PD (mm) after six weeks of treatment in favor of the antibiotic group compared to placebo (Median (IQR) of 3.45 (3.24 to 3.69) mm SDD versus 3.78 (3.52 to 4.2) mm Placebo, p = 0.034, n = 36 participants (18 per group)). A fourth trial [30] assessed the antibiotic effect at six months and one year but found no significant difference between groups (data not reported). A fifth trial [32] reported the mean percent of sites with low (0–3mm) and high (>=6mm) pocket depth in the four treatment groups at baseline, one, three, and six months. Since the study authors did not report the pocket depth (in mm), their results are not reported here.

3.6.2. Clinical Attachment Level (CAL)

Nine trials reported CAL [13,15,21,23,24,27,30,33,34]. Five trials [15,23,30,33,34] measured CAL (mm) at three months and a random effects meta-analysis of their results showed no significant difference in CAL(mm) (MD −0.16, 95% CI: −0.35 to 0.03, n = 217 participants, 5 trials, Figure 5) and there was no significant heterogeneity between trials (Chi^2 = 1.69, df = 4, p = 0.79, I^2 = 0%). One trial [23] also measured CAL (mm) at four months and found a significant reduction in favor of the antibiotic group (MD −0.30, 95%CI: −0.55 to −0.05, 50 participants). However, another trial [30] did not find significant difference between treatment groups at both month 6 (MD −0.30, 95%CI: −0.77 to 0.17, 56 participants) and month 12 (MD −0.40, 95%CI: −0.87 to 0.07, 56 participants, Figure 5).

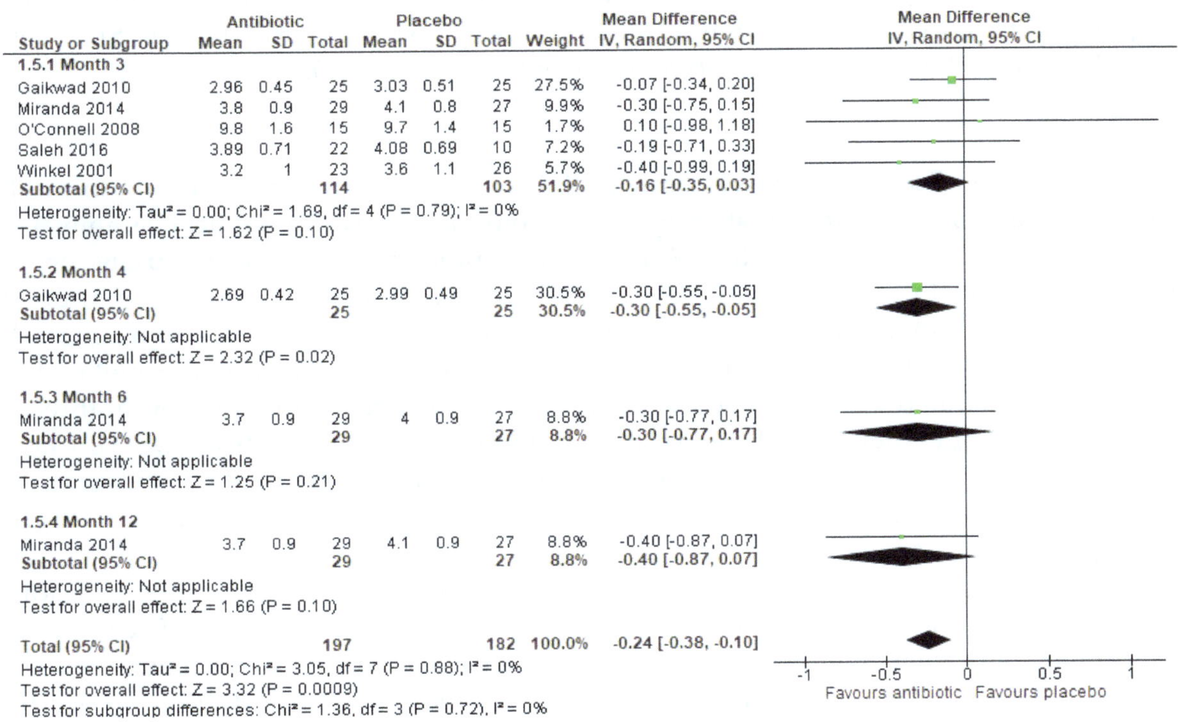

Figure 5. Meta-analysis of clinical attachment level (mm) after three months for studies assessing mechanical debridement with antibiotics in the treatment of periodontitis.

Two studies [21,27] measured the reduction in mean CAL (mm). The first study [27] found no significant differences between the treatment groups at month 1 (MD 0.11, 95%CI: −0.20 to 0.42, 28 participants). A meta-analysis of these two studies also found no significant differences between the treatment groups at month 3 (MD 0.17, 95%CI: −0.02 to 0.37, 75 participants, 2 studies) and month

6 (MD 0.00, 95%CI: −0.19 to 0.20, 75 participants, 2 studies); there was no significant heterogeneity between the two studies ($I^2 = 0\%$) (Figure 6).

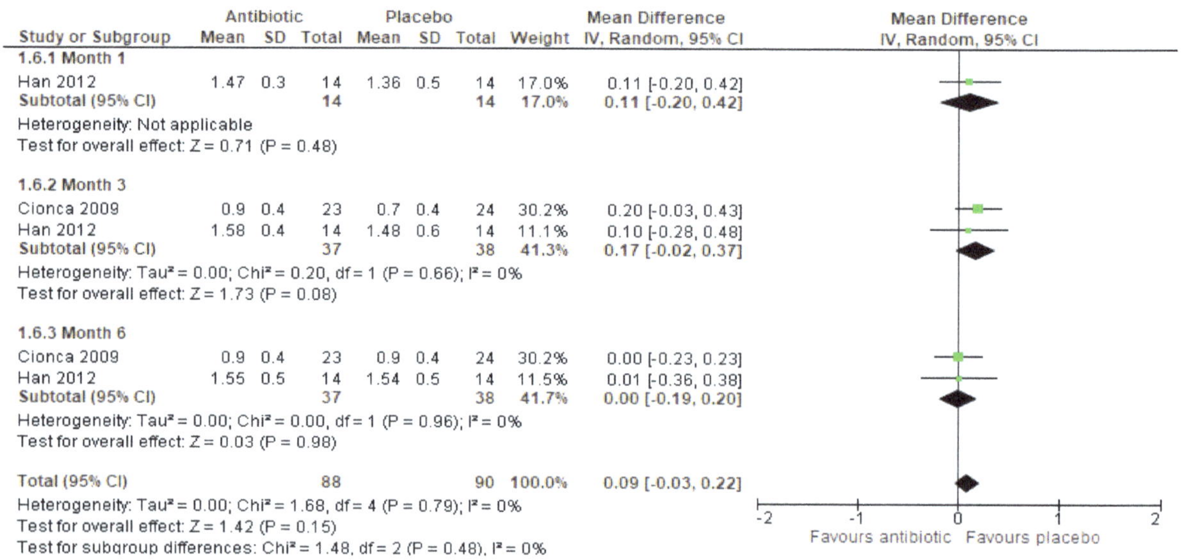

Figure 6. Meta-analysis of reduction in mean clinical attachment level (mm) after three months for studies assessing mechanical debridement with antibiotics in the treatment of periodontitis.

One study [24] found no significant difference in CAL between groups (values only given in a figure) and another study [13] found no significant difference in CAL (mm) between the antibiotic and placebo groups after six weeks of treatment (Median (IQR) of 3.97 (3.75 to 4.10) mm SDD versus 4.0 (3.66 to 4.46) mm Placebo, p = 0.521, n = 36 participants (18 per group)).

4. Discussion

We assessed the effectiveness of systemic antibiotics as an adjunctive therapy to mechanical debridement in the changes of inflammatory systemic biomarkers as well as clinical parameters among adult patients with chronic periodontitis. We included 18 randomized controlled trials consisting of 1350 adult participants in this systematic review and we found very little impact of antibiotics on changes in blood levels of inflammatory biomarkers such as MMPs, TiMPs, Cytokines/Interleukins (IL-1β, IL-6, and IL-8), CRP, HbA1c, and clinical attachment level. However, a meta-analysis of eight studies demonstrated a mean reduction of 0.26 mm in the periodontal pockets at three months (moderate certainty of evidence) in favor of the antibiotics. In meta-analyses, we did not detect substantial heterogeneity between studies and the studies generally had either unclear or low risk of bias. The majority of the studies were conducted in developed countries, mainly in Europe and the USA.

To our knowledge, this is the first systematic review to determine the effects of adjunctive antibiotics on systemic biomarkers. Several systematic reviews have assessed the effects of adjunctive antibiotics among patients with periodontitis; however, they assessed clinical outcomes only. From the two most recently published systematic reviews [36,37], the first [36] assessed the effect of adjunctive systemic antimicrobials on clinical outcomes of periodontitis in randomized controlled trials with follow-up of at least six months; they found that systemic antibiotic therapy with metronidazole and amoxycillin significantly improved probing pocket depth as well as clinical attachment level. The other systematic review [37] assessed adjunctive antibiotics in patients with untreated chronic periodontitis and also found significant effects of systemic antibiotics on pocket depth reduction at 3, 6, and 12 months, as well as on clinical attachment level gain after three months of treatment. This is in agreement with our findings of a statistically significant reduction in pocket depth at three months; however, our results did not find significant effects in clinical attachment level. The difference in our results is probably because we excluded studies before the year 2000 and did not separate analyses for different types of antibiotics as done in the other two systematic reviews.

In this systematic review, we included adult participants aged 18 to 75 years with moderate to advanced chronic periodontitis with or without comorbidities mainly from developed countries. Only one study was from India and none were from the African continent. This therefore limits the generalizability of our findings to young people and other population groups and regions not included in this review. Numerous included studies did not report results in a clear, tabular form with separate results for intervention and control groups [13,19,20,22,24,27,29,31]. In our GRADE assessment, we downgraded the certainty of evidence due to the lack of generalizability and the poor reporting of results. Overall, there is insufficient evidence to make general conclusions on the effects of adjunctive antibiotics on systemic biomarkers in the treatment of periodontitis. The use of antibiotics as an adjunct to mechanical debridement is seen to be satisfactory even though their results have been deemed as having little difference between the antibiotic and placebo groups in the outcomes concerning pocket depth reduction (at three months), the reduction of HbA1c, MMP-8, and CRP. The fact that antibiotic treatment disrupts the inflammatory pathways of chronic periodontitis serves as a justification for the adjunctive use of antibiotics with scaling and root planing (SRP) even if the clinical benefit is minor. The adjunctive use of 400 mg or 250 mg of metronidazole plus 500 mg of amoxicillin for 14 days provided clinically relevant benefits over SRP exclusively in the treatment of generalized chronic periodontitis [38]. Antibiotics are not a panacea for all non-responsive situation; however, adjunctive antibiotic use together with mechanical debridement provides effective control in chronic periodontitis [39].

We minimized bias in the review process in a number of ways. We conducted a comprehensive literature search of all relevant electronic database and consulted experts to identify grey or unpublished literature and relevant information. Our search was not language-restricted and in fact, we included one French study for which we received professional translation [35]. We also screened reference lists of included articles to identify potentially eligible studies. At least two review authors independently scrutinized and selected articles for inclusion in the review using pre-specified eligibility criteria. Articles were assessed for risk of bias and data were extracted in duplicates. However, there were some potential biases in the process of this systematic review. For instance, we did not perform separate analyses of studies with and without comorbidities and we are therefore unable to determine if there are differences in effects of systemic antibiotics between individuals with and without comorbidities. There is a difference in the host response to antibiotics in a systemically healthy individual compared to an individual with a co-morbidity during periodontal treatment [40]. We also did not compare the effects of different antibiotics and different dosages on the outcomes. Therefore, the results from this review will need cautious interpretation because of the broad grouping of participants and interventions. Future updates of this systematic review will need to determine if such differences exist.

5. Conclusions

5.1. *Implications for Practice*

The limited available evidence shows that adjunctive administration of systemic antibiotics for a minimum of three months may improve pocket depth clinical parameters compared to mechanical debridement alone, among adults with chronic periodontitis. Similarly, the extended two-year duration of adjunctive SDD with mechanical debridement may improve systemic CRP and MMPs serum levels.

5.2. *Implications for Research*

The included trials reported on the following outcomes: Serum/blood levels of MMPs, TIMPs, Cytokines, CRP, IL-1β, IL-6, IL-8, CRP, HbA1c, PD, and CAL. Further rigorous large randomized controlled trials of high quality would be beneficial to assess the effect of adjunctive antibiotics administration on systemic biomarkers in chronic periodontitis. Most of the included trials are of poor methodological quality and the results were portrayed in graphic displays, making it difficult to extract the data accurately. This limits the applicability of the result in clinical evidence-based practice.

Author Contributions: S.L.M.: Developed the protocol, screened studies for inclusion, assessed risk of bias, extracted data, performed data analysis, data interpretation, and manuscript writing. E.B.T.: Screened studies for inclusion, assessed risk of bias, extracted data, and manuscript writing. U.M.E.C.: Provided initial conceptual framework and critical appraisal to all sections of the manuscript. A.M.: Assessed risk of bias, performed data analysis, data interpretation, and manuscript writing. All authors read and approved the final version of the manuscript.

Acknowledgments: We acknowledge Carla Pontes for giving content advice. SM acknowledges the MSc in Clinical Epidemiology programme, Faculty of Medicine and Health Sciences, Stellenbosch University, South Africa.

Abbreviations

ADD: Anti-microbial dose doxycycline; CAL: Clinical attachment level; CI: Confidence interval; CRP: C-reactive protein; CAD: Coronary artery disease; FMPS: Full mouth plaque score; GCF: Gingival crevicular fluid; GI: Gingival index; HbA1c: Glycosylated hemoglobin; GRADE: Grading of recommendations assessment, development, and evaluation; IL-1β: Interleukin-1-beta; IL-6: Interleukin-6; IL-8: Interleukin-8; IQR: Inter-quartile range; MD: Mean difference; MetS: Metabolic syndrome; MMP-8: Matrix metallo-proteinase-8; OR: Odds ratio; PD: Probing depth; PPD: Probing pocket depth; PI: Plaque index; RCT: Randomized controlled trial; SD: Standard deviation; SDD: Sub-antimicrobial dose doxycycline; SCP: Severe chronic periodontitis; SE: Standard error; SRP: scaling and root-planing; TIMP-1: tissue inhibitor metallo-proteinase-1; TNF-α: Tumor necrosis factor – alpha; USA: United States of America; WHO: World Health Organization.

References

1. WHO. Oral Health. Available online: https://www.who.int/news-room/fact-sheets/detail/oral-health (accessed on 5 May 2020).
2. Nazir, M.A. Prevalence of periodontal disease, its association with systemic diseases and prevention. *Int. J. Health Sci. Qassim* **2017**, *11*, 72–80.
3. Caton, J.G.; Armitage, G.; Berglundh, T.; Chapple, I.L.C.; Jepsen, S.; Kornman, K.S. A new classification scheme for periodontal and peri-implant diseases and conditions—Introduction and key changes from the 1999 classification. *J. Clin. Periodontol.* **2018**, *45* (Suppl. 20), S1–S8. [CrossRef]
4. WHO. Oral Health. What Is the Burden of Oral Disease? Available online: https://www.who.int/oral_health/disease_burden/global/en/ (accessed on 5 May 2020).
5. Eke, P.I.; Dye, B.A.; Wei, L.; Slade, G.D.; Thornton-Evans, G.O.; Borgnakke, W.S.; Taylor, G.W.; Page, R.C.; Beck, J.D.; Genco, R.J. Update on Prevalence of Periodontitis in Adults in the United States: NHANES 2009 to 2012. *J. Periodontol.* **2015**, *86*, 611–622. [CrossRef]
6. Kassebaum, N.J.; Bernabé, E.; Dahiya, M.; Bhandari, B.; Murray, C.J.; Marcenes, W. Global burden of severe periodontitis in 1990–2010: A systematic review and meta-regression. *J. Dent. Res.* **2014**, *93*, 1045–1053. [CrossRef]
7. Bolerázska, B.; Mareková, M.; Markovská, N. Trends in Laboratory Diagnostic Methods in Periodontology. *Acta Med. Hradec Kralove* **2016**, *59*, 3–9. [CrossRef] [PubMed]
8. Kepic, T.J.; O'Leary, T.J.; Kafrawy, A.H. Total calculus removal: An attainable objective? *J. Periodontol.* **1990**, *61*, 16–20. [CrossRef]
9. Hinrichs, J.E.; Wolff, L.F.; Pihlstrom, B.L.; Schaffer, E.M.; Liljemark, W.F.; Bandt, C.L. Effects of scaling and root planing on subgingival microbial proportions standardized in terms of their naturally occurring distribution. *J. Periodontol.* **1985**, *56*, 187–194. [CrossRef] [PubMed]
10. Matthews, D.C. Prevention and treatment of periodontal diseases in primary care. *Evid. Based Dent.* **2014**, *15*, 68–69. [CrossRef] [PubMed]
11. Montebugnoli, L.; Servidio, D.; Miaton, R.A.; Prati, C.; Tricoci, P.; Melloni, C.; Melandri, G. Periodontal health improves systemic inflammatory and haemostatic status in subjects with coronary heart disease. *J. Clin. Periodontol.* **2005**, *32*, 188–192. [CrossRef]
12. Iwamoto, Y.; Nishimura, F.; Soga, Y.; Takeuchi, K.; Kurihara, M.; Takashiba, S.; Murayama, Y. Antimicrobial periodontal treatment decreases serum C-reactive protein, tumor necrosis factor-alpha, but not adiponectin levels in patients with chronic periodontitis. *J. Periodontol.* **2003**, *74*, 1231–1236. [CrossRef]

13. Heitz-Mayfield, L. Systemic antibiotics in periodontal therapy. *Aust. Dent. J.* **2009**, *54*, S96–S101. [CrossRef] [PubMed]
14. Tüter, G.; Kurtiş, B.; Serdar, M.; Aykan, T.; Okyay, K.; Yücel, A.; Toyman, U.; Pinar, S.; Cemri, M.; Çengel, A.; et al. Effects of scaling and root planing and sub-antimicrobial dose doxycycline on oral and systemic biomarkers of disease in patients with both chronic periodontitis and coronary artery disease. *J. Clin. Periodontol.* **2007**, *34*, 673–681. [CrossRef] [PubMed]
15. Emingil, G.; Gürkan, A.; Atilla, G.; Kantarci, A. Subantimicrobial-dose doxycycline and cytokine-chemokine levels in gingival crevicular fluid. *J. Periodontol.* **2011**, *82*, 452–461. [CrossRef]
16. O'Connell, P.A.; Taba, M., Jr.; Nomizo, A.; Foss Freitas, M.C.; Suaid, F.A.; Uyemura, S.A.; Trevisan, G.L.; Novaes, A.B., Jr.; Souza, S.L.S.; Palioto, D.B.; et al. Effects of periodontal therapy on glycemic control and inflammatory markers. *J. Periodontol.* **2008**, *79*, 774–783. [CrossRef] [PubMed]
17. Higgins, J.P.; Altman, D.G. Assessing risk of bias in included studies. In *Cochrane Handbook for Systematic Reviews of Interventions;* Cochrane: London, UK, 2008; pp. 187–241.
18. Guyatt, G.; Oxman, A.D.; Akl, E.A.; Kunz, R.; Vist, G.; Brozek, J.; Norris, S.; Falck-Ytter, Y.; Glasziou, P.; de Beer, H.; et al. GRADE guidelines: 1. Introduction-GRADE evidence profiles and summary of findings tables. *J. Clin. Epidemiol.* **2011**, *64*, 383–394. [CrossRef] [PubMed]
19. Almaghlouth, A.A.; Cionca, N.; Cancela, J.A.; Décaillet, F.; Courvoisier, D.S.; Giannopoulou, C.; Mombelli, A. Effect of periodontal treatment on peak serum levels of inflammatory markers. *Clin. Oral. Investig.* **2014**, *18*, 2113–2121. [CrossRef]
20. Botero, J.E.; Yepes, F.L.; Ochoa, S.P.; Hincapie, J.P.; Roldan, N.; Ospina, C.A.; Castrillon, C.A.; Becerra, M.A. Effects of periodontal non-surgical therapy plus azithromycin on glycemic control in patients with diabetes: A randomized clinical trial. *J. Periodontal. Res.* **2013**, *48*, 706–712. [CrossRef]
21. Cionca, N.; Giannopoulou, C.; Ugolotti, G.; Mombelli, A. Amoxicillin and metronidazole as an adjunct to full-mouth scaling and root planing of chronic periodontitis. *J. Periodontol.* **2009**, *80*, 364–371. [CrossRef]
22. Engebretson, S.P.; Hey-Hadavi, J. Sub-Antimicrobial doxycycline for periodontitis reduces hemoglobin A1c in subjects with type 2 diabetes: A pilot study. *Pharmacol. Res.* **2011**, *64*, 624–629. [CrossRef]
23. Gaikwad, S.P.; Gurav, A.N.; Shete, A.R.; Desarda, H.M. Effect of scaling and root planing combined with systemic doxycycline therapy on glycemic control in diabetes mellitus subjects with chronic generalized periodontitis: A clinical study. *J. Periodontal. Implant Sci.* **2013**, *43*, 79–86. [CrossRef]
24. Gilowski, L.; Kondzielnik, P.; Wiench, R.; Płocica, I.; Strojek, K.; Krzemiński, T.F. Efficacy of short-term adjunctive subantimicrobial dose doxycycline in diabetic patients—Randomized study. *Oral Dis.* **2012**, *18*, 763–770. [CrossRef]
25. Golub, L.M.; McNamara, T.F.; Ryan, M.E.; Kohut, B.; Blieden, T.; Payonk, G.; Sipos, T.; Baron, H.H. Adjunctive treatment with subantimicrobial doses of doxycycline: Effects on gingival fluid collagenase activity and attachment loss in adult periodontitis. *J. Clin. Periodontol.* **2001**, *28*, 146–156. [CrossRef] [PubMed]
26. Golub, L.M.; Lee, H.M.; Stoner, J.A.; Sorsa, T.; Reinhardt, R.A.; Wolff, M.S.; Ryan, M.E.; Nummikoski, P.V.; Payne, J.B. Subantimicrobial-dose doxycycline modulates gingival crevicular fluid biomarkers of periodontitis in postmenopausal osteopenic women. *J. Periodontol.* **2008**, *79*, 140–218. [CrossRef] [PubMed]
27. Han, B.; Emingil, G.; Özdemir, G.; Tervahartiala, T.; Vural, C.; Atilla, G.; Baylas, H.; Sorsa, T. Azithromycin as an adjunctive treatment of generalized severe chronic periodontitis: Clinical, microbiologic, and biochemical parameters. *J. Periodontol.* **2012**, *83*, 1480–1491. [CrossRef]
28. Jones, J.A.; Miller, D.R.; Wehler, C.J.; Rich, S.E.; Krall-Kaye, E.A.; McCoy, L.C.; Christiansen, C.L.; Rothendler, J.A.; Garcia, R.I. Does periodontal care improve glycemic control? The Department of Veterans Affairs Dental Diabetes Study. *J. Clin. Periodontol.* **2007**, *34*, 46–52. [CrossRef] [PubMed]
29. López, N.J.; Quintero, A.; Casanova, P.A.; Ibieta, C.I.; Baelum, V.; López, R. Effects of periodontal therapy on systemic markers of inflammation in patients with metabolic syndrome: A controlled clinical trial. *J. Periodontol.* **2012**, *83*, 267–278. [CrossRef]
30. Miranda, T.S.; Feres, M.; Perez-Chaparro, P.J.; Faveri, M.; Figueiredo, L.C.; Tamashiro, N.S.; Ferreira Bastos, M.; Mendes Duarte, P. Metronidazole and amoxicillin as adjuncts to scaling and root planing for the treatment of type 2 diabetic subjects with periodontitis: 1-Year outcomes of a randomized placebo-controlled clinical trial. *J. Clin. Periodontol.* **2014**, *41*, 890–899. [CrossRef]

31. Payne, J.B.; Golub, L.M.; Stoner, J.A.; Lee, H.M.; Reinhardt, R.A.; Sorsa, T.; Stepian, M.J. The effect of subantimicrobial-dose-doxycycline periodontal therapy on serum biomarkers of systemic inflammation: A randomized, double-masked, placebo-controlled clinical trial. *J. Am. Dent. Assoc.* **2011**, *142*, 262–273. [CrossRef]
32. Rooney, J.; Wade, W.G.; Sprague, S.V.; Newcombe, R.G.; Addy, M. Adjunctive effects to non-surgical periodontal therapy of systemic metronidazole and amoxycillin alone and combined. A placebo controlled study. *J Clin. Periodontol.* **2002**, *29*, 342–350. [CrossRef]
33. Saleh, A.; Rincon, J.; Tan, A.; Firth, M. Comparison of adjunctive azithromycin and amoxicillin/metronidazole for patients with chronic periodontitis: Preliminary randomized control trial. *Aust. Dent. J.* **2016**, *61*, 469–481. [CrossRef]
34. Winkel, E.G.; Van Winkelhoff, A.J.; Timmerman, M.F.; Van der Velden, U.; Van der Weijden, G.A. Amoxicillin plus metronidazole in the treatment of adult periodontitis patients. A double-blind placebo-controlled study. *J. Clin. Periodontol.* **2001**, *28*, 296–305. [CrossRef]
35. Soto-Franco, J.E.; Aldana, H.F.; Navia, J.M.; Peláez, M.; Quisoboni, J.; O'Meara, M.A.; Contreras, A. Efectos del raspaje y alisado radicular a boca completa con azitromicina sobre los niveles de proteina C reactiva ultra sensible, parametros clínicos y microbiológicos periodontales. Ensayo clinico aleatorizado. *Rev. Estomatol.* **2016**, *24*, 14–25. [CrossRef]
36. Teughels, W.; Feres, M.; Oud, V.; Martín, C.; Matesanz, P.; Herrera, D. Adjunctive effect of systemic antimicrobials in periodontitis therapy. A systematic review and meta-analysis. *J. Clin. Periodontol.* **2020**. [CrossRef] [PubMed]
37. Keestra, J.A.; Grosjean, I.; Coucke, W.; Quirynen, M.; Teughels, W. Non-Surgical periodontal therapy with systemic antibiotics in patients with untreated chronic periodontitis: A systematic review and meta-analysis. *J. Periodontal. Res.* **2015**, *50*, 294–314. [CrossRef] [PubMed]
38. Borges, I.; Faveri, M.; Figueiredo, L.C.; Duarte, P.M.; Retamal-Valdes, B.; Montenegro, S.C.L.; Feres, M. Different antibiotic protocols in the treatment of severe chronic periodontitis: A 1-year randomized trial. *J. Clin. Periodontol.* **2017**, *44*, 822–832. [CrossRef] [PubMed]
39. Shaddox, L.M.; Walker, C. Microbial testing in periodontics: Value, limitations and future directions. *Periodontology 2000* **2009**, *50*, 25–38. [CrossRef] [PubMed]
40. Cohen, J.J. Programmed cell death in the immune system. In *Advances in Immunology*; Elsevier: Amsterdam, The Netherlands, 1991; Volume 50, pp. 55–85.

4

Immunological and Microbiological Profiling of Cumulative Risk Score for Periodontitis

Joonas Liukkonen [1,*], Ulvi K. Gürsoy [1], Eija Könönen [1,2], Ramin Akhi [3,4,5], Aino Salminen [6], John M. Liljestrand [6], Pratikshya Pradhan-Palikhe [6], Milla Pietiäinen [6], Timo Sorsa [6,7], G. Rutger Persson [8,9], Päivi Mäntylä [6,10,11], Kåre Buhlin [6,7], Susanna Paju [6], Juha Sinisalo [12], Sohvi Hörkkö [3,4,5] and Pirkko J. Pussinen [1,6,*]

1 Institute of Dentistry, University of Turku, 20100 Turku, Finland; ulvi.gursoy@utu.fi (U.K.G.); eija.kononen@utu.fi (E.K.)
2 Oral Health Care, Welfare Division, 20100 Turku, Finland
3 Medical Microbiology and Immunology, Research Unit of Biomedicine, University of Oulu, 90100 Oulu, Finland; ramin.akhi@oulu.fi (R.A.); sohvi.horkko@oulu.fi (S.H.)
4 Medical Research Center, Oulu University Hospital and University of Oulu, 90100 Oulu, Finland
5 Nordlab, Oulu University Hospital, 90100 Oulu, Finland
6 Oral and Maxillofacial Diseases, University of Helsinki and Helsinki University Hospital, 00100 Helsinki, Finland; aino.m.salminen@helsinki.fi (A.S.); john.liljestrand@helsinki.fi (J.M.L.); pratikshya.pp@gmail.com (P.P.-P.); milla.pietiainen@helsinki.fi (M.P.); timo.sorsa@helsinki.fi (T.S.); paivi.mantyla@uef.fi (P.M.); kare.buhlin@ki.se (K.B.); susanna.paju@helsinki.fi (S.P.)
7 Department of Periodontology, Institute of Odontology, Karolinska Institutet, 12343 Huddinge, Sweden
8 Departments of Periodontics and Oral Medicine, University of Washington, Seattle, WA 98101, USA; rper@uw.edu
9 Department of Periodontology, University of Bern, 3001 Bern, Switzerland
10 Institute of Dentistry, University of Eastern Finland, 70100 Kuopio, Finland
11 Oral and Maxillofacial Diseases, Kuopio University Hospital, 70100 Kuopio, Finland
12 HUCH Heart and Lung Center, Helsinki University Central Hospital, 00100 Helsinki, Finland; juha.sinisalo@hus.fi
* Correspondence: joonas.liukkonen@utu.fi (J.L.); pirkko.pussinen@helsinki.fi (P.J.P.)

Abstract: The cumulative risk score (CRS) is a mathematical salivary diagnostic model to define an individual's risk of having periodontitis. In order to further validate this salivary biomarker, we investigated how periodontal bacteria, lipopolysaccharide (LPS), and systemic and local host immune responses relate to CRS. Subgingival plaque, saliva, and serum samples collected from 445 individuals were used in the analyses. Plaque levels of 28 microbial species, especially those of *Aggregatibacter actinomycetemcomitans*, *Porphyromonas gingivalis*, *Porphyromonas endodontalis*, *Prevotella intermedia*, and *Tannerella forsythia*, and serum and salivary levels of IgA and IgG against these five species were determined. Additionally, LPS activity was measured. High CRS associated strongly with all IgA/IgG antibody and LPS levels in saliva, whereas in serum the associations were not that obvious. In the final logistic regression model, the best predictors of high CRS were saliva IgA burden against the five species (OR 7.04, 95% CI 2.25–22.0), IgG burden (3.79, 1.78–8.08), LPS (2.19, 1.38–3.47), and the sum of 17 subgingival Gram-negative species (6.19, 2.10–18.3). CRS is strongly associated with microbial biomarker species of periodontitis and salivary humoral immune responses against them.

Keywords: biomarkers; bacteria; lipopolysaccharides; saliva; serum

---

1. Introduction

Periodontitis, an infection-driven chronic inflammation in tooth-supporting tissues, is highly common in adults and a major cause of tooth loss. High levels of periodontitis-associated subgingival bacteria and the humoral immune response to periodontal infection are considered important factors for the initiation and progression of periodontal disease [1]. In addition to dysbiosis-associated Gram-negative periodontal pathogens *Aggregatibacter actinomycetemcomitans*, *Porphyromonas gingivalis*, *Prevotella intermedia*, and *Tannerella forsythia* [2,3], increasing knowledge of polymicrobial synergy and the development of sequencing techniques have resulted in the discovery of new potential periodontal pathogens, e.g., *Porphyromonas endodontalis* [4,5]. Lipopolysaccharide (LPS) of Gram-negative bacteria is a classical trigger for septic shock, and an independent risk factor for chronic cardiometabolic disorders [6]. Circulating LPS leads to systemic low-grade inflammation [7]. It has been suggested that a significant part of the circulating LPS is originated from the oral cavity and that circulating LPS activity may be a link between periodontitis and coronary artery disease (CAD) [8].

Besides detecting periodontal pathogens directly in saliva or subgingival plaque, the odds for the pathogen's presence can be evaluated by measuring the levels of serum or saliva antibodies [1,9–11]. Immunoglobulin A and G (IgA/IgG) are usually determined in this context. Elevated levels of systemic antibodies against periodontal bacteria have been found in individuals with periodontitis [11–16] and, thus, serum antibody levels are considered potential diagnostic markers of the disease. According to our previous studies, IgA and IgG levels in serum associate with *P. gingivalis* and *A. actinomycetemcomitans* carriage in saliva, and the combination of serum antibody levels and salivary pathogen levels improves the detection of periodontitis [11,17,18]. Due to the local production of antibodies, the antibody levels against periodontal bacteria are higher in gingival crevicular fluid than in serum. Elevated IgA levels against *A. actinomycetemcomitans* and *P. gingivalis* [10] and IgG levels against *A. actinomycetemcomitans* leukotoxins [19] have been observed in the saliva of individuals suffering from periodontitis.

The fluctuating nature of periodontal pathogenesis limits the use of single biomarkers with established thresholds in the detection of periodontitis [20]. The cumulative risk score (CRS) is a mathematical model to define an individual's risk of having periodontitis [21]. Three selected salivary biomarkers, namely, *P. gingivalis*, interleukin (IL)-1β, and matrix metalloproteinase (MMP)-8, represent three components of the periodontal inflammatory process: microbial pathogen burden, cytokine production, and tissue degradation, respectively. Our previous results indicate that high CRS is significantly associated with clinical and radiological signs of periodontitis [21–23]. In the present study, our aim was to validate further the CRS by analyzing its associations with subgingival microbial biomarker species and salivary humoral immune responses against them.

2. Materials and Methods

2.1. Study Population

The Corogene study is a prospective cohort including Finnish patients who underwent coronary angiography between June 2006 and March 2008 at the Helsinki University Central Hospital [24]. The Parogene is a sub-study of 508 subjects, who received clinical and radiographic oral health examinations. As described in detail elsewhere [25,26], these examinations were performed by calibrated dental specialists. The information of dental hygiene and smoking habits were gathered with a questionnaire. All subjects signed an informed consent, and the study was approved by the Helsinki University Central Hospital ethics committee (approval reference number 106/2007, approved on the 1 August 2007). The present study population consists of the Parogene study patients based on the availability of their saliva determinations ($n = 445$, 87.6% of the Parogene cohort).

2.2. Serum and Saliva Samples

Serum samples were drawn from the arterial line during the coronary angiography and stored at −80 °C until further analyses [24]. Saliva samples were collected before the oral examination between 8 a.m. and 3 p.m. Study participants chewed a piece of paraffin for 5 min, and at least 2 mL of stimulated whole saliva was collected and stored at −70 °C until further use. The samples were analyzed blindly in the laboratory. After thawing, the samples were centrifuged at 9300× *g* for 5 min. The pellets from the process were used for the bacterial analyses, whereas the supernatant was used for the antibody determinations.

2.3. Measurement of Serum and Saliva Antibodies Against Periodontal Pathogens

An enzyme-linked immunosorbent assay (ELISA) [11,27] was used to determine serum levels of IgA and IgG against whole cell antigens of *A. actinomycetemcomitans*, *P. gingivalis*, *P. endodontalis*, *P. intermedia*, and *T. forsythia*. The details of these analyses are described elsewhere [18,28]. Salivary levels of IgA/IgG against the same whole cell antigens of the same species were analyzed using a chemiluminescence immunoassay as described in detail elsewhere [29]. The antigens used in the assays, dilutions, and inter-assay variations are presented in Supplementary Table (Table S1).

2.4. Subgingival Bacteria

Pooled subgingival plaque samples were collected from the deepest pocket of each jaw quadrant [30]. Checkerboard DNA–DNA hybridization was used to determine the levels of 28 bacterial species, and of these, the levels of the same five species used for the antibody determinations were selected for detailed analyses [31,32]. Additionally, a sum level of 17 Gram-negative (*P. gingivalis*, *T. forsythia*, *T. denticola*, *A. actinomycetemcomitans* (strains Y4 plus ATCC 29523), *P. intermedia*, *Fusobacterium nucleatum* ssp. *naviforme*, *F. nucleatum* ssp. *nucleatum*, *F. nucleatum* ssp. *polymorphum*, *F. periodonticum*, *Campylobacter rectus*, *C. gracilis*, *C. showae*, *Veillonella parvula*, *Capnocytophaga gingivalis*, *C. sputigena*, *C. ochracea*, and *Eikenella corrodens*) and 11 Gram-positive species (*Parvimonas micra*, *Actinomyces odontolyticus*, *A. israelii*, *A. naeslundii*, *A. neuii*, *Streptococcus mitis*, *S. oralis*, *S. sanguinis*, *S. gordonii*, *S. intermedius*, and *S. constellatus*) [32] were used in the statistical analyses.

2.5. LPS Activity in Serum and Saliva Samples

After diluting the samples with endotoxin-free water, the LPS activity was determined from the serum samples (1:5, *v*/*v*) and the saliva supernatant (1:40.000, *v*/*v*) by a commercially available assay, Limulus amebocyte lysate coupled with a chromogenic substrate (Hycult Biotec, Uden, The Netherlands). The inter-assay coefficient of variation was 5.5% for serum and 6.8% for the saliva samples.

2.6. CRS Determination

The CRS values of the present study population have been described previously [23]. Briefly, the concentrations of IL-1β and aMMP-8 were determined from the saliva supernatants and the quantity of *P. gingivalis* from the saliva pellets. IL-1β concentrations were determined with a flow cytometry-based technique (MILLIPLEX® Map Kit, Human Cytokine/Chemokine panel MPXHCYTO-60K, Millipore, Billerica, MA, USA and Luminex® xMAP™ technique, Luminex Corporation, Austin, TX, USA), and MMP-8 concentrations with a time-resolved immunofluorometric assay (IFMA), as described by Gürsoy et al. [33] A qPCR-based technique was used to quantitate *P. gingivalis* in saliva and the concentrations were calculated as genomic equivalents (GE)/mL [28]. All concentrations were divided into tertiles to achieve a cumulative sub-score for each study subject. These sub-scores were further multiplied with each other and used to categorize the study population with "low (CRS I), moderate (CRS II), or high (CRS III) risk of having periodontitis". A detailed methodological description of CRS and its diagnostic abilities to detect periodontitis has been published elsewhere [21,23].

2.7. Statistical Analyses

Statistical analyses were performed with the statistical program (SPSS version 21.0; SPSS Inc., Chicago, IL, USA). The data were not normally distributed and therefore are presented in medians with interquartile range (IQR). The chi-square test was used when examining the relation of gender, proportion of edentulous, ever smoked, and diabetes mellitus (type 1 and 2) to CRS I–III. The Jonckheere–Terpstra test was used when examining the linear relation of CRS I–III with age, number of teeth, serum or saliva IgA/IgG, LPS activity, and subgingival bacterial levels. Logistic regression models were used when the association of high CRS (III vs. CRS I–II) with serum or saliva IgA/IgG and LPS activity, and subgingival bacteria levels was examined. Firstly, the models were adjusted for age, gender, and number of remaining teeth, and, if found significant, they were additionally adjusted for the subgingival level of the corresponding bacterial species. The associations of high CRS (CRS III vs. CRS I–II) with antibody, LPS, and bacterial levels were analyzed in multiple logistic regression models adjusted for age, sex, number of teeth, and smoking (ever vs. never). To standardize the values, all models were performed for logarithmically (10-base) transformed results. The p-value < 0.05 was considered significant.

3. Results

Table 1 shows the characteristics of the population in relation to CRS I–III. As expected, there were statistically significant differences in the number of teeth and periodontal status between the CRS groups.

Table 1. Characteristics of the study population divided into three groups on the basis of cumulative risk score (CRS) I–III.

	CRS I	CRS II	CRS III	
		Median (IQR)		p-Value [1]
Age (years)	66 (10)	64 (14)	63 (13)	0.054
Number of teeth	21 (18)	24 (11)	24 (8)	**0.001**
		n (%)		p-Value [2]
Sex (% of men)	70 (58.8)	119 (71.3)	114 (66.3)	0.091
Ever smoked	57 (48.3)	96 (57.5)	89 (51.7)	0.286
Diabetes	26 (21.8)	33 (20.2)	51 (30.0)	0.089
Periodontal and dental status [3]				**<0.001**
No to mild periodontitis	88 (74.6)	125 (74.0)	102 (59.3)	
Moderate to severe periodontitis	15 (12.7)	36 (21.3)	67 (39.0)	
Edentulous	15 (12.7)	8 (4.7)	3 (1.7)	

[1] p-values from the Jonckheere–Terpstra test; [2] chi-square tests; [3] the classification is based on alveolar bone loss and periodontal probing pocket depth as reported in our previous study [23]. Results are presented as median values with interquartile range (IQR). Significant p-values are indicated in bold face.

Serum antibody and LPS activity levels in relation to CRS I–III are presented in Table 2. Elevating IgA levels against *P. gingivalis*, *P. endodontalis*, and *P. intermedia* and elevating IgG levels against *P. gingivalis*, *P. endodontalis*, and *P. intermedia* were found with increasing CRS, whereas the *T. forsythia* antibody levels or serum LPS activity did not differ between CRS I–III. In regression analyses, after adjusting for age, sex, and number of teeth (Model 1), high CRS (III) associated significantly with the IgA levels against *A. actinomycetemcomitans*, *P. gingivalis*, *P. endodontalis*, and *P. intermedia* and the IgG levels against *P. gingivalis*, *P. endodontalis*, and *P. intermedia*. When the models were further adjusted for the corresponding subgingival bacterial level, *A. actinomycetemcomitans* IgA, *P. gingivalis* IgG, *P. endodontalis* IgA/IgG, and *P. intermedia* IgA remained significantly associated with CRS III.

Saliva antibody and LPS activity levels in relation to CRS are presented in Table 3. The IgA/IgG antibody levels against all tested bacteria and LPS activity were elevating with increasing CRS. In logistic regression analyses adjusted for age, sex, and number of teeth (Model 1), high CRS (III) associated significantly with all IgA/IgG and LPS activity levels. These associations remained significant when the models were adjusted further for the corresponding subgingival bacterial level (the antibodies) or the sum of Gram-negative bacteria (LPS).

Subgingival bacterial levels in relation to CRS I–III are presented in Table 4. The counts of all examined bacteria, and the sum of 11 subgingival Gram-positive and 17 subgingival Gram-negative species increased with increasing CRS. In the association analyses adjusted for age, gender, and number of remaining teeth, high CRS (III) associated significantly with all examined bacterial species, and with the sum of 11 subgingival Gram-positive and 17 subgingival Gram-negative species.

Table 2. Serum antibody levels in response to five periodontal pathogens and lipopolysaccharide (LPS) levels according to the CRS.

Antigen/Measure	Antibody Class	CRS I $n = 117$	CRS II $n = 162$	CRS III n = 166	p-Value [1]	OR for High CRS (95% CI), p-Value [2]	
			Median (IQR)			Model 1	Model 2
Aggregatibacteractinomycetemcomitans	IgA	0.61 (0.61)	0.59 (0.67)	0.69 (0.69)	**0.037**	2.22 (1.19–4.18), **0.012**	2.39 (1.27–4.52), **0.007**
	IgG	0.60 (0.50)	0.69 (0.80)	0.73 (0.77)	**0.043**	1.66 (0.92–3.00), 0.094	
Porphyromonas gingivalis	IgA	0.24 (0.98)	0.33 (0.91)	0.86 (1.41)	**<0.001**	2.88 (1.89–4.38) **<0.001**	1.47 (0.92–2.35), 0.106
	IgG	0.84 (1.47)	0.95 (1.37)	1.71 (1.88)	**<0.001**	7.34 (3.65–14.7), **<0.001**	2.32 (1.04–5.18), **0.040**
Porphyromonas endodontalis	IgA	0.33 (0.55)	0.45 (0.61)	0.65 (1.26)	**<0.001**	3.52 (2.03–6.09), **<0.001**	2.95 (1.66–5.21), **<0.001**
	IgG	0.97 (1.31)	1.12 (1.17)	1.79 (1.66)	**<0.001**	7.41 (3.36–16.3), **<0.001**	6.08 (2.94–12.3), **<0.001**
Prevotellaintermedia	IgA	0.56 (0.41)	0.56 (0.44)	0.68 (0.60)	**0.013**	3.11(1.43–6.74), **0.004**	2.59 (1.15–5.81), **0.021**
	IgG	0.44 (0.35)	0.42 (0.28)	0.46 (0.35)	0.295	2.30 (1.01–5.22), **0.047**	1.87 (0.79–4.42), 0.154
Tannerella forsythia	IgA	0.23 (0.16)	0.18 (0.12)	0.19 (0.14)	0.114	1.28 (0.65–2.53), 0.474	
	IgG	0.12 (0.13)	0.10 (0.11)	0.10 (0.12)	0.203	1.06 (0.57–1.97), 0.855	
LPS		0.46 (0.43)	0.54 (0.62)	0.53 (0.58)	0.123	1.23 (0.68–2.22), 0.497	

[1] Jonckheere–Terpstra test; [2] logistic regression models, dependent variable CRS III vs. CRSI–II, odds ratio (OR) is presented/10-base logarithmically transformed unit; Model 1, adjusted for age, gender, and number of remaining teeth; Model 2, additionally adjusted for the subgingival level of the species. The antibody levels are presented as absorbance units, AU. The LPS activity is presented as endotoxin units, EU/mL. Statistically significant p-values are indicated by bold face.

Table 3. Saliva antibody levels in response to five periodontal pathogens and lipopolysaccharide (LPS) levels according to the CRS.

Antigen/Measure	Antibody Class	CRS I $n = 108$	CRS II $n = 155$	CRS III $n = 157$	p-Value [1]	OR for High CRS (95% CI), p-Value [2]	
			Median (IQR)			Model 1	Model 2
A. actinomycetemcomitans	IgA	2843 (2221)	3413 (3065)	4403 (5569)	**<0.001**	6.02 (3.06–11.8), **<0.001**	6.24 (3.11–12.5), **<0.001**
	IgG	4160 (4669)	7642 (15,265)	14,154 (40,410)	**<0.001**	3.28 (2.22–4.87), **<0.001**	3.26 (2.17–4.89), **<0.001**
P. gingivalis	IgA	3587 (5609)	5217 (5642)	9340 (12,507)	**<0.001**	6.72 (3.74–12.1), **<0.001**	4.50 (2.41–8.41), **<0.001**
	IgG	1500 (2254)	2647 (4725)	6111 (11,734)	**<0.001**	5.97 (3.72–9.61), **<0.001**	3.76 (2.26–6.25), **<0.001**
P. endodontalis	IgA	4809 (3249)	6971 (6315)	10,146 (9454)	**<0.001**	16.8 (7.50–37.5), **<0.001**	14.5 (6.36–32.8), **<0.001**
	IgG	1511 (1377)	2482 (2445)	4546 (5769)	**<0.001**	13.9 (7.11–27.3), **<0.001**	13.7 (6.89–27.4), **<0.001**
P. intermedia	IgA	2014 (1880)	3026 (2637)	3878 (4885)	**<0.001**	5.90 (3.04–11.4), **<0.001**	5.97 (3.01–11.8), **<0.001**
	IgG	1069 (637)	1534 (1755)	2547 (3284)	**<0.001**	10.2 (5.16–20.6), **<0.001**	10.0 (5.03–20.1), **<0.001**
T. forsythia	IgA	5893 (4254)	7849 (6614)	8359 (6605)	**<0.001**	5.43 (2.39–12.3), **<0.001**	6.92 (2.87–16.5), **<0.001**
	IgG	1448 (1069)	2208 (2712)	3956 (4397)	**<0.001**	7.83 (4.13–14.8), **<0.001**	8.81 (4.44–17.5), **<0.001**
LPS activity		3991 (8406)	4825 (10,816)	9065 (14,866)	**<0.001**	2.40 (1.600–3.591), **0.001**	2.42 (1.568–3.728), **<0.001** [3]

[1] Jonckheere–Terpstra test; [2] logistic regression models, dependent variable CRS III vs. CRSI–II, OR is presented/10-base logarithmically transformed unit; Model 1, adjusted for age, sex, and number of teeth; Model 2, additionally adjusted for the subgingival level of the species; [3] additionally adjusted for the sum of 17 Gram-negative subgingival species. The antibodies are presented as relative light units, RLU/100 ms. The LPS activity is presented as endotoxin units, EU/mL. Statistically significant p-values are indicated by bold face.

Table 4. Subgingival bacterial levels according to the CRS groups.

Species (Counts × 10^5)	CRS I	CRS II	CRS III	*p*-Value [1]	OR for High CRS (95% CI), *p*-Value [4]
		Median (IQR)			
A. actinomycetemcomitans	0.32 (1.12)	0.45 (1.58)	0.79 (1.92)	**<0.001**	1.85 (1.43–2.39), **<0.001**
P. gingivalis	0.26 (0.77)	0.38 (1.71)	2.95 (12.7)	**<0.001**	2.70 (2.11–3.46), **<0.001**
P. endodontalis	0.07 (0.94)	0.22 (1.31)	1.10 (4.30)	**<0.001**	1.97 (1.57–2.47), **<0.001**
P. intermedia	0.47 (1.42)	0.57 (1.98)	1.55 (3.07)	**<0.001**	1.95 (1.53–2.49), **<0.001**
T. forsythia	1.95 (9.28)	3.47 (11.1)	12.9 (24.8)	**<0.001**	2.00 (1.63–2.46), **<0.001**
Sum of Gram positive species [2]	4.24 (8.71)	4.75 (14.3)	9.82 (12.5)	**<0.001**	2.25 (1.52–3.34), **<0.001**
Sum of Gram negative species [3]	25.0 (48.9)	35.0 (67.1)	70.6 (67.6)	**<0.001**	3.28 (2.10–5.13), **<0.001**

[1] Jonckheere–Terpstra test; [2] sum of 11 subgingival species; [3] sum of 17 subgingival species; [4] logistic regression model, dependent variable CRS III vs. CRSI–II, OR is presented/10-base logarithmically transformed unit, adjusted for age, sex, and number of teeth. Statistically significant *p*-values are indicated by bold face.

Table 5 summarizes the associations of high CRS (III) with antibody and bacterial levels in a regression model that was adjusted for age, gender, number of teeth, and smoking. Salivary IgA burden against the five species, salivary IgG burden against the five species, salivary LPS, and the sum of subgingival Gram-negative species associated with high CRS. The odds ratios were 7.04 ($p = 0.001$), 3.79 ($p = 0.001$), 2.19 ($p = 0.001$), and 6.19 ($p = 0.001$), respectively.

Table 5. Association of high CRS with antibody and subgingival bacterial levels.

		Variable	Unit	OR (95% CI) for High CRS	*p*-Value [1]
Covariates		Age	years	0.997 (0.975–1.019)	0.779
		Sex	male	0.965 (0.640–1.455)	0.865
		Number of teeth	number	1.034 (1.008–1.061)	**0.011**
		Smoking	ever	1.055 (0.703–1.583)	0.796
Model	Serum	Serum IgA burden [2]	EU	0.910 (0.259–3.197)	0.883
		Serum IgG burden [2]	EU	2.949 (0.536–16.23)	0.214
		Serum LPS	EU/mL	1.396 (0.681–2.860)	0.362
	Saliva	Saliva IgA burden [2]	RLU/100 ms	7.043 (2.252–22.03)	**0.001**
		Saliva IgG burden [2]	RLU/100 ms	3.788 (1.777–8.077)	**0.001**
		Saliva LPS	EU/mL	2.191 (1.384–3.468)	**0.001**
	Subgingival	Sum of Gram-positive species [3]	count × 10^5	0.641 (0.266–1.547)	0.322
		Sum of Gram-negative species [4]	count × 10^5	6.191 (2.098–18.27)	**0.001**

[1] Logistic regression model, dependent variable CRS III vs. CRS I–II, model is adjusted for covariates presented above. For the bacteria, Ig, and LPS levels, OR is presented/10-base logarithmically transformed unit; [2] sum of antibody levels in response to *A. actinomycetemcomitans*, *P. gingivalis*, *P. endodontalis*, *P. intermedia*, and *T. forsythia*; [3] sum of 11 subgingival species; [4] sum of 17 subgingival species; [5] presented as counts × 10^5 EU, ELISA units; EU/mL, endotoxin units/mL; RLU, relative light units. Statistically significant *p*-values are indicated by bold face.

4. Discussion

Here we present a strong association of salivary IgA burden, salivary IgG burden, salivary LPS, and the sum of subgingival Gram-negative species with high CRS. Due to its associations with subgingival periodontal bacteria and the salivary humoral immune response to them, the present findings produce additional evidence on the diagnostic strength of CRS.

Our study shows for the first time that LPS activity in saliva associates with a risk of having periodontitis, based on CRS. We used the Limulus Amebocyte lysate assay to measure LPS activity in saliva and serum, because it is the most sensitive and most widely used method [34]. The assay is not targeted to any specific bacterial species but determines the overall biological activity of a mixture of endotoxins produced by Gram-negative bacteria. It has been shown that serum LPS correlates with periodontal status and serum LPS activity decreases after periodontal treatment [35–37]. A significant part of circulating LPS may originate from the oral cavity. There is supporting evidence that there is a correlation between serum and saliva LPS activity levels [8]. Moreover, a study performed with mice estimated that oral administration of *P. gingivalis* could change the gut microbiome and lead to elevated serum endotoxin levels [38]. In investigations on structural alterations in lipid-A-derived 3-OH fatty acid profiles or using a bioassay for Toll-like receptors 2 and 4, stimulants indicate that there are differences in saliva between individuals with and without periodontal disease [39,40]. These methods differ from the LAL assay and do not measure the activity level of LPS. Based on our previous data on LPS activity in saliva, LPS activity correlates with the number of remaining teeth and the amount of alveolar bone loss; however, no relation to clinical periodontal parameters was found [8,28,41]. Similarly, in the present study, no association between serum LPS and CRS was observed.

To date, findings on IgA/IgG binding to periodontal bacteria in saliva are limited to *A. actinomycetemcomitans*, *P. gingivalis*, *T. denticola*, *P. intermedia*, and *F. nucleatum* [10,42–44]. In the present population, we also determined the salivary antibodies against *T. forsythia* and *P. endodontalis* [28,45]. Elevated salivary levels of IgA antibodies against *A. actinomycetemcomitans* and *P. gingivalis* [10] and salivary IgG levels against *A. actinomycetemcomitans* leukotoxins [19] have been detected in periodontitis patients. Since all determined salivary antibody levels associated with CRS, we calculated their sum to be used in further statistical analyses and to strengthen the association. Notably, salivary IgA/IgG burden against these microbial biomarker species presented an independent and strong association with CRS even in models where the bacterial subgingival levels were used as covariates. This indicates immune hyperresponsiveness to dysbiosis, typical for the pathogenesis of periodontitis [46].

Elevated levels of systemic antibodies against periodontal bacteria are common in periodontitis patients [12,14–16,47]. Conceivably, it can be assumed that there is a connection between CRS and systemic IgA/IgG response. In this study, high CRS (III) associated significantly with the serum IgA levels against *A. actinomycetemcomitans*, *P. endodontalis*, and *P. intermedia* and with the IgG levels against *P. gingivalis* and *P. endodontalis*. Based on the association analyses, these serum antibody levels were also independent of the subgingival bacterial level. Interestingly, the most significant association with high CRS was observed with antibodies against *P. gingivalis* and *P. endodontalis*. An obvious explanation is that CRS already includes *P. gingivalis* concentration and, in the case of *P. endodontalis*, cross-reactivity of antibodies to *P. endodontalis* and closely related species cannot be excluded. The results regarding serum antibodies and CRS are in line with our previous observations on the associations with serum IgA/IgG levels of *P. gingivalis* and *A. actinomycetemcomitans* and their carriage in saliva, whereas periodontitis proved to have merely a modest modifying effect [11]. Furthermore, the impact of the variation of serum antibody response between individuals in relation to genetic and immunological background, previous exposure to periodontal bacteria, and immunogenic characteristics of the antigenic challenge have been discussed [48]. IgG antibodies with a long half-life represent exposure to the bacteria; however, these antibodies are extremely stable in plasma and do not allow an estimation of the time of the exposure [13,49]. Instead, IgA antibodies with a short half-time represent a recent or continuous exposure to the indicated pathogen [50]. Therefore, it seems that saliva, in comparison to serum, would be a more suitable specimen type to recognize biomarkers of active periodontal inflammation.

The relatively large sample size (n = 445) and verified background data on general and oral health are the major strengths of the present study. The suitability of CRS for the evaluation of the risk of having periodontitis is established in previous studies [21–23]. Here we demonstrated the connection of CRS with subgingival bacterial levels as well as with antibodies against periodontal bacteria and LPS activity in saliva samples. On the other hand, a weakness of the present research is that the study population consists of patients with symptomatic heart disease, including stable coronary artery disease, acute coronary syndrome, stable or atypical chest pains, valvular heart disease, or cardiomyopathy. Thus, especially when evaluating the levels of serum antibodies, the results may not be fully applicable to a general population. Additionally, the subgingival plaque sample collected from each dental quadrant was pooled into one sample per patient. While the samples were taken from the deepest pockets, the pool may not necessarily represent the whole mouth.

5. Conclusions

Our new findings suggest that CRS is a reliable and suitable diagnostic tool for periodontitis. The results reveal how the salivary biomarker combination, CRS, reflects the presence of dysbiotic subgingival biofilms and the local host response to periodontal pathogens and, further, validate CRS in saliva-based diagnostics on the road to more personalized dentistry.

Author Contributions: Designed the original study and collected the material: P.J.P., J.S., K.B., P.M., S.P. Clinical examinations: K.B., P.M., S.P., J.S. Laboratory analyses: U.K.G., R.A., A.S., J.M.L., P.P.-P., M.P., T.S., G.R.P., S.H. Designed the present study, performed the data analysis: J.L., U.K.G., E.K., P.J.P. Wrote the manuscript: J.L. All authors have read and agreed to the published version of the manuscript.

References

1. Ebersole, J.L.; Dawson, D.R., 3rd; Morford, L.A.; Peyyala, R.; Miller, C.S.; González, O.A. Periodontal disease immunology: 'Double indemnity' in protecting the host. *Periodontology 2000* **2013**, *62*, 163–202. [CrossRef] [PubMed]

2. Sanz, M.; Beighton, D.; Curtis, M.A.; Cury, J.A.; Dige, I.; Dommisch, H.; Ellwood, R.; Giacaman, R.A.; Herrera, D.; Herzberg, M.C.; et al. Role of microbial biofilms in the maintenance of oral health and in the development of dental caries and periodontal diseases. Consensus report of group 1 of the Joint EFP/ORCA workshop on the boundaries between caries and periodontal disease. *J. Clin. Periodontol.* **2017**, *44*, S5–S11. [CrossRef] [PubMed]
3. Socransky, S.S.; Haffajee, A.D.; Cugini, M.; Smith, C.; Kent, R.L. Microbial complexes in subgingival plaque. *J. Clin. Periodontol.* **1998**, *25*, 134–144. [CrossRef]
4. Perez-Chaparro, P.; Goncalves, C.; Figueiredo, L.C.; Faveri, M.; Lobao, E.; Tamashiro, N.; Duarte, P.; Feres, M. Newly Identified Pathogens Associated with Periodontitis. *J. Dent. Res.* **2014**, *93*, 846–858. [CrossRef] [PubMed]
5. Hajishengallis, G.; Lamont, R.J. Beyond the red complex and into more complexity: The polymicrobial synergy and dysbiosis (PSD) model of periodontal disease etiology. *Mol. Oral Microbiol.* **2012**, *27*, 409–419. [CrossRef] [PubMed]
6. Munford, R.S. Endotoxemia-menace, marker, or mistake? *J. Leukoc. Biol.* **2016**, *100*, 687–698. [CrossRef]
7. Pussinen, P.J.; Tuomisto, K.; Jousilahti, P.; Havulinna, A.S.; Sundvall, J.; Salomaa, V. Endotoxemia, Immune Response to Periodontal Pathogens, and Systemic Inflammation Associate with Incident Cardiovascular Disease Events. *Arter. Thromb. Vasc. Biol.* **2007**, *27*, 1433–1439. [CrossRef]
8. Liljestrand, J.; Paju, S.; Buhlin, K.; Persson, G.R.; Sarna, S.; Nieminen, M.S.; Sinisalo, J.; Mäntylä, P.; Pussinen, P.J. Lipopolysaccharide, a possible molecular mediator between periodontitis and coronary artery disease. *J. Clin. Periodontol.* **2017**, *44*, 784–792. [CrossRef]
9. Kinane, D.F.; Mooney, J.; Ebersole, J.L. Humoral immune response to Actinobacillus actinomycetemcomitans and Porphyromonas gingivalis in periodontal disease. *Periodontology 2000* **1999**, *20*, 289–340. [CrossRef]
10. Plombas, M.; Gobert, B.; De March, A.K.; Sarda, M.N.K.; Sixou, M.; Bene, M.C.; Miller, N.; Faure, G.C. Isotypic Antibody Response to Plaque Anaerobes in Periodontal Disease. *J. Periodontol.* **2002**, *73*, 1507–1511. [CrossRef]
11. Pussinen, P.J.; Könönen, E.; Paju, S.; Hyvärinen, K.; Gursoy, U.K.; Huumonen, S.; Knuuttila, M.; Suominen, A.L. Periodontal pathogen carriage, rather than periodontitis, determines the serum antibody levels. *J. Clin. Periodontol.* **2011**, *38*, 405–411. [CrossRef]
12. Ebersole, J.L.; Taubman, M.A.; Smith, D.J.; Frey, D.E.; Haffajee, A.D.; Socransky, S.S. Human serum antibody responses to oral microorganisms IV. Correlation with homologous infection. *Oral Microbiol. Immunol.* **1987**, *2*, 53–59. [CrossRef]
13. Papapanou, P.N.; Neiderud, A.M.; Disick, E.; Lalla, E.; Miller, G.C.; Dahlén, G. Longitudinal stability of serum immunoglobulin G responses to periodontal bacteria. *J. Clin. Periodontol.* **2004**, *31*, 985–990. [CrossRef]
14. Dye, B.A.; Herrera-Abreu, M.; Lerche-Sehm, J.; Vlachojannis, C.; Pikdöken, L.; Pretzl, B.; Schwartz, A.; Papapanou, P.N. Serum Antibodies to Periodontal Bacteria as Diagnostic Markers of Periodontitis. *J. Periodontol.* **2009**, *80*, 634–647. [CrossRef]
15. Kudo, C.; Naruishi, K.; Maeda, H.; Abiko, Y.; Hino, T.; Iwata, M.; Mitsuhashi, C.; Murakami, S.; Nagasawa, T.; Nagata, T.; et al. Assessment of the Plasma/Serum IgG Test to Screen for Periodontitis. *J. Dent. Res.* **2012**, *91*, 1190–1195. [CrossRef]
16. Buhlin, K.; Holmer, J.; Gustafsson, A.; Hörkkö, S.; Pockley, A.; Johansson, A.; Paju, S.; Klinge, B.; Pussinen, P.J. Association of periodontitis with persistent, pro-atherogenic antibody responses. *J. Clin. Periodontol.* **2015**, *42*, 1006–1014. [CrossRef]
17. Liljestrand, J.; Gursoy, U.K.; Hyvärinen, K.; Sorsa, T.; Suominen, A.L.; Könönen, E.; Pussinen, P.J. Combining Salivary Pathogen and Serum Antibody Levels Improves Their Diagnostic Ability in Detection of Periodontitis. *J. Periodontol.* **2014**, *85*, 123–131. [CrossRef]
18. Liljestrand, J.M.; Paju, S.; Pietiäinen, M.; Buhlin, K.; Persson, G.R.; Nieminen, M.S.; Sinisalo, J.; Mäntylä, P.; Pussinen, P. Immunologic burden links periodontitis to acute coronary syndrome. *Atherosclerosis* **2018**, *268*, 177–184. [CrossRef]
19. Engstrom, P.-E.; George, M.; Larsson, P.; Lally, E.T.; Taichman, N.S.; Norhagen, E.G. Oral and systemic immunoglobulin G-subclass antibodies to Actinobacillus actinomycetemcomitans leukotoxin. *Oral Microbiol. Immunol.* **1999**, *14*, 104–108. [CrossRef]

20. Kinney, J.; Morelli, T.; Braun, T.; Ramseier, C.; Herr, A.E.; Sugai, J.; Shelburne, C.; Rayburn, L.; Singh, A.; Giannobile, W.V. Saliva/pathogen biomarker signatures and periodontal disease progression. *J. Dent. Res.* **2011**, *90*, 752–758. [CrossRef]
21. Gursoy, U.K.; Könönen, E.; Pussinen, P.J.; Tervahartiala, T.; Hyvärinen, K.; Suominen, A.L.; Uitto, V.-J.; Paju, S.; Sorsa, T. Use of Host- and Bacteria-Derived Salivary Markers in Detection of Periodontitis: A Cumulative Approach. *Dis. Markers* **2011**, *30*, 299–305. [CrossRef] [PubMed]
22. Gursoy, U.K.; Pussinen, P.J.; Salomaa, V.; Syrjäläinen, S.; Könönen, E. Cumulative use of salivary markers with an adaptive design improves detection of periodontal disease over fixed biomarker thresholds. *Acta Odontol. Scand.* **2018**, *76*, 493–496. [CrossRef] [PubMed]
23. Salminen, A.; Gürsoy, U.K.; Paju, S.; Hyvärinen, K.; Mäntylä, P.; Buhlin, K.; Könönen, E.; Nieminen, M.S.; Sorsa, T.; Sinisalo, J.; et al. Salivary biomarkers of bacterial burden, inflammatory response, and tissue destruction in periodontitis. *J. Clin. Periodontol.* **2014**, *41*, 442–450. [CrossRef] [PubMed]
24. Vaara, S.; Nieminen, M.S.; Lokki, M.-L.; Perola, M.; Pussinen, P.J.; Allonen, J.; Parkkonen, O.; Sinisalo, J. Cohort Profile: The Corogene study. *Int. J. Epidemiol.* **2011**, *41*, 1265–1271. [CrossRef]
25. Buhlin, K.; Mäntylä, P.; Paju, S.; Peltola, J.S.; Nieminen, M.S.; Sinisalo, J.; Pussinen, P.J. Periodontitis is associated with angiographically verified coronary artery disease. *J. Clin. Periodontol.* **2011**, *38*, 1007–1014. [CrossRef]
26. Kallio, K.A.E.; Marchesani, M.; Vlachopoulou, E.; Mäntylä, P.; Paju, S.; Buhlin, K.; Suominen, A.L.; Contreras, J.; Knuuttila, M.; Hernandez, M.; et al. Genetic Variation on theBAT1-NFKBIL1-LTARegion of Major Histocompatibility Complex Class III Associates with Periodontitis. *Infect. Immun.* **2014**, *82*, 1939–1948. [CrossRef]
27. Pussinen, P.J.; Vilkuna-Rautiainen, T.; Alfthan, G.; Mattila, K.; Asikainen, S. Multiserotype Enzyme-Linked Immunosorbent Assay as a Diagnostic Aid for Periodontitis in Large-Scale Studies. *J. Clin. Microbiol.* **2002**, *40*, 512–518. [CrossRef]
28. Hyvärinen, K.; Mäntylä, P.; Buhlin, K.; Paju, S.; Nieminen, M.S.; Sinisalo, J.; Pussinen, P. A common periodontal pathogen has an adverse association with both acute and stable coronary artery disease. *Atherosclerosis* **2012**, *223*, 478–484. [CrossRef]
29. Akhi, R.; Wang, C.; Nissinen, A.E.; Kankaanpää, J.; Bloigu, R.; Paju, S.; Mäntylä, P.; Buhlin, K.; Sinisalo, J.; Pussinen, P.; et al. Salivary IgA to MAA-LDL and Oral Pathogens Are Linked to Coronary Disease. *J. Dent. Res.* **2019**, *98*, 296–303. [CrossRef]
30. Mäntylä, P.; Buhlin, K.; Paju, S. Subgingival Aggregatibacter actinomycetemcomitans associates with the risk of coronary artery disease. *J. Clin. Periodontol.* **2013**, *40*, 583–590. [CrossRef]
31. Socransky, S.S.; Haffajee, A.D.; Smith, C.; Martin, L.; Haffajee, J.A.; Uzel, N.G.; Goodson, J.M. Use of checkerboard DNA-DNA hybridization to study complex microbial ecosystems. *Oral Microbiol. Immunol.* **2004**, *19*, 352–362. [CrossRef]
32. Pradhan-Palikhe, P.; Mäntylä, P.; Paju, S.; Buhlin, K.; Persson, G.R.; Nieminen, M.S.; Sinisalo, J.; Pussinen, P.J. Subgingival Bacterial Burden in Relation to Clinical and Radiographic Periodontal Parameters. *J. Periodontol.* **2013**, *84*, 1809–1817. [CrossRef]
33. Gursoy, U.K.; Könönen, E.; Pradhan-Palikhe, P.; Tervahartiala, T.; Pussinen, P.J.; Suominen-Taipale, L.; Sorsa, T. Salivary MMP-8, TIMP-1, and ICTP as markers of advanced periodontitis. *J. Clin. Periodontol.* **2010**, *37*, 487–493. [CrossRef]
34. Manco, M.; Putignani, L.; Bottazzo, G.F. Gut Microbiota, Lipopolysaccharides, and Innate Immunity in the Pathogenesis of Obesity and Cardiovascular Risk. *Endocr. Rev.* **2010**, *31*, 817–844. [CrossRef]
35. Pussinen, P.J.; Vilkuna-Rautiainen, T.; Alfthan, G.; Palosuo, T.; Jauhiainen, M.; Sundvall, J.; Vesanen, M.; Mattila, K.; Asikainen, S. Severe Periodontitis Enhances Macrophage Activation via Increased Serum Lipopolysaccharide. *Arter. Thromb. Vasc. Biol.* **2004**, *24*, 2174–2180. [CrossRef]
36. Paju, S.; Pussinen, P.J.; Sinisalo, J.; Mattila, K.; Dogan, B.; Ahlberg, J.; Valtonen, V.; Nieminen, M.S.; Asikainen, S. Clarithromycin reduces recurrent cardiovascular events in subjects without periodontitis. *Atherosclerosis* **2006**, *188*, 412–419. [CrossRef]
37. Masi, S.; Orlandi, M.; Parkar, M.; Bhowruth, D.; Kingston, I.; O'Rourke, C.; Virdis, A.; Hingorani, A.D.; Hurel, S.J.; Donos, N.; et al. Mitochondrial oxidative stress, endothelial function and metabolic control in patients with type II diabetes and periodontitis: A randomised controlled clinical trial. *Int. J. Cardiol.* **2018**, *271*, 263–268. [CrossRef]

36. Paju, S.; Pussinen, P.J.; Sinisalo, J.; Mattila, K.; Dogan, B.; Ahlberg, J.; Valtonen, V.; Nieminen, M.S.; Asikainen, S. Clarithromycin reduces recurrent cardiovascular events in subjects without periodontitis. *Atherosclerosis* **2006**, *188*, 412–419. [CrossRef]
37. Masi, S.; Orlandi, M.; Parkar, M.; Bhowruth, D.; Kingston, I.; O'Rourke, C.; Virdis, A.; Hingorani, A.D.; Hurel, S.J.; Donos, N.; et al. Mitochondrial oxidative stress, endothelial function and metabolic control in patients with type II diabetes and periodontitis: A randomised controlled clinical trial. *Int. J. Cardiol.* **2018**, *271*, 263–268. [CrossRef]
38. Sato, K.; Takahashi, N.; Kato, T.; Matsuda, Y.; Yokoji, M.; Yamada, M.; Nakajima, T.; Kondo, N.; Endo, N.; Yamamoto, R.; et al. Aggravation of collagen-induced arthritis by orally administered Porphyromonas gingivalis through modulation of the gut microbiota and gut immune system. *Sci. Rep.* **2017**, *7*, 6955. [CrossRef]
39. Lappin, D.F.; Sherrabeh, S.; Erridge, C. Stimulants of Toll-like receptors 2 and 4 are elevated in saliva of periodontitis patients compared with healthy subjects. *J. Clin. Periodontol.* **2011**, *38*, 318–325. [CrossRef]
40. Buduneli, N.; Larsson, L.; Bıyıkoğlu, B.; Renaud, D.E.; Bagaitkar, J.; Scott, D.A. Fatty Acid Profiles in Smokers with Chronic Periodontitis. *J. Dent. Res.* **2010**, *90*, 47–52. [CrossRef]
41. Liukkonen, J.; Gursoy, U.K.; Pussinen, P.J.; Suominen, A.L.; Könönen, E. Salivary Concentrations of Interleukin (IL)-1β, IL-17A, and IL-23 Vary in Relation to Periodontal Status. *J. Periodontol.* **2016**, *87*, 1484–1491. [CrossRef] [PubMed]
42. Sandholm, L.; Tolo, K.; Olsen, I. Salivary IgG, a parameter of periodontal disease activity? High responders to Actinobacillus actinomycetemcomitans Y4 in juvenile and adult periodontitis. *J. Clin. Periodontol.* **1987**, *14*, 289–294. [CrossRef] [PubMed]
43. Hägewald, S.; Bernimoulin, J.-P.; Köttgen, E.; Kage, A. Total IgA and Porphyromonas gingivalis-reactive IgA in the saliva of patients with generalised early-onset periodontitis. *Eur. J. Oral Sci.* **2000**, *108*, 147–153. [CrossRef] [PubMed]
44. Hagewald, S.; Bernimoulin, J.-P.; Kottgen, E.; Kage, A. Salivary IgA subclasses and bacteria-reactive IgA in patients with aggressive periodontitis. *J. Periodontal Res.* **2002**, *37*, 333–339. [CrossRef] [PubMed]
45. Pietiäinen, M.; Liljestrand, J.; Akhi, R.; Buhlin, K.; Johansson, A.; Paju, S.; Salminen, A.; Mäntylä, P.; Sinisalo, J.; Tjäderhane, L.; et al. Saliva and Serum Immune Responses in Apical Periodontitis. *J. Clin. Med.* **2019**, *8*, 889. [CrossRef] [PubMed]
46. Kinane, D.F.; Stathopoulou, P.G.; Papapanou, P.N. Periodontal diseases. *Nat. Rev. Dis. Primers* **2017**, *3*, 17038. [CrossRef] [PubMed]
47. Papapanou, P.N.; Neiderud, A.-M.; Papadimitriou, A.; Sandros, J.; Dahlén, G. "Checkerboard" Assessments of Periodontal Microbiota and Serum Antibody Responses: A Case-Control Study. *J. Periodontol.* **2000**, *71*, 885–897. [CrossRef]
48. Beck, J.; Eke, P.; Heiss, G. Periodontal Disease and Coronary Heart Disease: A Reappraisal of the Exposure. *ACC Curr. J. Rev.* **2005**, *14*, 17. [CrossRef]
49. Lakio, L.; Antinheimo, J.; Paju, S.; Buhlin, K.; Pussinen, P.J.; Alfthan, G. Tracking of plasma antibodies againstAggregatibacter actinomycetemcomitansandPorphyromonas gingivalisduring 15 years. *J. Oral Microbiol.* **2009**, *1*, 1. [CrossRef]
50. Boillot, A.; Rangé, H.; Danchin, N.; Kotti, S.; Cosler, G.; Czernichow, S.; Meilhac, O.; Puymirat, E.; Zeller, M.; Tchetche, D.; et al. Periodontopathogens antibodies and major adverse events following an acute myocardial infarction: Results from the French Registry of Acute ST-Elevation and Non-ST-Elevation Myocardial Infarction (FAST-MI). *J. Epidemiol. Community Health* **2016**, *70*, 1236–1241. [CrossRef]

5

Salivary Extracellular DNA and DNase Activity in Periodontitis

Barbora Konečná [1], Alexandra Gaál Kovalčíková [2], Alexandra Pančíková [3], Bohuslav Novák [4], Eva Kovaľová [5], Peter Celec [1,6,7] and Ľubomíra Tóthová [1,*]

1 Institute of Molecular Biomedicine, Faculty of Medicine, Comenius University in Bratislava, 811 08 Bratislava, Slovakia; basa.konecna@gmail.com (B.K.); petercelec@gmail.com (P.C.)
2 Department of Pediatrics, National Institute of Children's Diseases and Faculty of Medicine, Comenius University in Bratislava, 831 01 Bratislava, Slovakia; alexandra.kovalcikova114@gmail.com
3 School of Biological Sciences, University of Edinburgh, Edinburgh EH9 3FF, UK; apancikova@gmail.com
4 Department of Stomatology and Maxillofacial Surgery, Faculty of Medicine, Comenius University, 811 08 Bratislava, Slovakia; bohuslav.novak@fmed.uniba.sk
5 Department of Maxillofacial Surgery and Dental Hygiene of J.A. Reiman Hospital in Prešov, 080 01 Prešov, Slovakia; kovalova@nextra.sk
6 Institute of Pathophysiology, Faculty of Medicine, Comenius University in Bratislava, 811 08 Bratislava, Slovakia
7 Department of Molecular Biology, Faculty of Natural Sciences, Comenius University in Bratislava, 841 04 Bratislava, Slovakia
* Correspondence: lubomira.tothova@imbm.sk

Abstract: Extracellular DNA (ecDNA) is a potential marker and predictor in several inflammatory diseases. Periodontitis, a chronic inflammatory disease, is associated with epithelial cell death and could lead to release of DNA. Our aim was to analyze salivary DNA concentration and deoxyribonuclease (DNase) activity in periodontitis patients. We hypothesized that salivary ecDNA will be higher than in controls and could serve as a marker of periodontitis severity. Samples of saliva were collected from 25 patients with chronic periodontitis and 29 age-matched controls. DNA was quantified fluorometrically in whole saliva, as well as in supernatants after centrifugation (depletion of cells at 1600× *g*) and in double-centrifuged supernatants (depletion of cell debris at 1600× *g* and 16,000× *g*). The subcellular origin of ecDNA was assessed using real-time PCR. In comparison to controls, patients with periodontitis had twofold higher salivary DNA ($p < 0.01$), higher mitochondrial DNA in centrifuged supernatants ($p < 0.05$) and lower nuclear ecDNA in double-centrifuged samples ($p < 0.05$). No correlations were found between salivary DNA and oral health status, but mitochondrial DNA positively correlated with papillary bleeding index in centrifuged samples. Salivary DNase activity was comparable between the groups. In conclusion, we proved that salivary DNA is higher in periodontitis. The source of the higher mitochondrial DNA in cell-free saliva and the causes of lower nuclear ecDNA remain to be elucidated. Further studies should focus on the role of mitochondrial DNA as a potential driver of inflammation in periodontitis.

Keywords: cell free DNA; salivary biomarkers; gingivitis; oral diseases; apoptotic bodies; deoxyribonucleases

1. Introduction

Extracellular DNA (ecDNA), i.e., DNA outside of the cells, was first discovered in the plasma of pregnant women [1] and cancer patients [2]. EcDNA could trigger inflammation and worsen the state of patients during pregnancy complications or cancer. In plasma, ecDNA has been studied also as a potential biomarker of sepsis [3], trauma [4], diabetes mellitus or organ transplantation [5]. It has been hypothesized that plasmatic ecDNA could be used as a personalized cancer therapy [6]. Even though usually plasma serves as a source of ecDNA, despite the common difficulties, such as high fragmentation and high variability in the yield, saliva might be of special interest in oral diseases, since it reflects the local oral conditions. Also, ecDNA has been studied in saliva of head and neck cancer patients, and it has been shown that mitochondrial DNA concentration is increased in saliva in these patients when compared to control healthy group [7]. All of the above indicates that body fluids DNA or ecDNA are not a disease-specific marker, however, it points towards pathogeneses of diseases, which is not fully understood.

Periodontitis is a chronic multifactorial inflammatory oral disease. It starts with bacterial plaque concentrating near the gingival part followed by gingivitis. The oral microbiome indeed plays a role in this initial stage [8]. Under normal circumstances, there is a fragile balance between microbes that act as the nonharmful commensals and the oral health status [9]. The dysbiosis consequence includes plaque build-up consisting of immunogenic substances in the subgingival crevice of teeth, which leads to the further activation of the immune system. The resulting inflammation and neutrophils activation, as a nonspecific reaction, damages the surrounding healthy tissue releasing several other immunogenic substances, triggering thus immune overreaction and circulus vitiosus. In susceptible individuals, the untreated inflammation can later outgrow into loss of connective tissue and decline in bone support (periodontitis) and eventually a tooth loss [10,11] with permanent inflammation of surrounding tissue. Recently, neutrophil extracellular traps as weblike structures containing DNA were already described as potential immunogenic agents in periodontitis, and they were hypothesized to be involved in the pathogenesis of this disease [12–14]. Neutrophils are activated during inflammation, directed towards the location of inflammation, in our case the oral cavity, and the fight against bacteria forming the traps. Neutrophil extracellular traps consist of histone proteins and DNA, therefore they are one of the various sources of ecDNA among others such as apoptosis or necrosis [15]. Salivary ecDNA obtained by double-centrifugation, as well as DNA in whole and centrifuged saliva, as potential triggers of inflammation in periodontitis, are worth testing as possible indicators of the oral status. As in plasma, there are also nucleases in saliva, such as deoxyribonuclease (DNase) that is responsible for degradation of ecDNA [16,17]. Therefore, we think that, together with DNA concentrations and origin analysis, it is also important to specify activity of DNase in saliva. We hypothesize that salivary DNA will be increased in patients with worsened oral health and DNase activity could be also altered. Therefore, in this study, we investigated whether DNA in whole saliva, in centrifuged and double-centrifuged samples differs between periodontitis patients and healthy controls and whether salivary DNase activity is affected.

2. Methods

2.1. Patients

Total number of participants was 54 of whom 25 patients were diagnosed with periodontitis (11 women and 14 men) and 29 were aged matched without periodontitis (18 women and 11 men). The presence of clinical attachment loss of at least 3 mm in two or more nonadjacent teeth was considered to be periodontitis along with radiographically confirmed alveolar bone loss. For an accurate diagnosis, the examination of the periodontal status of subjects was performed using several clinical markers. Gingival index (GI)—qualitative changes of gingival soft tissue—was determined according to Loe [18]. Briefly, a score of 0 represents no changes of gingival soft tissue; a score of 1 means slight inflammation with the mild change of color and discrete edema without bleeding on probing (BOP); and a score of 3 describes severe inflammation, redness, edema with ulcerations and the presence of spontaneous bleeding.

Papillary bleeding index (PBI)—the bleeding after cautiously probing the sulcus—was determined by PBI as described formerly by Newbrun [19]. A score of 0 means no bleeding; score 1 means one bleeding point few seconds after probing; a score of 2 means intermediate bleeding from several points and a score of 3 represents profuse bleeding along the gingival sulcus even after gentle probing. The bleeding on probing at the bottom of the pocket is defined as BOP. The BOP was assessed using a standardized probe (WHO probe 550B, LM Dental, Finland) as described previously [20]. The patients were evaluated for six areas for all teeth (midbuccal, midlingual, mesiolingual, distolingual, mesiobuccal, and distobuccal). To consider differences in the number of teeth, all indexes were divided by the total number of teeth. All measurements were performed by a single trained examiner to avoid interindividual differences. The clinical evaluation of patients can be seen in Table 1.

Table 1. Oral health indexes of subjects.

	Group				
Parameter	**Healthy Women**	**Women with Periodontitis**	**Healthy Men**	**Men with Periodontitis**	**Disease Effect *p* Value**
Age (years)	43.6 ± 11.6	46.8 ± 9.5	40.7 ± 6.0	50.7 ± 10.8	
GI (score)	0.59 ±0.46	1.08 ± 0.35	0.82 ± 0.45	1.54 ± 0.66	<0.001
PBI (score)	0.36 ± 0.25	0.81 ± 0.47	0.83 ± 0.56	1.32 ± 0.48	<0.001
BOP (%)	0.00 ± 0.00	22.5 ± 14.96	0.00 ± 0.00	32.2 ± 21.26	<0.001

Gingival index (GI)—0–3 as qualitative changes of gingival soft tissue; 0—normal gingiva, 1—mild inflammation, 2—moderate inflammation, 3—severe inflammation. Papilla bleeding index (PBI)—(0, 1, 2, 3)—for bleeding after cautiously probing to the sulcus; 0 means no bleeding; 1 means one bleeding point few seconds after probing; 2 means intermediate bleeding in few points; 3 profuse bleeding along gingival sulcus as a reaction on slightest. Bleeding on probing (BOP)—number of sites where bleeding to the total number of available sites, expressed as percentage. Data are expressed as mean ± SD.

Prior to examination, all participants were asked not to eat, drink or brush their teeth 60 min before saliva sampling. All samples were collected at a dental clinic in Prešov, Slovakia. Sampling was performed in the morning (8:00–10:00) into sterile tubes. The whole unstimulated saliva samples were collected by passive drooling for 10 min and salivary flow was recorded. Whole saliva samples were aliquoted and stored; the rest of the whole saliva was centrifuged at 1600× *g* for 10 min to wash down the cell debris. The centrifuged supernatant was aliquoted and stored, followed by 16,000× *g* centrifugation of the rest of the supernatant for 10 min to obtain cellfree double-centrifuged supernatant [21]. Original saliva as well as samples after each centrifugation were measured by bicinchonic acid protein assay kit (Sigma-Aldrich, St. Louis, Missouri, United States) to determine the protein content and stored at −20 °C until further processes. Patients with a known extraoral systemic disease, taking any medications including vitamin supplements and smokers were excluded from this study. The study was approved by the Ethical Committee of the Department of Maxillofacial Surgery and Dental Hygiene of J.A. Reiman Hospital in Prešov. The clinical part of this study was performed according to the principles given in the Declaration of Helsinki. All participants signed written informed consent declarations.

2.2. DNA Isolation

DNA was isolated from 200 μL of all saliva samples using QIAamp DNA Blood Mini Kit (Qiagen, Hilden, Germany) according to the protocol of the manufacturer. Sixty μL of ultrapure water were used for the elution of DNA as the final step. DNA samples were stored at −20 °C until further analysis.

2.3. *Quantification of ecDNA*

Qubit Fluorometer and Qubit dsDNA HS Assay Kit (Invitrogen, Carlsbad, CA, USA) were used for the measurement of total cfDNA according to the protocol from the manufacturer. Real-time polymerase chain reaction (RT-PCR) was used for the quantification of nuclear DNA (ncDNA) and mitochondrial DNA (mtDNA) in saliva isolates. RT-PCR was performed on the Mastercycler realplex 4 (Eppendorf, Hamburg, Germany) using the SsoAdvanced Universal SYBR Green Supermix (Bio-Rad, Hercules, CA, USA) with the following program: one cycle of 3 min at 98 °C, followed by 40 cycles of 98 °C for 15 s for denaturation and annealing for 30 s at 51 °C for ncDNA and 47 °C for mtDNA and extension 30 s at 60 °C. Primers were designed for the amplification of human globin gene to quantify ncDNA (F: GCT TCT GAC ACA ACT GTG TTC, R: CAC CAA CTT CAT CCA CGT TCA) and D-loop to quantify mtDNA (F: CAT AAA AAC CCA ATC CAC ATC A, R: GAC GGG TGG CTT TGG AGT). All values were normalized to proteins.

2.4. *DNase Activity Measurement*

DNase activity was measured by single radial enzyme diffusion (SRED) method using 1% agarose gel (20 mM Tris–HCl, pH 7.5, 2 mM $MgCl_2$, 2 mM $CaCl_2$), which contained DNA isolated from chicken liver (7 mL of 5 mg/mL DNA into 100 mL of gel). From each saliva sample, 1 µL was pipetted into the gel and incubated over night at 37 °C in the dark. Dilutions of DNase I (Qiagen, Hilden, Germany) of known concentrations were used for creating the calibration curve. The diameters of circles were measured by ImageJ software. The values were normalized to proteins.

3. Statistical Analysis

Analysis was performed using GraphPad Prism 6.01 (GraphPad Software, San Diego, CA, USA). To compare the measured parameters between healthy controls and patients with periodontitis, unpaired t-test was performed. Correlations were performed as nonparametric using Spearman correlation. Level $\alpha = 0.05$ is considered as a limit level of significance.

4. Results

This study included 25 patients with periodontitis and 29 healthy controls. Patient characteristics are shown in Table 1. All patients were characterized using GI and PBI score as well as BOP expressed as a percentage. Individuals in the control group had no BOP and no sign of alveolar bone loss. Significantly higher values were observed in periodontitis patients in comparison to healthy controls according to GI, PBI and BOP (Table 1). No gender differences were observed in further analyses.

DNA concentration in whole saliva showed significantly higher values in periodontitis compared to healthy controls (504.6 ± 82.32 vs. 237.4 ± 26.66 ng/mg; $p < 0.01$) (Figure 1). Once the whole saliva was centrifuged, there were no differences observed in concentration of DNA between periodontitis patients and healthy controls (69.59 ± 13.37 vs. 54.22 ± 8.06 ng/mg; p = ns) (Figure 1). Similarly, in double-centrifuged samples, total ecDNA concentrations did not differ between the groups, periodontitis vs. healthy (13.54 ± 1.14 vs. 16.14 ± 2.54 ng/mg; p = ns; Figure 1). Determination of nuclear DNA in centrifuged samples showed no differences between groups, periodontitis vs. healthy (6629 ± 1727 vs. 5638 ± 2151 copy/mg; p = ns; Figure 2A). However mtDNA was significantly increased in periodontitis in comparison to healthy controls (10,656,989 ± 3,419,262 vs. 2,630,658 ± 809,983 copy/mg; $p < 0.05$; Figure 2B). In double-centrifuged samples, ncDNA concentration was significantly lower in the periodontitis group in comparison to the healthy group (788.8 ± 238.8 vs. 4947 ± 1508 copy/mg; $p < 0.01$) (Figure 2A), although mtDNA concentration was similar in both groups (14,608 ± 4809 vs. 11,957 ± 3296 copy/mg; p = ns; Figure 2B).

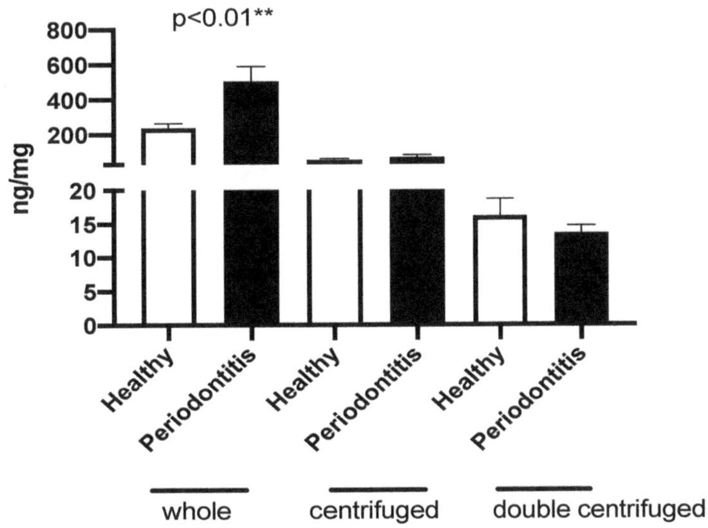

Figure 1. Total DNA in whole saliva, centrifuged saliva (1600× *g*) and double-centrifuged saliva (1600× *g* + 16,000× *g*). Results are expressed as mean + SEM. Salivary DNA is higher in periodontitis in whole saliva ($p < 0.01$**). No differences were found in centrifuged and double-centrifuged samples between the healthy and periodontitis group.

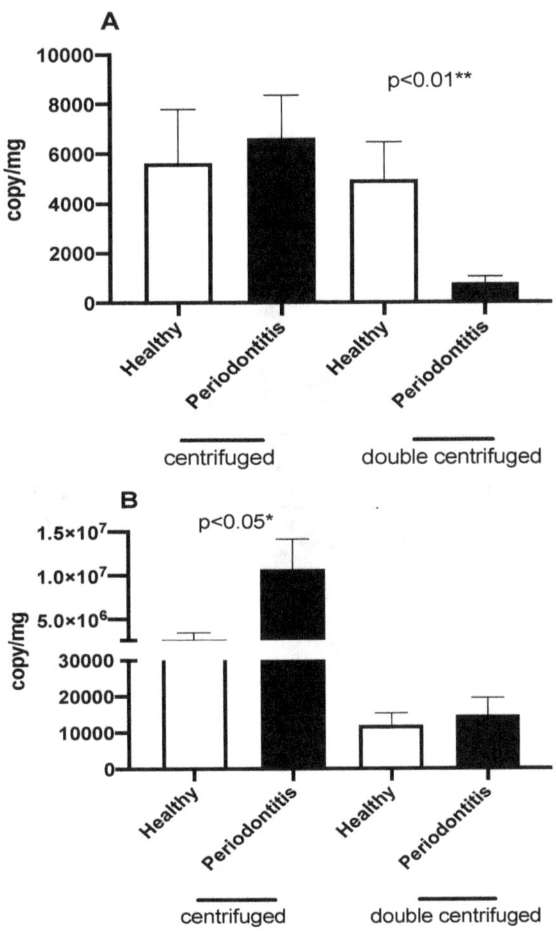

Figure 2. The effect of periodontitis on **A**: nuclear DNA (ncDNA). No differences were found in centrifuged samples. NcDNA was significantly lower in periodontitis in double-centrifuged samples ($p < 0.01$**). The effect of periodontitis on **B**: mitochondrial DNA (mtDNA). MtDNA was significantly higher in periodontitis in centrifuged samples. No differences were found in double-centrifuged samples. Results are expressed as mean + SEM.

Correlation analysis revealed that there is no linear association between concentration of total DNA, mtDNA, ncDNA and health indexes of periodontitis patients (Table 2). Only significant and positive correlation was observed between PBI and mtDNA in centrifuged samples (r = 0.62; Table 2). No significant differences were found in DNase activity between periodontitis samples and healthy controls either in centrifuged samples (0.54 ± 0.06 vs. 0.39 ± 0.05 KU/mg; p = ns) or in double-centrifuged samples (0.51 ± 0.03 vs. 0.53 ± 0.03 KU/mg; p = ns; Figure 3).

Table 2. Correlation between oral health indexes and total, nuclear DNA (ncDNA), and mitochondrial DNA (mtDNA) in whole saliva, centrifuged (1600× g) and double-centrifuged (1600× g + 16,000× g) samples.

Parameter	Centrifuged	Double Centrifuged
Total DNA		
GI (score)	r = 0.01	r = −0.01
PBI (score)	r = 0.24	r = −0.08
BOP (%)	r = −0.01	r = −0.1
Nuclear DNA		
GI (score)	r = 0.16	r = 0.25
PBI (score)	r = 0.35	r = 0.2
BOP (%)	r = 0.03	r = 0.28
Mitochondrial DNA		
GI (score)	r = 0.43	r = -0.09
PBI (score)	r = 0.62 *	r = 0.33
BOP (%)	r = −0.04	r = -0.12

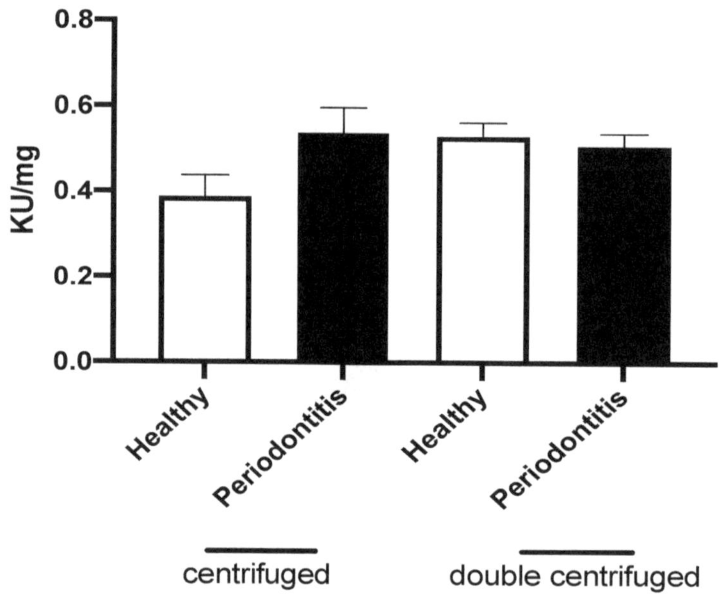

Figure 3. The effect of periodontitis on activity of DNase in centrifuged and double-centrifuged samples. Results are expressed as mean + SEM. No differences were found between healthy and periodontitis samples.

No significant correlations were found beside the positive significant correlation between PBI and mtDNA in centrifuged samples ($p < 0.05$*).

5. Discussion

Saliva and its content can reflect health status. As the latest research shows, saliva contains various markers helpful for the diagnosis and monitoring of many disorders such as cancer [22,23], neurological diseases [24], renal diseases [25], inflammatory bowel disease [26] or cardiovascular diseases [27]. The health status of the teeth, gingiva or salivary glands is also reflected in saliva [28]. Markers of inflammation, such as cytokines and inflammatory mediators, are produced as a result of bacterial infection and were proved to be higher in saliva of patients with periodontitis in comparison to healthy controls [29].

Based on the above-mentioned studies, total ecDNA or ecDNA of different origin were expected to be increased in periodontitis and could serve as a possible biomarker of periodontitis severity. However, as is defined by Jiang et al. [21], ecDNA is obtained after 16,000× *g* centrifugation, although they used plasma, not saliva. In our previously published study [30], we tried to determine the total DNA in whole saliva as well as in salivary supernatant. We hypothesized that we have analyzed ecDNA once the fluid is centrifuged and depleted of cells. However, no differences were found either in ecDNA between healthy and chronic periodontitis, and similarly no differences were observed between genders. These results were possibly obtained due to technical issues such as insufficient centrifuging while analyzing ecDNA. Therefore, we decided to repeat this observational study, in which we obtained ecDNA appropriately prepared using two-step centrifugation, 1600× *g* followed by 16,000× *g* according to Jiang et al. [21]. It is assumed that, after 1600× *g* centrifugation, only cells are spun down. However, generally, when talking about ecDNA, 16,000× *g* centrifugation is needed in order to spin down the bigger particles and cell debris. Based on this, we decided to analyze DNA in all three fractions, i.e., in whole saliva, centrifuged saliva and double-centrifuged saliva. According to our results, total DNA was higher in patients with periodontitis in whole saliva perhaps due to increased cell debris as a result of bleeding and worsened oral health. Once the whole saliva was centrifuged, the differences in total DNA were not observed anymore. Also, when we quantified separately ncDNA and mtDNA, we could observe differences in mtDNA, but not in ncDNA. Increased concentration of mtDNA in periodontitis indicates the presence of mitochondria, which could potentiate the inflammation in oral cavity [31]. Mitochondria are more likely to be still intact, because after the double-centrifugation, the mtDNA concentrations are same in both groups. EcDNA of mitochondrial origin is the same in healthy controls as well as in periodontitis, however ecDNA of nuclear origin is increased in healthy controls, even though there are no differences observed in total ecDNA. This could happen due to higher fragmentation of ncDNA in periodontitis [30], since short fragments are not detectable by qPCR but are visible by spectrofluorometry. Moreover, fragmented DNA could further potentiate inflammatory status [21,32,33], and thus worsen the course of disease. This hypothesis should be clarified by further studies. Nevertheless, if this hypothesis is proven correct, the ecDNA might become another therapeutic target.

We expected that altered DNase activity could be potentially associated with periodontitis. There was not significant change in DNase activity in our samples, however studying the activity of this enzyme is still in process as it is still not clear if the DNase activity is related with ecDNA concentrations. Even though the preliminary experiments on DNase activity have been already published [34], it is also not clear whether differences exist among genders under physiological circumstances [35]. However, it is important to remark that not all ecDNA is similarly sensitive to DNase activity. It has been found that the microbiome might influence DNase activity [36]. The shift of commensals to more pathogenic bacteria in gingivitis and periodontitis was shown to affect the DNase activity in saliva. However, we did not search for microbiota difference in our patients, which is the limitation of this study.

The collection of samples could not be done without freezing in our conditions, which is a limitation of many studies. It was shown that freezing of serum and plasma samples causes release of free nucleic acids from large circulating vesicles [37]. However, the uniqueness of our study is that saliva samples were processed right after sampling without freezing and thawing. Only the original samples intended for DNase activity measurement were frozen. In our preliminary unpublished data, we showed that DNase activity could decrease with longer storage period. Therefore, we can only hypothesize, that the measurement of DNase activity in fresh salivary samples could reveal its higher activity. Nevertheless, we measured the DNase activity within the period of two months from the collection.

In conclusion, we proved that worse periodontal status in patients and the presence of inflammation is associated with increased total and mtDNA concentrations in different fractions of saliva. Further studies should focus on the role of mtDNA as a potential driver of inflammation in periodontitis. It is also important to focus on DNA fragmentation as it shows that ecDNA originating in the nucleus seems to be decreased in periodontitis. This approach could lead to new treatment targets related to DNA origin, metabolism and recognition by immune cells.

Author Contributions: Conceptualization, P.C., B.N., E.K., and L'.T.; methodology, A.G.K., B.K., and P.C.; formal analysis, P.C. and L'.T.; investigation, B.K., E.K., and A.P.; data curation, B.K., A.G.K. and A.P.; writing—original draft preparation, B.K. and L'.T.; writing—review and editing, A.G.K., A.P., E.K., B.N., and P.C.; supervision, P.C., L'.T.", please turn to the CRediT taxonomy for the term explanation. All authors have read and agreed to the published version of the manuscript.

References

1. Lo, Y.D.; Corbetta, N.; Chamberlain, P.F.; Rai, V.; Sargent, I.L.; Redman, C.W.; Wainscoat, J.S. Presence of fetal DNA in maternal plasma and serum. *Lancet* **1997**, *350*, 485–487. [CrossRef]
2. Chen, X.Q.; Stroun, M.; Magnenat, J.L.; Nicod, L.P.; Kurt, A.M.; Lyautey, J.; Lederrey, C.; Anker, P. Microsatellite alterations in plasma DNA of small cell lung cancer patients. *Nat. Med.* **1996**, *2*, 1033–1035. [CrossRef] [PubMed]
3. Dwivedi, D.J.; Toltl, L.J.; Swystun, L.L.; Pogue, J.; Liaw, K.L.; Weitz, J.I.; Cook, D.J.; Fox-Robichaud, A.E.; Liaw, P.C.; Canadian Critical Care Translational Biology Group. Prognostic utility and characterization of cell-free DNA in patients with severe sepsis. *Crit. Care.* **2012**, *16*, R151. [CrossRef] [PubMed]
4. Lo, Y.M.; Rainer, T.H.; Chan, L.Y.; Hjelm, N.M.; Cocks, R.A. Plasma DNA as a prognostic marker in trauma patients. *Clin. Chem.* **2000**, *46*, 319–323. [CrossRef]
5. Butt, A.N.; Swaminathan, R. Overview of circulating nucleic acids in plasma/serum. *Ann. N. Y. Acad. Sci.* **2008**, *1137*, 236–242. [CrossRef] [PubMed]
6. Oellerich, M.; Schütz, E.; Beck, J.; Kanzow, P.; Plowman, P.N.; Weiss, G.J.; Walson, P.D. Using circulating cell-free DNA to monitor personalized cancer therapy. *Crit. Rev. Clin. Lab. Sci.* **2017**, *54*, 205–218. [CrossRef]
7. Jiang, W.W.; Masayesva, B.; Zahurak, M.; Carvalho, A.L.; Rosenbaum, E.; Mambo, E.; Zhou, S.; Minhas, K.; Benoit, N.; Westra, W.H.; et al. Increased mitochondrial DNA content in saliva associated with head and neck cancer. *Clin. Cancer Res.* **2005**, *11*, 2486–2491. [CrossRef]
8. Kinane, D.F.; Stathopoulou, P.G.; Papapanou, P.N. Periodontal diseases. *Nat. Rev. Dis. Primers.* **2017**, *3*, 17038. [CrossRef]
9. Nowicki, E.M.; Shroff, R.; Singleton, J.A.; Renaud, D.E.; Wallace, D.; Drury, J.; Zirnheld, J.; Colleti, B.; Ellington, A.D.; Lamont, R.J.; et al. Microbiota and Metatranscriptome Changes Accompanying the Onset of Gingivitis. *MBio* **2018**, *9*. [CrossRef]
10. Hajishengallis, G. Periodontitis: From microbial immune subversion to systemic inflammation. *Nat. Rev. Immunol.* **2015**, *15*, 30–44. [CrossRef]
11. Pihlstrom, B.L.; Michalowicz, B.S.; Johnson, N.W. Periodontal diseases. *Lancet* **2005**, *366*, 1809–1820. [CrossRef]
12. Konecna, B.; Sysak, R.; Kacerovsky, M.; Celec, P.; Vlkova, B. Deoxyribonuclease activity in plasma of pregnant women and experimental animals. *J. Matern. Fetal Neonatal Med.* **2018**, *31*, 1807–1809. [CrossRef] [PubMed]
13. White, P.; Sakellari, D.; Roberts, H.; Risafi, I.; Ling, M.; Cooper, P.; Milward, M.; Chapple, I. Peripheral blood neutrophil extracellular trap production and degradation in chronic periodontitis. *J. Clin. Periodontol.* **2016**, *43*, 1041–1049. [CrossRef] [PubMed]
14. White, P.C.; Chicca, I.J.; Cooper, P.R.; Milward, M.R.; Chapple, I.L. Neutrophil Extracellular Traps in Periodontitis: A Web of Intrigue. *J. Dent. Res.* **2016**, *95*, 26–34. [CrossRef]
15. Thierry, A.R.; El Messaoudi, S.; Gahan, P.B.; Anker, P.; Stroun, M. Origins, structures, and functions of circulating DNA in oncology. *Cancer Metastasis Rev.* **2016**, *35*, 347–376. [CrossRef]

16. Lauková, L.; Bertolo, E.M.J.; Zelinková, M.; Borbélyová, V.; Conka, J.; Kovalcíková, A.G.; Domonkos, E.; Vlková, B.; Celec, P. Early Dynamics of Plasma DNA in a Mouse Model of Sepsis. *Shock* **2019**, *52*, 257–263. [CrossRef]
17. Rathnayake, N.; Åkerman, S.; Klinge, B.; Lundegren, N.; Jansson, H.; Tryselius, Y.; Sorsa, T.; Gustafsson, A. Salivary biomarkers of oral health: A cross-sectional study. *J. Clin. Periodontol.* **2013**, *40*, 140–147. [CrossRef]
18. Loe, H. The Gingival Index, the Plaque Index and the Retention Index Systems. *J. Periodontol.* **1967**, *38*, 610–616. [CrossRef]
19. Newbrun, E. Indices to measure gingival bleeding. *J. Periodontol.* **1996**, *67*, 555–561. [CrossRef]
20. Pyysalo, M.J.; Pyysalo, L.M.; Hiltunen, J.; Järnstedt, J.; Helminen, M.; Karhunen, P.J.; Pessi, T. The dental infections in patients undergoing preoperative dental examination before surgical treatment of saccular intracranial aneurysm. *BMC Res. Notes.* **2018**, *11*, 600. [CrossRef] [PubMed]
21. Jiang, P.; Chan, C.W.; Chan, K.A.; Cheng, S.H.; Wong, J.; Wong, V.W.S.; Wong, G.L.; Chan, S.L.; Mok, T.S.; Chan, H.L.; et al. Lengthening and shortening of plasma DNA in hepatocellular carcinoma patients. *Proc. Natl. Acad. Sci. USA* **2015**, *112*, E1317–E1325. [CrossRef]
22. Nair, S.; Tang, K.D.; Kenny, L.; Punyadeera, C. Salivary exosomes as potential biomarkers in cancer. *Oral. Oncol.* **2018**, *84*, 31–40. [CrossRef] [PubMed]
23. Rapado-González, Ó.; Majem, B.; Muinelo-Romay, L.; Álvarez-Castro, A.; Santamaría, A.; Gil-Moreno, A.; López-López, R.; Suárez-Cunqueiro, M.M. Human salivary microRNAs in Cancer. *J. Cancer* **2018**, *9*, 638–649. [CrossRef] [PubMed]
24. Farah, R.; Haraty, H.; Salame, Z.; Fares, Y.; Ojcius, D.M.; Said Sadier, N. Salivary biomarkers for the diagnosis and monitoring of neurological diseases. *Biomed. J.* **2018**, *41*, 63–87. [CrossRef]
25. Kovalčíková, A.; Janšáková, K.; Gyurászová, M.; Podracká, L.; Šebeková, K.; Celec, P.; Tóthová, L. Salivary creatinine and urea are higher in an experimental model of acute but not chronic renal disease. *PLoS ONE* **2018**, *13*, e0200391. [CrossRef] [PubMed]
26. Zheng, X.; Chen, F.; Zhang, Q.; Liu, Y.; You, P.; Sun, S.; Lin, J.; Chen, N. Salivary exosomal PSMA7: A promising biomarker of inflammatory bowel disease. *Protein Cell* **2017**, *8*, 686–695. [CrossRef]
27. Abdul Rehman, S.; Khurshid, Z.; Hussain Niazi, F.; Naseem, M.; Al Waddani, H.; Sahibzada, H.A.; Sannam Khan, R. Role of Salivary Biomarkers in Detection of Cardiovascular Diseases (CVD). *Proteomes* **2017**, *5*, 21. [CrossRef]
28. Yoshizawa, J.M.; Schafer, C.A.; Schafer, J.J.; Farrell, J.J.; Paster, B.J.; Wong, D.T. Salivary biomarkers: Toward future clinical and diagnostic utilities. *Clin. Microbiol. Rev.* **2013**, *26*, 781–791. [CrossRef]
29. Ebersole, J.L.; Schuster, J.L.; Stevens, J.; Dawson, D.; Kryscio, R.J.; Lin, Y.; Thomas, M.V.; Miller, C.S. Patterns of salivary analytes provide diagnostic capacity for distinguishing chronic adult periodontitis from health. *J. Clin. Immunol.* **2013**, *33*, 271–279. [CrossRef]
30. Baňasová, L.; Kamodyová, N.; Janšáková, K.; Tóthová, L.; Stanko, P.; Turňa, J.; Celec, P. Salivary DNA and markers of oxidative stress in patients with chronic periodontitis. *Clin. Oral. Investig.* **2015**, *19*, 201–207. [CrossRef]
31. Missiroli, S.; Genovese, I.; Perrone, M.; Vezzani, B.; Vitto, V.A.M.; Giorgi, C. The Role of Mitochondria in Inflammation: From Cancer to Neurodegenerative Disorders. *J. Clin. Med.* **2020**, *9*, 740. [CrossRef]
32. Mouliere, F.; Robert, B.; Peyrotte, E.A.; Del Rio, M.; Ychou, M.; Molina, F.; Gongora, C.; Thierry, A.R. High fragmentation characterizes tumour-derived circulating DNA. *PLoS ONE* **2011**, *6*, e23418. [CrossRef]
33. Zhang, R.; Nakahira, K.; Guo, X.; Choi, A.M.; Gu, Z. Very Short Mitochondrial DNA Fragments and Heteroplasmy in Human Plasma. *Sci. Rep.* **2016**, *6*, 36097. [CrossRef] [PubMed]
34. Malíčková, K.; Ďuricová, D.; Bortlík, M.; Hrušková, Z.; Svobodová, B.; Machková, N.; Komárek, V.; Fučíková, T.; Janatková, I.; Zima, T.; et al. Impaired deoxyribonuclease I activity in patients with inflammatory bowel diseases. *Autoimmune Dis.* **2011**, *2011*, 945861. [CrossRef]
35. Janovicova, L.; Konecna, B.; Vokalova, L.; Laukova, L.; Vlkova, B.; Celec, P. Sex, Age, and Bodyweight as Determinants of Extracellular DNA in the Plasma of Mice: A Cross-Sectional Study. *Int. J. Mol. Sci.* **2019**, *20*, 4163. [CrossRef] [PubMed]
36. Palmer, L.J.; Chapple, I.L.; Wright, H.J.; Roberts, A.; Cooper, P.R. Extracellular deoxyribonuclease production by periodontal bacteria. *J. Periodontal Res.* **2012**, *47*, 439–445. [CrossRef]
37. Muller, L.; Hong, C.S.; Stolz, D.B.; Watkins, S.C.; Whiteside, T.L. Isolation of biologically-active exosomes from human plasma. *J. Immunol. Methods* **2014**, *411*, 55–65. [CrossRef] [PubMed]

6

Effects of Initial Periodontal Therapy on Heat Shock Protein 70 Levels in Gingival Crevicular Fluid from Periodontitis Patients

Nobuhisa Furuse [1], Hideki Takai [1,2] and Yorimasa Ogata [1,2,*]

1 Department of Periodontology, Nihon University School of Dentistry at Matsudo, Matsudo, Chiba 271-8587, Japan; furuse-dental@jcom.zaq.ne.jp (N.F.); takai.hideki@nihon-u.ac.jp (H.T.)
2 Research Institute of Oral Science, Nihon University School of Dentistry at Matsudo, Matsudo, Chiba 271-8587, Japan
* Correspondence: ogata.yorimasa@nihon-u.ac.jp

Abstract: Periodontitis is an inflammatory disease of periodontium which is caused by periodontopathic bacteria. Moreover, various cytokines such as interleukin-1β (IL-1β), tumor necrosis factor-α (TNF-α), and IL-6 are expressed in the inflamed periodontium. Heat shock proteins (HSPs) protect cells from abnormal conditions including inflammation, microbial infection and diseases. The 70-kDa HSPs (HSP70s) are major HSPs that express in the inflamed tissues. In this study, an enzyme-linked immunosorbent assay was applied to measure the levels of HSP70 in gingival crevicular fluid (GCF) from two periodontal pockets in each of 10 patients with Stage III, Grade B periodontitis. Sites with probing pocket depth (PPD) of ≤3 mm were named the healthy control (HC) sites, and sites with PPD of ≥5 mm were named the diseased sites. HSP70 levels in GCF were expressed higher at diseased sites than at HC sites, and decreased after initial periodontal therapy at diseased sites. These results suggest the association of HSP70 with the stage of periodontitis.

Keywords: 70-kDa heat shock proteins; gingival crevicular fluid; heat shock protein; periodontitis

---

1. Introduction

Periodontitis, a common disease, is the inflammation of periodontium caused by oral microorganisms [1]. Numerous cytokines have been detected in the gingival crevicular fluid (GCF). Interleukin-1β (IL-1β) and tumor necrosis-α (TNF-α) levels have been found in increased GCF from inflamed gingival tissues [2,3]. IL-1β, matrix metalloproteinase-8, and IL-8 levels in GCF were significantly higher in diseased sites than in healthy subjects, and those levels in GCF were significantly decreased after periodontal treatment [4]. In a recent study, GCF volume and IL-1β levels in GCF reflected the disease severity, and these parameters were suggested to be better than probing pocket depth (PPD) and bleeding on probing (BOP) as markers of gingival inflammation [5]. Therefore, it could be helpful to investigate the inflammatory cytokine levels in GCF for diagnosis of the active phase of periodontal disease.

Heat shock proteins (HSPs) act as molecular chaperones, which are enhanced proteins for protecting cells immediately after cells are exposed to heat shock stress [6]. The 70-kDa HSPs (HSP70s) comprising various isoforms are involved in a number of human pathologies, ranging from cancer to neurodegenerative diseases [7,8]. HSP70 levels were higher in protein extract from inflamed gingiva collected during periodontal surgery, and HSP60 and HSP65 levels were higher in serum from the patients with periodontitis [9]. In addition, expression levels of IL-1β, IL-8, and HSP70 were increased in GCF from patients with periodontitis compared to healthy subjects [10]. Serum concentration of chitinase-3-like-1 (YKL-40), which is a novel marker of acute and chronic inflammation, was significantly higher in patients with periodontitis and diabetes compared to healthy groups. However, GCF concentration of YKL-40 was similar in patients with periodontitis, patients with diabetes, and healthy subjects. YKL-40 levels were significantly increased in diabetes patients with periodontitis [11]. Therefore, HSP70 can be considered potentially as a marker for the severity of periodontal disease. However, there is no report on changes in HSP70 concentration in GCF before and after initial periodontal therapy, or its correlation with clinical parameters. The aim of this study was to elucidate the HSP70 levels in GCF from patients with periodontitis, and to compare their concentrations in GCF at first visit, after initial periodontal therapy, and at a three month follow-up.

2. Materials and Methods

2.1. Study Population

Ten patients with Stage III, Grade B periodontitis (mean age, 53.9 ± 3 years) at Nihon University Hospital School of Dentistry at Matsudo, Japan were recruited and then received initial periodontal therapy, including oral hygiene instruction, scaling and root planing, and professional mechanical tooth cleaning. The stage of periodontitis was assessed clinically based on clinical attachment loss (CAL), radiographic bone loss (BL), periodontal history of tooth loss (PTL), PPD, BOP, furcation involvement (Class II or III), plaque index (PlI), and gingival index (GI) [12–14]. A CP11 probe (Hu-Friedy, Chicago, IL, USA) was used to measure the PPD and CAL. They were diagnosed when BL affected the middle third of the root or beyond and CAL was 5 mm or more. If PTL was four teeth or less, then the diagnosis was stage III. When the patient's previous periodontal records were available, the rate of periodontitis progression in the previous five years could be estimated. If progression was <2 mm, then the diagnosis was Grade B periodontitis [15]. GCF samples were taken from two periodontal PPD sites (shallow PPD of ≤3 mm were named the healthy control (HC) sites and deep PPD of ≥5 mm were named the diseased sites) for each patient.

This study was approved by the ethics committee at Nihon University School of Dentistry at Matsudo (EC17-017; 6Dec2017, EC18-17-017-1; 31, August, 2018). Written informed consent was obtained from all patients after all of the details of the investigative approach had been explained to them. Ten patients were confirmed physically healthy and had no experience of periodontal treatment or antibiotic treatment for at least three months prior to participation in this study. None of the patients were smokers.

2.2. Sample Size

Sample size was determined by the statistical software Easy R (EZR) on R commander Ver.1.27 (Tokyo, Japan) [16]. It was calculated that six samples (samples were taken from two sites per patient) were necessary for each group (HC and diseased sites) to reach 80% power at 5% level of significance. Therefore, the number of samples taken was appropriate.

2.3. Clinical Protocol

Clinical examinations were performed three times (first visit (1st), second examination (2nd) after initial periodontal therapy, and third examination (3rd) at a three month follow-up after initial periodontal therapy) by two periodontal specialists (H.T. and Y.O.). Average period of initial periodontal therapy was three months. At the point of each examination (1st, 2nd, and 3rd), GCF was collected using Periopaper subsequent to removal of supragingival plaque with a sterile curette. The GCF volume (μL) was measured using a Periotron 4000 (Oraflow, New York, NY, USA). GCF samples for the second visit data were taken before the periodontal therapy on the same day. Periopaper was then inserted into the pocket for 30 s each time. GCF samples were kept in Eppendorf tubes from two periodontal sites (≥5 mm (deep diseased site) and ≤3 mm (shallow healthy control site; HC)) from each patient and stored at −80 °C until measurement of HSP70 levels [17].

2.4. Enzyme-Linked Immunosorbent Assay (ELISA)

Concentrations of HSP70 in GCF samples were measured by ELISA using the Human HSPA4 (HSP70) ELISA kit (Invitrogen) according to the manufacturer's instructions. GCF samples were dissolved in 300 μL of Sample Diluent C in the ELISA kit. Diluted samples (100 μL) were incubated for 2.5 h in an anti-human HSP70 pre-coated 96-well strip plate. After a wash, biotinylated antibody was added to the wells for 1 h. After a wash, streptavidin-HRP solution was added to the wells for 45 min. After washing, TMB substrate was added to the wells for 30 min. Color development was stopped and the optical density at 450 nm of each well was measured within 30 min using a microplate reader. All measurements were performed in duplicate and the concentrations of HSP70 were expressed in ng/mL.

2.5. Statistical Analysis

Clinical parameters are shown as mean ± standard error (SE) in Table 1. The significant differences between each examination (1st, 2nd, and 3rd) for clinical parameters, GCF volume, and HSP70 levels among the groups were determined by one-way ANOVA. Difference in BOP at the 1st to 3rd examinations were analyzed by a Chi-squared test. The level of significance was adjusted at 5%. Four steps Ekuseru-Toukei (the publisher OMS Ltd.) was used for statistical analyses.

Table 1. Patient characteristics.

	HC Sites	Diseased Sites
Age	53.9 ± 3	
Gender (male/female)	2/8	
PPD	2.7 ± 0.2	6.5 ± 0.5
CAL	3.9 ± 0.4	7.7 ± 0.7
PlI	1.1 ± 0.2	1.1 ± 0.2
GI	0.3 ± 0.2	1.7 ± 0.2
BOP	0 (0%)	8 (80%)

HC, healthy control; PPD, probing pocket depth; CAL, clinical attachment loss; PlI, plaque index; GI, gingival index; BOP, bleeding on probing; mean ± SE (n = 10).

3. Results

The patient characteristics such as age, sex, PPD, CAL, PlI, GI, and BOP distributions for the 10 patients in this study are listed in Table 1. Average PPD and CAL at the HC sites (PPD ≤ 3 mm) were 2.7 ± 0.2 mm and 3.9 ± 0.4 mm, and at the diseased sites (PPD ≥ 5 mm) were 6.5 ± 0.5 mm and 7.7 ± 0.7 mm, respectively. GI and BOP scores at the diseased sites (1.7 ± 0.2 and 80%) were higher than those at the HC sites (0.3 ± 0.2 and 0%). PlI at the HC and diseased sites were the same score (1.1 ± 0.2).

The concentrations of HSP70 in GCF from the HC and diseased sites at each point of examination during initial periodontal therapy are shown in Table 2. The average HSP70 level at the 1st visit in GCF from diseased sites was significantly higher than HC sites. Moreover, the concentration of HSP70 at diseased sites was significantly decreased at 3rd examination (a three month follow-up after initial periodontal therapy) as compared to the 1st examination. The concentration of HSP70 at HC sites did not change through the periodontal therapy (1st, 2nd, and 3rd examinations) (Table 2).

Table 2. Changes in the concentrations of HSP70 in GCF collected from HC and diseased sites during the periodontal therapy.

Concentration (ng/mL)	1st	2nd	3rd
HC sites	18 ± 4.99 *	16.73 ± 6.37	6.64 ± 3.46
Diseased sites	64.36 ± 13.74	35.1 ± 6.67	5.69 ± 1.78 **

GCF, gingival crevicular fluid; HC, healthy control; 1st, first visit; 2nd, after initial periodontal therapy; 3rd, a three month follow-up after initial periodontal therapy; mean ± SE (n = 10), * $p < 0.05$, ** $p < 0.01$.

Changes in five kinds of clinical parameters (PPD, CAL, PlI, GI, and BOP scores) at the HC and diseased sites during initial periodontal therapy are listed in Tables 3 and 4. At HC sites, PlIs were significantly decreased at the 2nd and 3rd examinations as compared to the 1st examination (Table 3). On the other hand, PPD and PlI at diseased sites were significantly decreased at the 2nd and 3rd examinations compared to the 1st examination. Furthermore, GI and BOP scores at diseased sites were significantly decreased at the 3rd examination compared to the 1st examination. GCF volumes from HC and diseased sites were measured by Periotron 4000 during the course of periodontal therapy (Table 5). GCF volumes from HC and diseased sites did not change during the periodontal therapy, however, the volumes of GCF from the diseased sites were significantly higher than those in the HC sites at the 1st and 2nd visits (Table 5).

Table 3. Changes in clinical parameters at HC sites.

	1st	2nd	3rd
PPD	2.7 ± 0.2	2.5 ± 0.2	2.5 ± 0.2
CAL	3.9 ± 0.4	3.6 ± 0.5	3.6 ± 0.4
PlI	1.1 ± 0.2	0.6 ± 0.2 *	0.6 ± 0.2 *
GI	0.3 ± 0.2	0	0.4 ± 0.3
BOP	0 (0%)	0 (0%)	2 (20%)

HC, healthy control; 1st, first visit; 2nd, after initial periodontal therapy; 3rd, a three month follow-up after initial periodontal therapy; PPD, probing pocket depth; CAL, clinical attachment loss; PlI, plaque index; GI, gingival index; BOP, bleeding on probing; mean ± SE ($n = 10$), * $p < 0.05$.

Table 4. Changes in clinical parameters at diseased sites.

	1st	2nd	3rd
PPD	6.5 ± 0.5	4.3 ± 0.4 *	4.3 ± 0.5 *
CAL	7.7 ± 0.7	6.2 ± 0.9	5.9 ± 0.7
PlI	1.1 ± 0.2	0.5 ± 0.2 *	0.6 ± 0.2 *
GI	1.7 ± 0.2	1.2 ± 0.3	0.9 ± 0.3 *
BOP	8 (80%)	5 (50%)	4 (40%) *

1st, first visit; 2nd, after initial periodontal therapy; 3rd, a three month follow-up after initial periodontal therapy; PPD, probing pocket depth; CAL, clinical attachment loss; PlI, plaque index; GI, gingival index; BOP, bleeding on probing; mean ± SE ($n = 10$), * $p < 0.05$.

Table 5. Changes in GCF volume at HC and diseased sites during the periodontal therapy.

GCF (μL)	1st	2nd	3rd
HC sites	0.92 ± 0.2	0.47 ± 0.2	0.66 ± 0.2
Diseased sites	2.41 ± 0.5 *	1.6 ± 0.3 *	1.31 ± 0.3

GCF, gingival crevicular fluid; HC, healthy control; 1st, first visit; 2nd, after initial periodontal therapy; 3rd, a three month follow-up after initial periodontal therapy; mean ± SE ($n = 10$), * $p < 0.05$.

4. Discussion

In this study, we have shown that there was a significant difference in HSP70 concentration in GCF between HC and diseased sites at the first visit. The concentration of HSP70 in GCF from diseased sites was significantly decreased at the three month follow-up after initial periodontal therapy (3rd examination; Table 2). At HC sites, PlI was significantly decreased at the 2nd and 3rd examinations (Table 3). At diseased sites, PPD and PlI were significantly decreased at the 2nd and 3rd examinations, whereas GI and BOP were significantly decreased only at the 3rd examination as compared to the 1st visit (Table 4). These results suggest that initial periodontal therapy is effective in improving inflammation of periodontal tissues and there is an association between the level of HSP70 and periodontitis. In addition, improvements of GI, BOP, and HSP70 levels were found to take longer than improvements of PPD and PlI.

Intracellular HSP levels are elevated immediately after exposed to stresses such as high temperature. HSPs are involved in the maintenance of cellular homeostasis and protein repair in damaged cells [18].

However, there are several unclear points in the relationship between HSPs and periodontitis. Inflammatory periodontal pockets have a higher temperature than healthy pockets [19]. Inflammatory cytokines, such as IL-1, TNF-α, and INF-γ, are produced in inflamed periodontal tissues [20], and they might act as stressors to induce the expression of HSPs. Lipopolysaccharide (LPS) and IL-1 increased hyperthermia-induced HSP70 in monocyte/macrophage-like RAW264.7 cells [21]. However, one study described how HSP70 dramatically down-regulated in the inflamed periodontal tissues [22]. Another study showed that GCF volume at the first visit decreased significantly after initial periodontal therapy [23]. However, in this study, GCF volumes from HC and diseased sites did not change during periodontal therapy (Table 5), although the GCF volumes from diseased sites at the 1st and 2nd visits were significantly higher than the GCF volumes from HC sites (Table 5). Therefore, further study is necessary to elucidate the involvement of HSP70 in the onset and progression of periodontitis.

Stress and smoking are environmental factors for periodontitis [24,25]. Several studies have shown that smoking has an adverse effect on the incidence and progression of periodontitis [25]. In the synovial tissues of smokers with rheumatoid arthritis (RA), HSP70 levels were significantly higher than in the synovial tissues of non-smokers with RA [26]. Therefore, smoking could increase the expression of HSP70. There are several studies describing the association between HSP70 and cancer. Malignant cells, such as osteosarcoma derived cells, expressed higher levels of HSP70 during tumor progression compared to normal cells [27]. Moreover, HSP70 has been assessed as a marker for oral epithelial dysplasia such as oral leukoplakia [28]. Therefore, various studies have been conducted to develop the HSP70 inhibitors for cancer therapy [29]. We have previously shown that the anti-HSP70 antibody levels were significantly higher in GCF from HC sites than diseased sites, and the anti-HSP70 antibody levels were increased after initial periodontal therapy in both HC and diseased sites [30]. Therefore, these results suggest that anti-HSP70 antibody may reduce inflammation of periodontal tissues via decreasing the HSP70 levels.

In conclusion, GCF volumes from the diseased sites were significantly higher than those in the HC sites at the 1st and 2nd visits. HSP70 concentration in GCF from diseased sites was significantly higher than the concentration of HSP70 from HC sites at the 1st visit. Moreover, the HSP70 concentration at the 1st visit was significantly decreased at the three month follow-up after initial periodontal therapy together with clinical parameters, such as PPD, GI, PlI, and BOP. These results suggest that the HSP70 concentration could become an appropriate indicator for the healing process of periodontitis.

Author Contributions: Conceptualization, H.T. and Y.O.; methodology, N.F., H.T. and Y.O.; manuscript preparation, H.T. and Y.O. All authors have read and agreed to the published version of the manuscript.

Abbreviations

BOP	bleeding on probing
CAL	clinical attachment loss
GCF	gingival crevicular fluid
GI	gingival index
HC	healthy control
HSP	Heat shock protein
IL-1β	interleukin-1β
PlI	plaque index
PPD	probing pocket depth
SE	standard error
TNF-α	tumor necrosis factor-α

References

1. Page, R.C.; Kornman, K.S. The pathogenesis of human periodontitis: An introduction. *Periodontology 2000* **1997**, *14*, 9–11. [CrossRef] [PubMed]
2. Perozini, C.; Chibebe, P.C.; Leao, M.V.; Queiroz, C.S.; Pallos, D. Gingival crevicular fluid biochemical markers in periodontal disease: A cross-sectional study. *Quintessence Int.* **2010**, *41*, 877–883.

3. Stashenko, P.; Jandinski, J.J.; Fujiyoshi, P.; Rynar, J.; Socransky, S.S. Tissue levels of bone resorptive cytokines in periodontal disease. *J. Periodontol.* **1991**, *62*, 504–509. [PubMed]
4. Konopka, L.; Pietrzak, A.; Brzezińska-Błaszczyk, E. Effect of scaling and root planing on interleukin-1b, interleukin-8 and MMP-8 levels in gingival crevicular fluid from chronic periodontitis patients. *J. Periodontal Res.* **2012**, *47*, 681–688. [CrossRef]
5. Oh, H.; Hirano, J.; Takai, H.; Ogata, Y. Effects of initial periodontal therapy on interleukin-1β level in gingival crevicular fluid and clinical periodontal parameters. *J. Oral Sci.* **2015**, *57*, 67–71. [CrossRef]
6. Schlesinger, M.J. Heat shock proteins. *J. Biol. Chem.* **1990**, *265*, 12111–12114. [PubMed]
7. Milićević, Z.T.; Petković, M.Z.; Drndarević, N.C.; Pavlović, M.D.; Todorović, V.N. Expression of Heat Shock Protein 70 (HSP70) in Patients with Colorectal Adenocarcinoma–Immunohistochemistry and Western Blot Analysis. *Neoplasma* **2007**, *54*, 37–45.
8. Lackie, R.E.; Maciejewski, A.; Ostapchenko, V.G.; Marques-Lopes, J.; Choy, W.Y.; Duennwald, M.L.; Prado, V.F.; Prado, M.A.M. The Hsp70/Hsp90 Chaperone Machinery in Neurodegenerative Diseases. *Front. Neurosci.* **2017**, *11*, 254. [CrossRef]
9. Ando, T.; Kato, T.; Ishihara, K.; Ogiuchi, H.; Okuda, K. Heat shock proteins in the human periodontal disease process. *Microbiol. Immunol.* **1995**, *39*, 321–327. [CrossRef]
10. Tsybikov, N.N.; Baranov, S.V.; Kuznik, B.I. Serum, oral and gingival fluid levels of heat shock protein-70, cytokines and their autoantibodies by periodontal disease. *Stomatologiia (MosK)* **2014**, *93*, 16–18.
11. Kumar, P.A.; Kripal, K.; Chandrasekaran, K.; Bhavanam, S.R. Estimation of YKL-40 Levels in Serum and Gingival Crevicular Fluid in Chronic Periodontitis and Type 2 Diabetes Patients among South Indian Population: A Clinical Study. *Contemp. Clin. Dent.* **2019**, *10*, 304–310. [PubMed]
12. Loe, H.; Silness, J. Periodontal disease in pregnancy. I. Prevalence and severity. *Acta Odontol. Scand.* **1963**, *21*, 533–551. [CrossRef] [PubMed]
13. Silness, J.; Loe, H. Periodontal disease in pregnancy. II. Correlation between oral hygiene and periodontal condition. *Acta Odontol. Scand.* **1964**, *22*, 122–135. [CrossRef]
14. Tonetti, M.S.; Greenwell, H.; Kornman, K.S. Staging and grading of periodontitis: Framework and proposal of a new classification and case definition. *J. Periodontol.* **2018**, *89* (Suppl. 1), S15–S172. [CrossRef] [PubMed]
15. Tonetti, M.S.; Sanz, M. Implementation of the new classification of periodontal diseases: Decision-making algorithms for clinical practice and education. *J. Clin. Periodontol.* **2019**, *46*, 398–405. [CrossRef] [PubMed]
16. Kanda, Y. Investigation of the freely available easy-to-use software 'EZR' for medical statistics. *Bone Marrow Transpl.* **2013**, *48*, 452–458. [CrossRef]
17. Ito, H.; Numabe, Y.; Sekino, S.; Murakashi, E.; Iguchi, H.; Hashimoto, S.; Sasaki, D.; Yaegashi, T.; Kunimatsu, K.; Takai, H.; et al. Evaluation of bleeding on probing and gingival crevicular fluid enzyme activity for detection of periodontally active sites during supportive periodontal therapy. *Odontology* **2014**, *102*, 50–56. [CrossRef]
18. Rokutan, K.; Hirakawa, T.; Teshima, S.; Nakano, Y.; Miyoshi, M.; Kawai, T.; Konda, E.; Morinaga, H.; Nikawa, T.; Kishi, K. Implications of heat shock/stress proteins for medicine and disease. *J. Med. Investig.* **1998**, *44*, 137–147.
19. Fedi, P.F., Jr.; Killoy, W.J. Temperature differences at periodontal sites in health and disease. *J. Periodontol.* **1992**, *63*, 24–27. [CrossRef]
20. Alexander, M.B.; Damoulis, P.D. The role of cytokines in the pathogenesis of periodontal disease. *Curr. Opin. Periodontol.* **1994**, 39–53.
21. Aditi, G.; Zachary, A.C.; Mohan, E.T.; Ratnakar, P.; Tapan, M.; Jeffrey, D.H.; Ishwar, S.S. Toll-like Receptor Agonists and Febrile Range Hyperthermia Synergize to Induce Heat Shock Protein 70 Expression and Extracellular Release. *J. Biol. Chem.* **2013**, *288*, 2756–2766.
22. Seo, B.; Coates, D.E.; Seymour, G.J.; Rich, A.M. Unfolded protein response-related gene regulation in inflamed periodontal tissues with and without Russell bodies. *Arch. Oral Biol.* **2016**, *69*, 1–6. [CrossRef] [PubMed]
23. Rossi, V.; Romagna, R.; Angst, P.D.M.; Gomes, S.C. Gingival crevicular fluid response to protocols of non-surgical periodontal therapy: A longitudinal evaluation. *Ross. Indian J. Dent. Res.* **2019**, *30*, 736–741.
24. Alex, S.S.; Alessandra, N.P.; Tereza, A.D.V.S.; Jose, R.C.; Fernando, O.C.; Sheila, C.C.; Álvaro, F.B. Effects of two chronic stress models on ligature-induced periodontitis in Wistar rats. *Archs. Oral Biol.* **2012**, *57*, 66–72.
25. Leite, F.R.M.; Nascimento, G.G.; Scheutz, F.; López, R. Effect of Smoking on Periodontitis: A Systematic Review and Meta-regression. *Am. J. Prev. Med.* **2018**, *54*, 831–841. [CrossRef]

26. Ospelt, C.; Camici, G.G.; Engler, A.; Kolling, C.; Vogetseder, A.; Gay, R.E.; Michel, B.A.; Gay, S. Smoking induces transcription of the heat shock protein system in the joints. *Ann. Rheum. Dis.* **2014**, *73*, 1423–1426. [CrossRef] [PubMed]
27. Ciocca, D.R.; Calderwood, S.K. Heat shock proteins in cancer: Diagnostic, prognostic, predictive, and treatment implications. *Cell Stress Chaperones* **2005**, *10*, 86–103. [CrossRef]
28. Seoane, J.M.; Varela-Centelles, P.I.; Ramirez, J.R.; Cameselle-Teijeiro, J.; Romero, M.A.; Aguirre, J.M. Heat shock proteins (HSP70 and HSP27) as markers of epithelial dysplasia in oral leukoplakia. *Am. J. Dermatopathol.* **2006**, *28*, 417–422. [CrossRef]
29. Yun, C.W.; Kim, H.J.; Lim, J.H.; Lee, S.H. Heat Shock Proteins: Agents of Cancer Development and Therapeutic Targets in Anti-Cancer Therapy. *Cells* **2019**, *9*, 60. [CrossRef]
30. Takai, H.; Furuse, N.; Ogata, Y. Anti-heat shock protein 70 levels in gingival crevicular fluid of Japanese patients with chronic periodontitis. *J. Oral Sci.* **2020**, *62*, 281–284. [CrossRef]

7

Saliva and Serum Immune Responses in Apical Periodontitis

Milla Pietiäinen [1,*], John M. Liljestrand [1,*], Ramin Akhi [2,3,4,*], Kåre Buhlin [1,5], Anders Johansson [6], Susanna Paju [1], Aino Salminen [1], Päivi Mäntylä [7,8], Juha Sinisalo [9], Leo Tjäderhane [1], Sohvi Hörkkö [2,3,4] and Pirkko J. Pussinen [1]

1 Oral and Maxillofacial Diseases, University of Helsinki and Helsinki University Hospital, FI-00014 Helsinki, Finland; kare.buhlin@ki.se (K.B.); susanna.paju@helsinki.fi (S.P.); aino.m.salminen@helsinki.fi (A.S.); leo.tjaderhane@helsinki.fi (L.T.); pirkko.pussinen@helsinki.fi (P.J.P.)
2 Medical Microbiology and Immunology, Research Unit of Biomedicine, University of Oulu, FI-90014 Oulu, Finland; sohvi.horkko@nordlab.fi
3 Medical Research Center, Oulu University Hospital and University of Oulu, FI-90014 Oulu, Finland
4 Nordlab, Oulu University Hospital, FI-90220 Oulu, Finland
5 Division of Periodontology, Department of Dental Medicine, Karolinska Institutet, S-141 04 Huddinge, Sweden
6 Department of Odontology, Molecular Periodontology Research, Umeå University, S-901 87 Umeå, Sweden; anders.p.johansson@umu.se
7 Institute of Dentistry, University of Eastern Finland, FI-70211 Kuopio, Finland; paivi.mantyla@uef.fi
8 Kuopio University Hospital, Oral and Maxillofacial Diseases, FI-70029 Kuopio, Finland
9 HUCH Heart and Lung Center, Helsinki University Hospital, FI-00029 Helsinki, Finland; juha.sinisalo@hus.fi
* Correspondence: milla.pietiainen@helsinki.fi (M.P.); john.liljestrand@helsinki.fi (J.M.L.); ramin.akhi@oulu.fi (R.A.)

Abstract: Apical periodontitis is an inflammatory reaction at the apex of an infected tooth. Its microbiota resembles that of marginal periodontitis and may induce local and systemic antibodies binding to bacteria- and host-derived epitopes. Our aim was to investigate the features of the adaptive immune response in apical periodontitis. The present Parogene cohort (n = 453) comprises patients with cardiac symptoms. Clinical and radiographic oral examination was performed to diagnose apical and marginal periodontitis. A three-category endodontic lesion score was designed. Antibodies binding to the bacteria- and host-derived epitopes were determined from saliva and serum, and bacterial compositions were examined from saliva and subgingival samples. The significant ORs (95% CI) for the highest endodontic scores were observed for saliva IgA and IgG to bacterial antigens (2.90 (1.01–8.33) and 4.91 (2.48–9.71)/log10 unit), saliva cross-reacting IgG (2.10 (1.48–2.97)), serum IgG to bacterial antigens (4.66 (1.22–10.1)), and Gram-negative subgingival species (1.98 (1.16–3.37)). In a subgroup without marginal periodontitis, only saliva IgG against bacterial antigens associated with untreated apical periodontitis (4.77 (1.05–21.7)). Apical periodontitis associates with versatile adaptive immune responses against both bacterial- and host-derived epitopes independently of marginal periodontitis. Saliva immunoglobulins could be useful biomarkers of oral infections including apical periodontitis—a putative risk factor for systemic diseases.

Keywords: apical periodontitis; adaptive immunity; saliva; serum; antibody

---

1. Introduction

Apical periodontitis (AP) is an inflammatory disease that affects the tissues surrounding the apex of the tooth. It is triggered by oral pathogens infecting root canal. Both acute (abscess) and chronic inflammatory reaction (periapical granuloma and radicular cyst) can develop depending on the intensity of the bacterial infection and the host immune responses. Primary apical periodontitis usually develops when the bacteria in a caries lesion enter through enamel and dentin and cause microbial colonization of the pulp and eventually necrosis of the pulp tissue. Secondary apical periodontitis arises from a persistent infection of previously treated root canals or leakage of the filling in a root canal-treated tooth. Apical periodontitis is diagnosed from radiographs as an evident radiolucent area (referred to as endodontic lesion) at the tip of the root. Even slight radiographically evident widening of the periapical space is associated with an infection in the tooth [1]. AP is treated with root canal treatment where infection is eliminated chemomechanically and the root canal is filled.

Apical periodontitis is a highly common and underdiagnosed disease. It is estimated that approximately 10% of all teeth are endodontically treated, 5% have periapical radiolucencies [2], and the prevalence of apical periodontitis varies between 24 and 86% in different populations [3]. Up to 78% of endodontically treated teeth have root canal fillings with poor quality and ~36% of the root canal-treated teeth present apical periodontitis [2], suggesting that recurrent or persistent endodontic infections are common. Apical periodontitis is usually symptomless, and it can be diagnosed only by radiography.

Endodontic infections are polymicrobial and the structure of the intracanal biofilm may evolve toward obligate aerobes and Gram-negative anaerobes as the infection progresses. More than 400 different microbial taxa have been identified in endodontic samples from teeth with different forms of apical periodontitis [4]. Several studies have also shown that distinct bacterial communities are found in primary and secondary AP [5–8]. Despite the high interindividual variability in endodontic microbial community composition, the most often encountered phyla in the intracanal samples include Firmicutes, Actinobacteria, Bacteroidetes, Proteobacteria, and Fusobacteria. Genera such as Prevotella, Fusobacterium, Parvimonas, Lactobacillus, Streptococcus, and Porphyromonas are highly prevalent in intracanal samples [9]. Several members of these genera are also considered etiological pathogens for marginal periodontitis and the microbial profiles of these two conditions resemble each other [10].

Microbial antigens stimulate innate immune responses in periapical tissue aiming to restrict the infection. The expression of proinflammatory cytokines, prostaglandins, and proteolytic enzymes are markedly increased in the areas of tissue destruction [11]. As one antimicrobial strategy, apical periodontitis is also associated with oxidative stress [12]. Some studies suggest a modest contribution of endodontic infections to the plasmatic inflammatory markers [13,14], while a recent study found a significant association between endodontic lesions and systemic inflammatory burden in young adults [15].

Additionally, adaptive immune responses are activated to prevent the microbial invasion into the tissues surrounding teeth or into circulation. High concentrations of local immunoglobulins IgG and IgA and lesser amounts of IgM and secretory IgA are present in the inflamed tissues [16–19]. The levels of systemic immunoglobulins, including total IgA, IgG, and IgM, are increased in patients with AP [13]. We recently showed that subgingival *Porphyromonas endodontalis* levels and serum IgG against it were associated with a higher endodontic lesion score [20]. Several oral pathogens are also known to be able to induce cross-reactive antibodies, which may influence inflammatory responses. The cross-reactive antibodies are part of an immunological process called molecular mimicry, in which bacterial antigens sufficiently resembling human proteins are able to induce the production of antibodies reacting with human epitopes. The most studied epitopes include those present in the heat shock proteins (HSPs) and in oxidized low-density lipoproteins (oxLDL) [21].

The association of marginal periodontitis with several systemic conditions such as cardiovascular diseases (CVDs) is well established [22]. Due to similarities in the inflammatory and microbial profiles between marginal periodontitis and AP, it is also suggested that there could be a link between AP and CVDs [23,24]. Even though the possible association of apical periodontitis with systemic diseases has been of high interest, the adaptive immune response against the disease has not been investigated in detail. In this study we aimed to investigate serum and saliva antibodies against several oral pathogens associated with apical periodontitis and the role of cross-reactive antibodies in the disease.

2. Experimental Section

2.1. Population

The Corogene is a prospective cohort of Finnish patients who had an indication to coronary angiography between June 2006 and March 2008 at the Helsinki University Hospital [25]. The present study comprises the Parogene, which is a substudy of 508 patients with clinical and radiographic oral health examinations. The details of the examinations have been described elsewhere [26]. The information of smoking habits was collected with a questionnaire before the oral examination. The presence of diabetes (type I and II) was obtained from medical records. All subjects signed an informed consent and the study was approved by the Helsinki University Hospital ethics committee (approval reference number 106/2007). Patients with antibody measurements from serum and saliva samples were included (n = 453, 89.2% of the whole cohort). The number of dentate patients and subgingival samples was 426 (n of edentulous 27, 6.0%).

2.2. Oral Diagnosis

Endodontic lesions were diagnosed from the radiographs as described in detail earlier [20]. The recorded findings included root canal fillings, widened periapical space indicating irreversible pulpitis or precursors for endodontic lesions [1], and apical periodontitis seen as periradicular destruction in the tip of the root. An endodontic lesion score was defined to describe the severity of apical periodontitis [20]. Score I included patients without endodontic lesions (n = 162, 38.2%); score II, patients with ≥1 widened periapical space and/or 1 tooth with apical periodontitis (n = 194, 45.2%); and score III, patients with ≥2 teeth with apical periodontitis (n = 68, 16.0%). In addition, another subgrouping—the endodontic treatment score—was designed according to treated/untreated apical periodontitis: I, no endodontic lesions (n = 352, 77.7%); II, teeth with apical periodontitis, all with root canal fillings (n = 51, 11.3%); and III, apical periodontitis in tooth/teeth without root canal fillings (n = 50, 11.0%). Number of teeth and implants, presence of carious teeth, and inadequate root canal fillings were also recorded from the radiographs.

Diagnosis for marginal periodontitis was based on alveolar bone loss (ABL) detected in the radiographs and bleeding on probing (BOP) registered in the clinical examination from four sites of each tooth. Patient was considered periodontally healthy, when no ABL and <25% BOP was present; with gingivitis, when no ABL but ≥25% BOP; and with periodontitis, when ABL was present [27].

2.3. Bacterial Analyses

Subgingival plaque samples were collected from the deepest pathological periodontal pocket (≥ 4 mm) in each dentate quadrant as described earlier [28]. The microbiome analysis including 79 taxa was performed by using the checkerboard DNA-DNA hybridization assay [29] and the data was analyzed as described in our earlier article [28]. In the present work, we summed up the results of Gram-positive taxa (n = 45) and Gram-negative taxa (n = 34), which are presented in Supplementary Table S1.

Saliva samples were collected after stimulation by chewing for 5 min, and a minimum of 2 mL of saliva was collected by expectoration. The methods for sample processing and quantitative real-time PCR have been described in detail earlier [30]. Saliva concentration of four bacterial species associated with periodontitis was analyzed: *Aggregatibacter actinomycetemcomitans*, *Porphyromonas gingivalis*, *Tannerella forsythia*, and *Prevotella intermedia*.

2.4. Antibody Determinations

Serum IgA- and IgG-class antibody levels against seven bacterial species—*A. actinomycetemcomitans*, *P. gingivalis*, *T. forsythia*, *P. intermedia*, *Campylobacter rectus*, *Fusobacterium nucleatum*, and *P. endodontalis*—were determined with ELISA as described earlier [31]. The antigens were composed of formalin-killed whole cells and two dilutions in duplicate were measured [32]. After all antibody levels were determined, the absorbances were normalized according to the reference applied on each plate and the results were expressed as continuous ELISA-units (EU). The list of the antigens, sample dilutions, and coefficients of interassay variations are presented earlier [31].

Saliva IgA- and IgG-class antibody levels against five species—*A. actinomycetemcomitans*, *P. gingivalis*, *T. forsythia*, *P. intermedia*, *and P. endodontalis*—were determined from saliva supernatants obtained after centrifugation at 9300× *g* for 3 min. The target antigens used in the assays were either heat-killed whole bacterial cells or oxidized LDL epitope malondialdehyde acetaldehyde modification (MAA-LDL), copper-oxidized LDL (CuOx-LDL) [33], recombinant *P. gingivalis* virulence factor gingipain (Rgp44) [34], and 60-kDa *A. actinomycetemcomitans* heat shock protein (Aa-HSP60) [35]. Levels of salivary IgA and IgG antibodies to oxidized LDL and bacterial epitopes were determined by chemiluminescence immunoassay as previously described in detail [36,37]. The saliva samples were diluted accordingly: 1:250 for total IgA and IgG, 1:50 for IgA to oxidized antigens, 1:20 for Aa-HSP60, and 1:10 for bacterial antigens. For IgG measurements, saliva samples were diluted 1:10 for all antigens. Each saliva sample was measured as triplicates. Immunoassay results were presented as relative light units (RLU) per 100 milliseconds (ms).

2.5. Calculations of Cross-Reactive Antibodies and Antibodies Binding to Bacterial Antigens

In addition to the mean levels of antibodies against each specific antigen, the combined antibody levels of saliva and serum IgA and IgG were calculated. The bacterial antigens included *A. actinomycetemcomitans*, *P. gingivalis*, *P. intermedia*, *P. endodontalis*, and *T. forsythia* (referred as IgA/IgG against bacteria). The epitopes recognized in *P. gingivalis* and *A. actinomycetemcomitans* giving rise to cross-reactive antibodies with MAA-LDL included Rgp-44 and Aa-HSP60 (referred as cross-reacting IgA/IgG).

2.6. Statistical Methods

The characteristics are presented as mean values with standard deviations (SD) or 95% confidence intervals. For clarity, standard error is displayed in the figures as error bars. In the supplementary tables, the bacterial levels are presented as medians and interquartile ranges (IQR). Before statistical comparisons, the antibody and bacterial levels were transformed with 10-base logarithm. The significance of the differences was tested by using *t*-test, ANOVA, Chi-square, or Mann–Whitney, when appropriate. The weighted linear terms were examined with ANOVA and Jonckheere–Terpstra test for normally distributed and skewed data, respectively. The associations were analyzed by using linear and logistic regression models adjusted for age, sex, marginal periodontitis (healthy, gingivitis, and periodontitis), number of teeth, and smoking (never/ever). When the dependent variable was composed of several subgroups, multinomial regression was used. When the associations were examined in the subgroup of patients without marginal periodontitis, the confounders were limited to age, sex, and smoking (never/ever).

3. Results

Characteristics of the dentate population are presented in Table 1. The mean (SD) age was 62.9 (9.1) years and 67% were males. The mean number of teeth was 21.4 (7.5), and caries and apical periodontitis were common findings, in 47.4% and 23.8% of the population, respectively. Also, marginal periodontitis ranging from mild to severe was present in most patients (75.5%).

Table 1. Characteristics of the population.

	Character	Mean (SD)
	Age (years)	62.9 (9.1)
	BMI (kg/m^2)	27.8 (5.1)
	Number of teeth	21.4 (7.5)
		Mean (95% CI)
	Number of implants	0.12 (0.05–0.18)
	Carious teeth	0.99 (0.84–1.14)
	Root canal fillings	2.17 (1.96–2.39)
	Inadequate root fillings	1.08 (0.95–1.20)
	Widened periapical space	0.80 (0.71–0.89)
	Apical periodontitis	0.36 (0.27–0.45)
	With root canal fillings	0.16 (0.12–0.21)
	Without root canal fillings	0.19 (0.11–0.27)
		N (%)
	Gender (males)	284 (67.0)
	Smoking (ever)	220 (51.9)
	Hypertension	266 (62.9)
	Diabetes (type I or II)	92 (21.9)
	Dyslipidemia	340 (80.6)
	Carious teeth	198 (47.4)
	Root canal fillings	304 (71.7)
	Widened periapical spaces	224 (53.8)
	Apical periodontitis	101 (23.8)
Endodontic lesion score	No endodontic lesions	162 (38.2)
	≥1 tooth with widened periapical space or one tooth with apical periodontitis	194 (45.8)
	≥2 teeth with apical periodontitis	68 (16.0)
Endodontic treatment score	No endodontic lesions	323 (76.2)
	Apical periodontitis in teeth with root canal fillings	51 (12.0)
	Apical periodontitis in teeth without root canal fillings	50 (11.8)
Marginal periodontitis	Healthy	42 (9.9)
	Gingivitis	61 (14.4)
	Periodontitis	320 (75.5)

The endodontic findings registered included root canal fillings, widened periapical space, and apical periodontitis. Mean antibody levels in serum and saliva against specific antigens, as well as the saliva and subgingival bacterial levels according to the endodontic findings are presented in supplementary tables (Supplementary Tables S2 and S3).

Among serum or saliva IgA-class antibody levels only sporadic significant differences were observed between patients with and without endodontic findings, whereas among IgG-class antibodies several significant differences were found. The antigens producing these differences included *A. actinomycetemcomitans*, *P. gingivalis*, *P. intermedia*, *P. endodontalis*, *C. rectus*, *F. nucleatum*, and *T. forsythia*, as well as Aa-HSP60, rgp44, MAA-LDL, and CuOx-LDL (Table S2). Among the salivary or subgingival bacterial concentrations, significant differences were mostly found between patients with and without widened periapical spaces (Table S3).

For further analyses, the microbial biomarkers were combined, and the mean levels are presented in Figures 1 and 2. The combinations included antibody level against bacteria, cross-reactive antibodies, salivary bacteria, and subgingival bacteria. Similarly as above, the mean saliva IgG-class antibody levels against bacteria and the cross-reactive antibodies as well as saliva and subgingival bacterial levels were higher in patients with endodontic findings. From the serum antibody levels, the IgG against bacteria were higher only in patients with widened periapical spaces ($p = 0.015$). In these patients, the increase of subgingival bacterial levels was due to both Gram-positive ($p = 0.022$) and Gram-negative ($p = 0.005$) species.

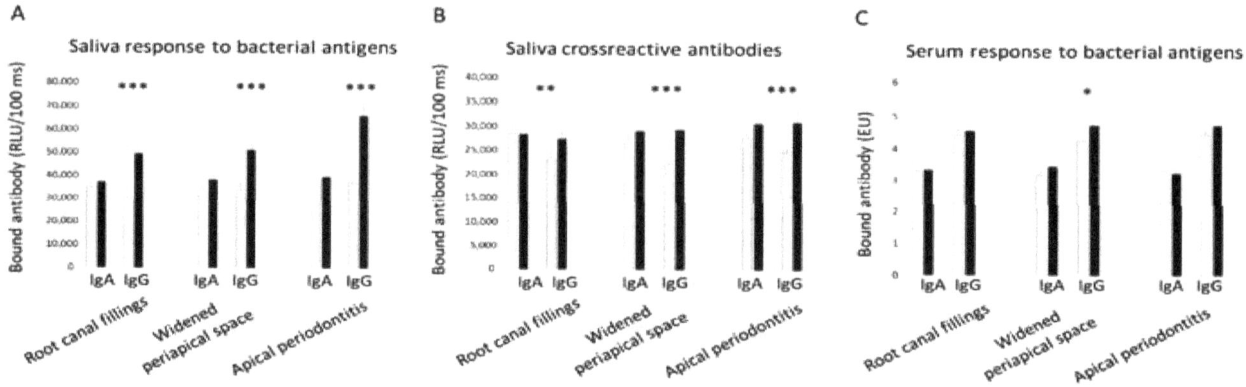

Figure 1. Saliva and serum antibody levels according to endodontic findings. The patients were divided into groups according to the presence of root canal fillings, widened periapical spaces, and apical periodontitis. Saliva (A, B) and serum (C) IgA- and IgG-class antibodies were determined. The bacterial antigens included *A. actinomycetemcomitans, P. gingivalis, P. intermedia, P. endodontalis,* and *T. forsythia*. The antigens giving rise to cross-reactive antibodies included MAA-LDL, Rgp-44, and Aa-HSP60. White columns depict the absence of the endodontic finding and black columns depict the presence of the endodontic finding. Means and standard errors are shown. The asterisks depict statistical significance between the groups defined by the *t*-test after logarithmic transformation: * $p < 0.05$, ** $p < 0.01$. *** $p < 0.001$.

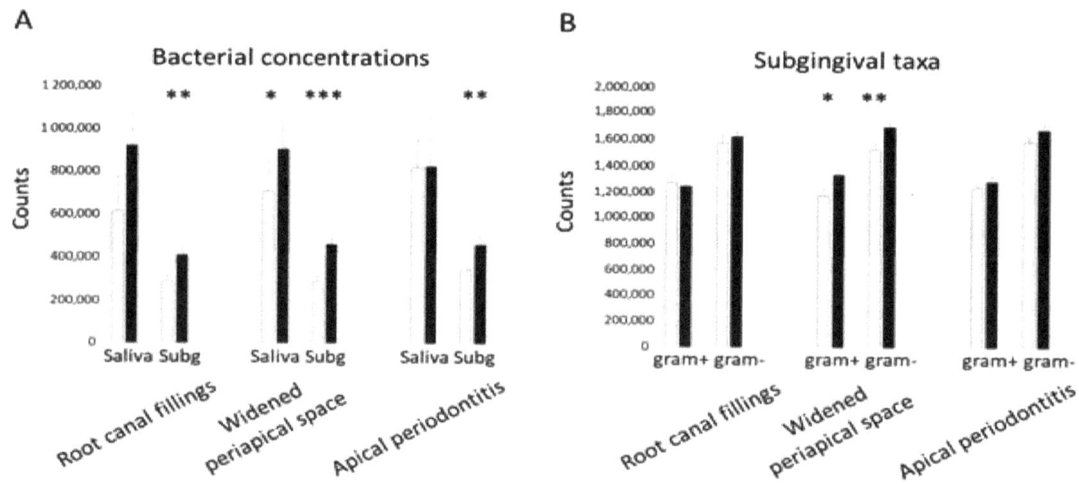

Figure 2. Saliva and subgingival bacteria according to endodontic findings. The patients were divided into groups according to the presence of root canal fillings, widened periapical spaces, and apical periodontitis. Salivary bacterial concentrations of *A. actinomycetemcomitans, P. gingivalis, P. intermedia,* and *T. forsythia* were determined by qPCR, and subgingival *A. actinomycetemcomitans, P. gingivalis, P. intermedia, P. endodontalis,* and *T. forsythia* by checkerboard DNA–DNA hybridization (A). This method was also used to examine subgingival 79 taxa, which were divided into Gram-positive ($n = 45$) and Gram-negative ($n = 34$) (B). The white columns depict the absence, and black columns presence of the endodontic finding. Means and standard errors are shown. The asterisks depict statistical significance between the groups defined by the *t*-test after logarithmic transformation: * $p < 0.05$, ** $p < 0.01$. *** $p < 0.001$.

The associations of antibody and bacterial levels with endodontic findings are presented in Table 2 for the whole population calculated by using linear and logistic regression models adjusted for age, sex, number of teeth, smoking, and status of marginal periodontitis. The estimates are presented for a 10-fold increase in the antibody or bacterial levels, number of root canal-treated teeth associated with saliva IgA and IgG against bacteria, and cross-reacting IgG. Among these, only saliva IgG against bacteria associated with the presence of root canal-treated teeth with an OR (95% CI) 2.52 (1.43–4.43). Number of widened periapical spaces associated with saliva cross-reactive IgA and IgG, saliva IgG against bacteria, and subgingival bacteria in linear regression models. The presence of widened periapical spaces associated with saliva IgA and IgG against bacteria with ORs 2.09 (1.01–4.34) and 2.25 (1.40–3.61), respectively, and with cross-reacting IgG, 1.56 (1.22–1.99). Significant associations were also observed between the presence of widened periapical space and Gram-positive and Gram-negative subgingival bacteria with ORs 1.40 (1.02–1.92) and 1.45 (1.05–2.00). Number of teeth with apical periodontitis associated with saliva IgG against bacteria and cross-reacting IgG, which also presented significant ORs with the presence of apical periodontitis (2.90 (1.71–4.92) and 1.62 (1.24–2.11)).

A 3-category endodontic lesion score was designed for the severity of apical periodontitis. In addition, a 3-category endodontic treatment score was designed to investigate the contribution of treatment (root canal fillings) on the associations. The characteristics of the population are presented according to these scores in Table 3. Number of teeth, carious teeth, teeth with root canal fillings, and inadequate root canal fillings increased significantly with increasing scores. Also marginal periodontitis was more prevalent with high endodontic lesion ($p < 0.001$) or endodontic treatment ($p = 0.287$) score. Mean antibody levels in serum and saliva against specific antigens, as well as the saliva and subgingival bacterial levels according to these scores are presented in supplementary tables (Table S4 and S5). The association of the scores with the combined microbial biomarkers was analyzed by multinomial regression models for the $\log_{10}$-transforemed units (Figure 3). All measured parameters displayed positive trends with the increasing endodontic lesion score. Statistically significant associations (OR (95% CI)) with the highest endodontic scores were observed for saliva IgA (2.90 (1.01–8.33)) and IgG (4.91 (2.48–9.71)) against bacteria, saliva cross-reacting IgG (2.10 (1.48–2.97)), serum IgG against bacteria (4.66 (1.22–10.1)), subgingival species (1.15 (1.07–1.25)), and Gram-negative subgingival species (1.98 (1.16–3.37)). Regarding the treatment, only saliva IgG against bacteria, cross-reacting IgG, and serum IgA and IgG displayed increasing trends. Significant odds (OR (95%CI)) for untreated apical periodontitis were observed for saliva IgG against bacteria (5.32 (2.61–10.8)) and for cross-reacting IgG (2.04 (1.44–2.88)) (Figure 3).

The main results were reanalyzed in the subgroup of patients without marginal periodontitis ($n = 132$). There were no significant differences in the bacterial levels between groups divided according to the endodontic findings. Saliva IgG antibodies against bacteria and cross-reacting antibodies were higher in subjects with root canal fillings ($p = 0.003$ and 0.004), widened periapical spaces ($p = 0.008$ and 0.008), and apical periodontitis ($p = 0.012$ and 0.385). Both antibody levels increased in groups of patients with increasing endodontic scores (p for linear trend 0.009 and 0.020). The antibodies against bacteria (p for linear trend 0.007), but not the cross-reacting antibodies ($p = 0.569$), increased in patients with greater endodontic treatment scores. The associations of the saliva IgG class antibodies with endodontic lesion score and endodontic treatment score are presented in Table 4. Increasing trends were observed clearly only for saliva IgG against bacteria; the multivariate odds (OR (95% CI)) for having multiple teeth with apical periodontitis and for having teeth with untreated apical periodontitis were 3.45 (0.83–14.3) and 4.77 (1.05–21.7), respectively.

Table 2. Associations of endodontic findings with saliva and serum antibody levels and bacterial concentrations.

	Root Canal Fillings		Widened Periapical Space		Apical Periodontitis	
	Beta, *p*-Value	OR (95% CI), *p*	Beta, *p*-Value	OR (95% CI), *p*	Beta, *p*-Value	OR (95% CI), *p*
Saliva IgA against bacteria *	**0.096, 0.041**	2.162 (0.934–5.004), 0.072	0.062, 0.204	**2.090 (1.007–4.337), 0.048**	0.059, 0.235	1.995 (0.870–4.573), 0.103
Saliva IgG against bacteria *	**0.169, <0.001**	**2.519 (1.431–4.434), 0.001**	**0.138, 0.005**	**2.246 (1.397–3.611), 0.001**	**0.182, <0.001**	**2.904 (1.714–4.922), <0.001**
Serum IgA against bacteria *	0.031, 0.527	1.144 (0.516–2.539), 0.741	0.017, 0.738	1.513 (0.753–3.040), 0.245	0.037, 0.476	0.922 (0.421–2.018), 0.838
Serum IgG against bacteria *	0.010, 0.838	1.272 (0.443–3.656), 0.655	0.002, 0.963	2.048 (0.840–4.995), 0.115	0.083, 0.102	1.710 (0.615–4.754), 0.304
Saliva pathogen sum	0.012, 0.802	0.996 (0.932–1.064), 0.900	0.068, 0.163	1.046 (0.989–1.107), 0.117	0.079, 0.111	0.998 (0.936–1.064), 0.951
Subgingival pathogen sum	0.053, 0.273	0.991 (0.934–1.051), 0.760	0.086, 0.085	1.051 (0.999–1.105), 0.056	**0.098, 0.049**	1.047 (0.987–1.112), 0.127
45 gram-positive taxa	0.025, 0.603	0.754 (0.515–1.104), 0.147	**0.121, 0.014**	**1.395 (1.016–1.917), 0.040**	0.045, 0.375	1.096 (0.761–1.578), 0.622
33 gram-negative taxa	0.056, 0.237	0.945 (0.660–1.353), 0.757	**0.121, 0.014**	**1.446 (1.046–1.999), 0.026**	0.059, 0.238	1.249 (0.850–1.836), 0.257
Saliva cross-reactive IgA **	0.086, 0.067	1.248 (0.926–1.680), 0.146	**0.096, 0.049**	1.295 (0.995–1.685), 0.055	0.064, 0.196	1.327 (0.986–1.788), 0.062
Saliva cross-reactive IgG **	**0.128, 0.006**	1.240 (0.942–1.632), 0.125	**0.160, 0.001**	**1.555 (1.217–1.987), <0.001**	**0.159, 0.001**	**1.615 (1.237–2.108), <0.001**

The dependent variable in the linear regression was the number of findings and in the logistic regression the presence of findings. Adjusted for age, sex, marginal periodontitis (healthy, gingivitis, periodontitis), number of teeth, and smoking (never/ever). * Antibodies against *A. actinomycetemcomitans*, *P. gingivalis*, *P. intermedia*, *P. endodontalis*, and *T. forsythia*; ** Cross-reactive antibodies, antigens Pg-Rgp44, Aa-HSP60, and MAA-LDL.

Table 3. Characteristics of the population according to endodontic scores.

Character	Endodontic Lesion Score				Endodontic Treatment Score			
	Score I	Score II	Score III		Score I	Score II	Score III	
		Mean (SD)		P [1]		Mean (SD)		P [1]
Age (years)	63.3 (9.2)	63.1 (8.7)	63.7 (9.8	0.924	63.3 (9.0)	64.3 (9.0)	62.5 (9.5)	0.578
BMI (kg/m^2)	27.8 (5.0)	27.8 (5.1)	27.8 (4.4)	0.990	27.7 (5.0)	27.9 (4.8)	28.2 (4.8)	0.852
Number of teeth	18.1 (10.5)	21.5 (7.3)	22.0 (6.7)	**<0.001**	19.7 (9.3)	23.2 (6.0)	20.5 (8.0)	**0.031**
		Mean (95% CI)				Mean (95% CI)		
Number of implants	0.17 (0.04–0.29)	0.10 (0.01–0.20)	0.12 (0.04–0.28)	0.696	0.15 (0.06–0.23)	0.14 (0.07–0.35)	0.02 (0.02–0.06)	0.546
Carious teeth	0.68 (0.52–0.84)	0.97 (0.75–1.18)	1.74 (1.20–2.27)	**<0.001**	0.83 (0.69–0.98)	1.24 (0.76–1.71)	1.82 (1.10–2.53)	**<0.001**
Root canal fillings	0.95 (0.73–1.17)	2.54 (2.26–2.82)	3.91 (3.21–4.61)	**<0.001**	1.82 (1.61–2.02)	4.65 (3.84–5.45)	1.91 (1.28–2.54)	**<0.001**
Inadequate root fillings	0.41 (0.29–0.52)	1.26 (1.10–1.42)	2.07 (1.64–2.51)	**<0.001**	0.88 (0.76–1.00)	2.33 (1.83–2.84)	1.05 (0.65–1.44)	**<0.001**
		N (%)		P [2]		N (%)		P [2]
N (%)	189 (41.7)	196 (43.3)	68 (15.0)		352 (77.7)	51 (11.3)	50 (11.0)	
Sex (males)	123 (65.1)	132 (67.3)	47 (69.1)	0.803	234 (66.5)	33 (64.7)	35 (70.0)	0.842
Smoking (ever)	92 (48.9)	112 (57.1)	35 (51.5)	0.265	190 (54.1)	23 (45.1)	26 (52.0)	0.478
Hypertension	122 (64.6)	123 (63.4)	41 (61.2)	0.885	226 (64.6)	30 (58.8)	30 (61.2)	0.683
Diabetes (type I/II)	39 (20.9)	47 (24.2)	14 (21.2)	0.711	78 (22.4)	11 (22.0)	11 (22.4)	0.998
Dyslipidemia	148 (78.3)	165 (85.5)	49 (73.1)	0.050	285 (81.7)	42 (84.0)	35 (70.0)	0.121
Marginal periodontitis	111 (58.7)	154 (78.6)	56 (82.4)	**<0.001**	244 (69.3)	37 (72.5)	40 (80.0)	0.287

[1] ANOVA; [2] Chi-square test; Endodontic lesion score: score I, no endodontic lesions; score II, patients with ≥1 widened periapical space and/or 1 tooth with apical periodontitis; and score III, patients with ≥2 teeth with apical periodontitis. Endodontic treatment score: score I, no endodontic lesions; score II, apical periodontitis only in teeth with root canal fillings; score III, apical periodontitis in teeth without root canal fillings.

Table 4. Association of saliva IgG class antibody levels with endodontic scores in the subpopulation free from marginal periodontitis.

		OR (95% CI), *P*-Value			
		Saliva IgG Against Bacteria *		Saliva Cross-Reacting IgG **	
		Univariate	Multivariate [1]	Univariate	Multivariate [1]
Endodontic lesion score	No endodontic lesions	1.0	1.0	1.0	1.0
	≥1 tooth with widened periapical space or apical periodontitis	**2.92 (1.17–7.26), 0.022**	**2.67 (1.03–6.94), 0.044**	**2.06 (1.31–3.22), 0.002**	**1.97 (1.24–3.11), 0.004**
	≥2 teeth with apical periodontitis	**3.88 (0.99–15.5), 0.050**	3.45 (0.83–14.3), 0.088	1.32 (0.65–2.69), 0.435	1.30 (0.64–2.62), 0.472
Endodontic treatment score	No endodontic lesions	1.0	1.0	1.0	1.0
	Apical periodontitis in teeth with root canal fillings	2.52 (0.70–9.06), 0.157	2.44 (0.66–9.06), 0.184	1.11 (0.60–2.03), 0.746	1.12 (0.60–2.08), 0.731
	Apical periodontitis in teeth without root canal fillings	**5.88 (1.32–26.2), 0.020**	**4.77 (1.05–21.7), 0.043**	1.43 (0.73–2.80), 0.297	1.39 (0.70–2.78), 0.351

[1] Adjusted for age, sex, and smoking (never/ever). Multinomial logistic regression. * Antibodies against *A. actinomycetemcomitans*, *P. gingivalis*, *P. intermedia*, *P. endodontalis*, and *T. forsythia*; ** Cross-reactive antibodies, antigens Pg-Rgp44, Aa-HSP60, and MAA-LDL.

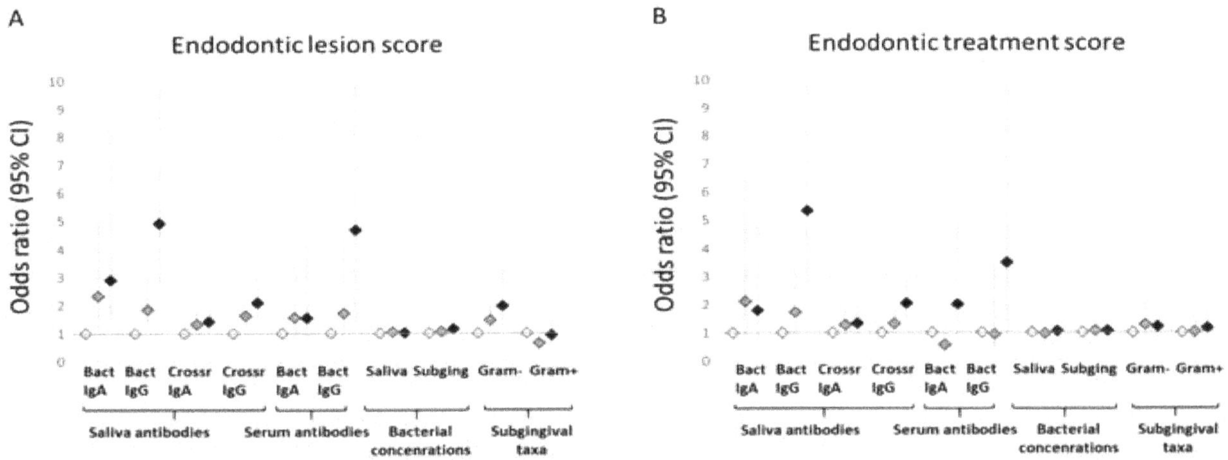

Figure 3. Associations of the antibody and bacterial levels with endodontic lesion score and endodontic treatment score. Endodontic lesion score (A): score I, no endodontic lesions; score II, patients with ≥1 widened periapical space and/or 1 tooth with apical periodontitis; and score III, patients with ≥2 teeth with apical periodontitis. Endodontic treatment score (B): score I, no endodontic lesions; score II, apical periodontitis only in teeth with root canal fillings; score III, apical periodontitis in teeth without root canal fillings. The associations were investigated by using multinomial regression models adjusted for age, sex, marginal periodontitis (healthy, gingivitis, periodontitis), number of teeth, and smoking (never/ever). The estimates for lowest (reference), middle, and highest scores are depicted with white, gray, and black diamonds, respectively.

4. Discussion

We showed that apical periodontitis is associated with elevated levels of saliva IgA and IgG and serum IgG against bacterial antigens and saliva cross-reacting IgG, which recognise both bacterial and host epitopes. The associations were independent of marginal periodontitis. The local antibody response may contribute to the systemic IgG levels, which associate with the severity of apical periodontitis and arise mainly from untreated apical infections. High salivary IgA was associated with the number of widened periapical spaces, most likely indicating early endodontic infection.

Elevated levels of salivary total IgG associated with endodontic findings including root canal treatments, widened periapical spaces and radiographically diagnosed apical periodontitis. Both the presence and number of endodontic findings were significantly associated with total salivary IgG levels. In the case of total salivary IgA, the presence of root canal fillings and the number of widened periapical spaces, but neither the presence nor the number of teeth with apical periodontitis, associated with higher antibody levels. In health, the saliva IgGs mainly derive from the circulation by transudation through the gingival crevice. They comprise less than 15 percent of the total salivary immunoglobulins, as the major salivary immunoglobulin is secretory IgA produced by the salivary glands in mucosal plasma cells [38,39]. However, high concentrations of IgG and IgA and smaller amounts of IgM and secretory IgA have been detected within the periapical granulomas, in periapical cysts, as well as in root canal exudates with periapically affected teeth [40]. In addition, the total IgG and IgA levels detected from the periapical exudate were shown to correlate with clinical findings of the infected teeth [41]. As the half-life of IgA-class antibodies is only a few days, they are considered to reflect either recent or repeated exposure to the pathogen, while IgG is more stable, thus indicating a past, and maybe chronic, infection. Widened periapical spaces reflect either symptomatic teeth with irreversible pulpitis or precursors for established AP in necrotic teeth [1]. Since all determined antibody levels and bacterial concentrations correlated with the endodontic score, our results support the suggestion that the widened periapical spaces are likely to reflect early endodontic lesions [20].

When antibody response was studied in more detail, it was observed that salivary IgG levels against all studied species (*A. actinomycetemcomitans*, *P. gingivalis*, *P. intermedia*, *P. endodontalis*, and *T. forsythia)* were significantly higher in the groups with endodontic findings. In addition, patients with widened periapical spaces had higher saliva IgA-antibodies against *P. endodontalis*. It is widely accepted that endodontic infections have a multimicrobial etiology [4], and several pathogens associated with marginal periodontitis, such as *P. intermedia*, *P. gingivalis*, *T. denticola* and *P. endodontalis*, are frequently detected in teeth with necrotic pulps [42–44]. As apical periodontitis is often restricted to the periapical tissues, it is not surprising that the amount of studied salivary and subgingival bacteria were not consistently associated with the endodontic findings. On the other hand, it is reported that in the case of combined endodontic-periodontal lesions, where apical periodontitis can be initiated either in the pulp or in the periodontium, the microbial profiles of apical lesions and periodontal pockets resemble each other [10]. In such cases, it is probable that bacteria enter the root canal from the periodontium via the apical foramen, dentinal tubules and accessory root canals [45].

Two major pathogens in marginal periodontitis, *A. actinomycetemcomitans* and *P. gingivalis*, express several virulence factors including *P. gingivalis*-specific gingipains degrading the extracellular matrix and bioactive peptides [46], as well as heat shock proteins (HSPs) produced by both species [47]. These proteins elicit strong antibody production and are also able to induce a variety of cross-reactive antibodies recognizing human epitopes such as HSPs and oxidized low-density lipoproteins (oxLDL). These cross-reactions are considered potential links between periodontitis and an increased risk of cardiovascular diseases [21]. The oxidation of LDL gives rise to various epitopes and a frequently used model of oxLDL include the immunodominant epitopes malondialdehyde (MDA) and malondialdehyde acetaldehyde (MAA). It is reported that the presence of antibodies binding to MDA-LDL is associated with both the progression of atherosclerosis and with the presence and severity of periodontitis [37,48–50]. A monoclonal IgM antibody to MDA-LDL recognizes *P. gingivalis* virulence factor gingipain (Rgp44) as an antigen [34] and *A. actinomycetemcomitans* heat shock protein 60 (Aa-HSP60) cross-reacts with MAA-LDL [35]. To our knowledge, this study is the first to show the association between apical periodontitis and salivary cross-reactive antibodies. Especially cross-reactive antibodies representing IgG-class were strongly associated with different endodontic conditions.

All measured parameters displayed positive trends with increasing number of endodontic findings as both the salivary IgA and IgG against bacterial antigens, as well as the cross-reacting IgG, were significantly associated with the highest endodontic score. In addition, the effect of endodontic treatment on antibody response was evident indicating that the levels of both saliva IgG against bacterial antigens and cross-reacting IgG were significantly higher in the patients with primary apical periodontitis compared to those who had apical periodontitis in teeth with root canal fillings. The aim of root canal treatment is to eradicate the biofilm from the infected root canal and prevent the recurrent infection. However, if the treatment is inadequately performed, some bacteria may survive and cause secondary infection. The microbiome of endodontically treated root canals consists of fewer bacterial species, and some of the species are more resilient to endodontic treatment [10]. This phenomenon may reflect to the levels of antibodies measured in this study.

The production of local IgGs is also enhanced in advanced marginal periodontitis by local plasma cells of the gingiva [51]. We repeated our main analyses in a subgroup of subjects without marginal periodontitis. Although the number of patients in this subgroup was low, the association between saliva IgG against bacterial antigens and primary apical periodontitis remained significant, suggesting further that IgG antibody response is independent of marginal periodontitis.

The main limitation of this study is that our study population consists of middle-aged and elderly participants, and thus the oral infections are very common. In addition, all participants had an initial indication for coronary angiography. Another restriction is the lack of intracanal bacterial samples; hence the bacterial analyses were only conducted from saliva and subgingival samples. Different methods were used for the detection of the antibody levels in serum and saliva, and not the same antibody panels were available. For instance, we did not have information on the serum cross-reactive antibodies, which will be an aim for future investigations. Also different methodologies were used for the bacterial analyses, since the subgingival samples were examined by checkerboard DNA–DNA hybridization and the saliva samples by qPCR.

Although apical periodontitis has been considered as a potential risk factor for systemic diseases such as coronary artery disease (CAD) [52], only a few studies have attempted to draw conclusions on the associations between apical periodontitis and systemic diseases. Evidence for the association between AP and CVDs, such as endothelial dysfunction [53], atherosclerosis [54], and coronary heart disease [55], has been reported in separate studies. However, recent systematic reviews suggest only modest participation of endodontic infection on the systemic levels of biomarkers and a moderate or low correlation between some systemic diseases and apical periodontitis [14,23,24,56]. In our recent study, we demonstrated a confounder-adjusted association between apical periodontitis and CAD [20]. In the present study, we showed that apical periodontitis may contribute to the levels of IgG in serum which link oral bacteria to CAD risk [31]. These serum antibodies have been repeatedly associated with prevalent and incident CVD as well as with subclinical atherosclerosis [57–60]. Also the saliva cross-reacting antibodies and immunoglobulins against bacterial antigens have been associated with increased risk for CAD [37].

Salivary immunoglobulins are potential biomarkers of oral infectious diseases, but the specific antigens should be selected carefully. This would be especially beneficial in the case of apical periodontitis, as the disease is often asymptomatic and remains undiagnosed. This study represents a limited set of antibodies against selected bacterial targets, and further research is needed to investigate the levels of antibodies against other bacterial species commonly found in infected root canals.

5. Conclusions

Our results suggest that the inflammatory condition caused by endodontic infections could be identified by the increased salivary IgG levels independently of marginal periodontitis. The levels of saliva IgG may have a small, but significant effect on the systemic levels of biomarkers, indicating the potential link between apical periodontitis and systemic diseases.

Author Contributions: Conceptualization, M.P. and P.J.P.; investigation—laboratory analyses, M.P., J.M.L., R.A., S.H., and P.J.P.; investigation—clinical examination, K.B., S.P., P.M., and J.S.; investigation—radiographic examination, J.M.L., K.B., S.P., A.S., P.M., and L.T.; formal analysis, M.P., A.S., and P.J.P.; writing—original draft preparation, M.P.; writing—review and editing, A.J., A.S., S.P., J.M.L., R.A., and P.J.P.; project administration, P.J.P; funding acquisition, S.P. and P.J.P.; supervision, P.J.P.

References

1. Carrotte, P. Endodontics: Part 3. Treatment of endodontic emergencies. *Br. Dent. J.* **2004**, *197*, 299–305. [CrossRef] [PubMed]
2. Pak, J.G.; Fayazi, S.; White, S.N. Prevalence of periapical radiolucency and root canal treatment: A systematic review of cross-sectional studies. *J. Endod.* **2012**, *38*, 1170–1176. [CrossRef] [PubMed]
3. Persoon, I.F.; Özok, A.R. Definitions and Epidemiology of Endodontic Infections. *Curr. Oral. Health Rep.* **2017**, *4*, 278–285. [CrossRef]
4. Siqueira, J.F., Jr.; Rôças, I.N. Distinctive features of the microbiota associated with different forms of apical periodontitis. *J. Oral. Microbiol.* **2009**, *1*. [CrossRef] [PubMed]
5. Hong, B.Y.; Lee, T.K.; Lim, S.M.; Chang, S.W.; Park, J.; Han, S.H.; Zhu, Q.; Safavi, K.E.; Fouad, A.F.; Kum, K.Y. Microbial analysis in primary and persistent endodontic infections by using pyrosequencing. *J. Endod.* **2013**, *39*, 1136–1140. [CrossRef] [PubMed]
6. Tzanetakis, G.N.; Azcarate-Peril, M.A.; Zachaki, S.; Panopoulos, P.; Kontakiotis, E.G.; Madianos, P.N.; Divaris, K. Comparison of Bacterial Community Composition of Primary and Persistent Endodontic Infections Using Pyrosequencing. *J. Endod.* **2015**, *41*, 1226–1233. [CrossRef] [PubMed]
7. Keskin, C.; Demiryürek, E.Ö.; Onuk, E.E. Pyrosequencing analysis of cryogenically ground samples from primary and secondary/persistent endodontic infections. *J. Endod.* **2017**, *43*, 1309–1316. [CrossRef] [PubMed]
8. Bouillaguet, S.; Manoil, D.; Girard, M.; Louis, J.; Gaïa, N.; Leo, S.; Schrenzel, J.; Lazarevic, V. Root Microbiota in Primary and Secondary Apical Periodontitis. *Front. Microbiol.* **2018**, *9*, 2374. [CrossRef] [PubMed]
9. Shin, J.M.; Luo, T.; Lee, K.H.; Guerreiro, D.; Botero, T.M.; McDonald, N.J.; Rickard, A.H. Deciphering Endodontic Microbial Communities by Next-generation Sequencing. *J. Endod.* **2018**, *44*, 1080–1087. [CrossRef]

10. Gomes, B.P.; Berber, V.B.; Kokaras, A.S.; Chen, T.; Paster, B.J. Microbiomes of Endodontic-Periodontal Lesions before and after Chemomechanical Preparation. *J. Endod.* **2015**, *4*, 1975–1984. [CrossRef] [PubMed]
11. Graunaite, I.; Lodiene, G.; Maciulskiene, V. Pathogenesis of apical periodontitis: A literature review. *J. Oral. Maxillofac. Res.* **2011**, *2*, e1. [CrossRef] [PubMed]
12. Hernández-Ríos, P.; Pussinen, P.J.; Vernal, R.; Hernández, M. Oxidative Stress in the Local and Systemic Events of Apical Periodontitis. *Front. Physiol.* **2017**, *1*, 869. [CrossRef] [PubMed]
13. Gomes, M.S.; Blattner, T.C.; Sant'Ana Filho, M.; Grecca, F.S.; Hugo, F.N.; Fouad, A.F.; Reynolds, M.A. Can apical periodontitis modify systemic levels of inflammatory markers? A systematic review and meta-analysis. *J. Endod.* **2013**, *39*, 1205–1217. [CrossRef] [PubMed]
14. Vidal, F.; Fontes, T.V.; Marques, T.V.; Gonçalves, L.S. Association between apical periodontitis lesions and plasmatic levels of C-reactive protein, interleukin 6 and fibrinogen in hypertensive patients. *Int. Endod. J.* **2016**, *49*, 1107–1115. [CrossRef] [PubMed]
15. Garrido, M.; Cárdenas, A.M.; Astorga, J.; Quinlan, F.; Valdés, M.; Chaparro, A.; Carvajal, P.; Pussinen, P.; Huamán-Chipana, P.; Jalil, J.E.; et al. Elevated Systemic Inflammatory Burden and Cardiovascular Risk in Young Adults with Endodontic Apical Lesions. *J. Endod.* **2019**, *45*, 111–115. [CrossRef] [PubMed]
16. Greening, A.B.; Schonfeld, S.E. Apical lesions contain elevated immunoglobulin G levels. *J. Endod.* **1980**, *12*, 867–869. [CrossRef]
17. Johannessen, A.C.; Nilsen, R.; Skaug, N. Deposits of immunoglobulins and complement factor C3 in human dental periapical inflammatory lesions. *Scand. J. Dent. Res.* **1983**, *91*, 191–199. [CrossRef]
18. Keudell, K.; Powel, G.; Berry, H. A review of microbial and immunologic aspects of endodontics. *J. Oral. Pathol. Med.* **1981**, *36*, 39–43.
19. Torres, J.O.C.; Torabinejad, M.; Matiz, R.A.R.; Mantilla, E.G. Presence of secretory IgA in human periapical lesions. *J. Endod.* **1994**, *20*, 87–89. [CrossRef]
20. Liljestrand, J.M.; Mäntylä, P.; Paju, S.; Buhlin, K.; Kopra, K.A.; Persson, G.R.; Hernandez, M.; Nieminen, M.S.; Sinisalo, J.; Tjäderhane, L.; et al. Association of Endodontic Lesions with Coronary Artery Disease. *J. Dent. Res.* **2016**, *95*, 1358–1365. [CrossRef]
21. Pietiäinen, M.; Liljestrand, J.M.; Kopra, E.; Pussinen, P.J. Mediators between oral dysbiosis and cardiovascular diseases. *Eur. J. Oral. Sci.* **2018**, *126* (Suppl. 1), 26–36. [CrossRef] [PubMed]
22. Lockhart, P.B.; Bolger, A.F.; Papapanou, P.N.; Osinbowale, O.; Trevisan, M.; Levison, M.E.; Taubert, K.A.; Newburger, J.W.; Gornik, H.L.; Gewitz, M.H.; et al. Periodontal disease and atherosclerotic vascular disease: Does the evidence support an independent association? A scientific statement from the American Heart Association. *Circulation* **2012**, *125*, 2520–2544. [CrossRef] [PubMed]
23. Khalighinejad, N.; Aminoshariae, M.R.; Aminoshariae, A.; Kulild, J.C.; Mickel, A.; Fouad, A.F. Association between systemic diseases and apical periodontitis. *J. Endod.* **2016**, *42*, 1427–1434. [CrossRef] [PubMed]
24. Berlin-Broner, Y.; Febbraio, M.; Levin, L. Association between apical periodontitis and cardiovascular diseases: A systematic review of the literature. *Int. Endod. J.* **2017**, *50*, 847–859. [CrossRef] [PubMed]
25. Vaara, S.; Nieminen, M.S.; Lokki, M.L.; Perola, M.; Pussinen, P.J.; Allonen, J.; Parkkonen, O.; Sinisalo, J. Cohort Profile: The Corogene study. *Int. J. Epidemiol.* **2012**, *41*, 1265–1271. [CrossRef] [PubMed]
26. Buhlin, K.; Mäntylä, P.; Paju, S.; Peltola, J.S.; Nieminen, M.S.; Sinisalo, J.; Pussinen, P.J. Periodontitis is associated with angiographically verified coronary artery disease. *J. Clin. Periodontol.* **2011**, *38*, 1007–1014. [CrossRef] [PubMed]
27. Liljestrand, J.M.; Paju, S.; Buhlin, K.; Persson, G.R.; Sarna, S.; Nieminen, M.S.; Sinisalo, J.; Mäntylä, P.; Pussinen, P.J. Lipopolysaccharide, a possible molecular mediator between periodontitis and coronary artery disease. *J. Clin. Periodontol.* **2017**, *44*, 784–792. [CrossRef]
28. Mäntylä, P.; Buhlin, K.; Paju, S.; Persson, G.R.; Nieminen, M.S.; Sinisalo, J.; Pussinen, P.J. Subgingival *Aggregatibacter actinomycetemcomitans* associates with the risk of coronary artery disease. *J. Clin. Periodontol.* **2013**, *40*, 583–590. [CrossRef]
29. Socransky, S.S.; Haffajee, A.D.; Smith, C.; Martin, L.; Haffajee, J.A.; Uzel, N.G.; Goodson, J.M. Use of checkerboard DNA-DNA hybridization to study complex microbial ecosystems. *Oral. Microbiol. Immunol.* **2004**, *19*, 352–362. [CrossRef]
30. Hyvärinen, K.; Mäntylä, P.; Buhlin, K.; Paju, S.; Nieminen, M.S.; Sinisalo, J.; Pussinen, P.J. A common periodontal pathogen has an adverse association with both acute and stable coronary artery disease. *Atherosclerosis* **2012**, *223*, 478–484. [CrossRef]

31. Liljestrand, J.M.; Paju, S.; Pietiäinen, M.; Buhlin, K.; Persson, G.R.; Nieminen, M.S.; Sinisalo, J.; Mäntylä, P.; Pussinen, P.J. Immunologic burden links periodontitis to acute coronary syndrome. *Atherosclerosis* **2018**, *268*, 177–184. [CrossRef] [PubMed]
32. Pussinen, P.J.; Könönen, E.; Paju, S.; Hyvärinen, K.; Gursoy, U.K.; Huumonen, S.; Knuuttila, M.; Suominen, A.L. Periodontal pathogen carriage, rather than periodontitis, determines the serum antibody levels. *J. Clin. Periodontol.* **2011**, *38*, 405–411. [CrossRef] [PubMed]
33. Hörkkö, S.; Bird, D.A.; Miller, E.; Itabe, H.; Leitinger, N.; Subbanagounder, G.; Berliner, J.A.; Friedman, P.; Dennis, E.A.; Curtiss, L.K.; et al. Monoclonal autoantibodies specific for oxidized phospholipids or oxidized phospholipid-protein adducts inhibit macrophage uptake of oxidized low-density lipoproteins. *J. Clin. Investig.* **1999**, *103*, 117–128. [CrossRef] [PubMed]
34. Turunen, S.P.; Kummu, O.; Harila, K.; Veneskoski, M.; Soliymani, R.; Baumann, M.; Pussinen, P.J.; Hörkkö, S. Recognition of *Porphyromonas gingivalis* gingipain epitopes by natural IgM binding to malondialdehyde modified low-density lipoprotein. *PLoS ONE* **2012**, *7*, e34910. [CrossRef]
35. Wang, C.; Kankaanpää, J.; Kummu, O.; Turunen, S.P.; Akhi, R.; Bergmann, U.; Pussinen, P.; Remes, A.M.; Hörkkö, S. Characterization of a natural mouse monoclonal antibody recognizing epitopes shared by oxidized lowdensity lipoprotein and chaperonin 60 of *Aggregatibacter actinomycetemcomitans*. *Immunol. Res.* **2016**, *64*, 699–710. [CrossRef] [PubMed]
36. Karvonen, J.; Päivänsalo, M.; Kesäniemi, Y.A.; Hörkkö, S. Immunoglobulin M type of autoantibodies to oxidized low-density lipoprotein has an inverse relation to carotid artery atherosclerosis. *Circulation* **2003**, *108*, 2107–2112. [CrossRef]
37. Akhi, R.; Wang, C.; Nissinen, A.E.; Kankaanpää, J.; Bloigu, R.; Paju, S.; Mäntylä, P.; Buhlin, K.; Sinisalo, J.; Pussinen, P.J.; et al. Salivary IgA to MAA-LDL and Oral Pathogens Are Linked to Coronary Disease. *J. Dent. Res.* **2019**, *98*, 296–303. [CrossRef]
38. Gao, X.; Jiang, S.; Koh, D.; Hsu, C.Y. Salivary biomarkers for dental caries. *Periodontology* **2000**, *70*, 128–141. [CrossRef]
39. Brandtzaeg, P. Secretory immunity with special reference to the oral cavity. *J. Oral. Microbiol.* **2013**, *5*, 20401. [CrossRef]
40. Marton, I.J.; Kiss, C. Protective and destructive immune reactions in apical periodontitis. *Oral. Microbiol. Immunol.* **2000**, *15*, 139–150. [CrossRef]
41. Matsuo, T.; Nakanishi, T.; Ebisu, S. Immunoglobulins in periapical exudates of infected root canals: Correlation with the clinical findings of the involved teeth. *Endod. Dent. Traumatol.* **1995**, *11*, 95–99. [CrossRef]
42. Gomes, B.P.; Jacinto, R.C.; Pinheiro, E.T.; Sousa, E.L.; Zaia, A.A.; Ferraz, C.C.; Souza-Filho, F.J. *Porphyromonas gingivalis, Porphyromonas endodontalis, Prevotella intermedia* and *Prevotella nigrescens* in endodontic lesions detected by culture and by PCR. *Oral. Microbiol. Immunol.* **2005**, *20*, 211–215. [CrossRef] [PubMed]
43. Tomazinho, L.F.; Avila-Campos, M.J. Detection of *Porphyromonas gingivalis*, *Porphyromonas endodontalis*, *Prevotella intermedia*, and *Prevotella nigrescens* in chronic endodontic infection. *Oral Surg. Oral Med. Oral Pathol. Oral Radiol. Endod.* **2007**, *103*, 285–288. [CrossRef] [PubMed]
44. Martinho, F.C.; Chiesa, W.M.; Leite, F.R.; Cirelli, J.A.; Gomes, B.P. Antigenic activity of bacterial endodontic contents from primary root canal infection with periapical lesions against macrophage in the release of interleukin-1beta and tumor necrosis factor alpha. *J. Endod.* **2010**, *36*, 1467–1474. [CrossRef]
45. Solomon, C.; Chalfin, H.; Kellert, M.; Weseley, P. The endodontic-periodontal lesion: A rational approach to treatment. *J. Am. Dent. Assoc.* **1995**, *126*, 473–479. [CrossRef] [PubMed]
46. Potempa, J.; Pike, R.; Travis, J. Titration and mapping of the active site of cysteine proteinases from *Porphyromonas gingivalis* (gingipains) using peptidyl chloromethanes. *Biol. Chem.* **1997**, *378*, 223–230. [CrossRef]
47. Ford, P.J.; Gemmell, E.; Hamlet, S.M.; Hasan, A.; Walker, P.J.; West, M.J.; Cullinan, M.P.; Seymour, G.J. Cross-reactivity of GroEL antibodies with human heat shock protein 60 and quantification of pathogens in atherosclerosis. *Oral. Microbiol. Immunol.* **2005**, *20*, 296–302. [CrossRef]
48. Montebugnoli, L.; Servidio, D.; Miaton, R.A.; Prati, C.; Tricoci, P.; Melloni, C.; Melandri, G. Periodontal health improves systemic inflammatory and haemostatic status in subjects with coronary heart disease. *J. Clin. Periodontol.* **2005**, *32*, 188–192. [CrossRef]
49. Monteiro, A.M.; Jardini, M.A.; Alves, S.; Giampaoli, V.; Aubin, E.C.; Figueiredo Neto, A.M.; Gidlund, M. Cardiovascular disease parameters in periodontitis. *J. Periodontol.* **2009**, *80*, 378–388. [CrossRef]

50. Buhlin, K.; Holmer, J.; Gustafsson, A.; Hörkkö, S.; Pockley, A.G.; Johansson, A.; Paju, S.; Klinge, B.; Pussinen, P.J. Association of periodontitis with persistent, pro-atherogenic antibody responses. *J. Clin. Periodontol.* **2015**, *42*, 1006–1014. [CrossRef]
51. Russell, M.W.; Hajishengallis, G.; Childers, N.K.; Michalek, S.M. Secretory Immunity in Defense against Cariogenic Mutans Streptococci. *Caries Res.* **1999**, *33*, 4–15. [CrossRef] [PubMed]
52. Mattila, K.J.; Nieminen, M.S.; Valtonen, V.V.; Rasi, V.P.; Kesäniemi, Y.A.; Syrjälä, S.L.; Jungell, P.S.; Isoluoma, M.; Hietaniemi, K.; Jokinen, M.J. Association between dental health and acute myocardial infarction. *BMJ* **1989**, *298*, 779–781. [CrossRef] [PubMed]
53. Cotti, E.; Dessi, C.; Piras, A.; Flore, G.; Deidda, M.; Madeddu, C.; Zedda, A.; Longu, G.; Mercuro, G. Association of endodontic infection with detection of an initial lesion to the cardiovascular system. *J. Endod.* **2011**, *37*, 1624–1629. [CrossRef] [PubMed]
54. Petersen, J.; Glaßl, E.M.; Nasseri, P.; Crismani, A.; Luger, A.K.; Schoenherr, E.; Bertl, K.; Glodny, B. The association of chronic apical periodontitis and endodontic therapy with atherosclerosis. *Clin. Oral Investig.* **2014**, *18*, 1813–1823. [CrossRef] [PubMed]
55. Pasqualini, D.; Bergandi, L.; Palumbo, L.; Borraccino, A.; Dambra, V.; Alovisi, M.; Migliaretti, G.; Ferraro, G.; Ghigo, D.; Bergerone, S.; et al. Association among oral health, apical periodontitis, CD14 polymorphisms, and coronary heart disease in middle-aged adults. *J. Endod.* **2012**, *38*, 1570–1577. [CrossRef] [PubMed]
56. Aminoshariae, A.; Kulild, J.C.; Fouad, A.F. The Impact of Endodontic Infections on the Pathogenesis of Cardiovascular Disease(s): A Systematic Review with Meta-analysis Using GRADE. *J. Endod.* **2018**, *44*, 1361–1366.e3. [CrossRef] [PubMed]
57. Pussinen, P.J.; Jousilahti, P.; Alfthan, G.; Palosuo, T.; Asikainen, S.; Salomaa, V. Antibodies to periodontal pathogens are associated with coronary heart disease. *Arterioscler. Thromb. Vasc. Biol.* **2003**, *23*, 1250–1254. [CrossRef]
58. Pussinen, P.J.; Alfthan, G.; Rissanen, H.; Reunanen, A.; Asikainen, S.; Knekt, P. Antibodies to periodontal pathogens and stroke risk. *Stroke* **2004**, *35*, 2020–2023. [CrossRef]
59. Pussinen, P.J.; Nyyssönen, K.; Alfthan, G.; Salonen, R.; Laukkanen, J.A.; Salonen, J.T. Serum antibody levels to *Actinobacillus actinomycetemcomitans* predict the risk for coronary heart disease. *Arterioscler. Thromb. Vasc. Biol.* **2005**, *25*, 833–838. [CrossRef]
60. Beck, J.D.; Eke, P.; Heiss, G.; Madianos, P.; Couper, D.; Lin, D.; Moss, K.; Elter, J.; Offenbacher, S. Periodontal disease and coronary heart disease: A reappraisal of the exposure. *Circulation* **2005**, *112*, 19–24. [CrossRef]

8

Effect of Periodontal Disease on Diabetic Retinopathy in Type 2 Diabetic Patients

Yuko Yamamoto [1], Toshiya Morozumi [2,*], Takahisa Hirata [2], Toru Takahashi [3], Shinya Fuchida [4], Masami Toyoda [5], Shigeru Nakajima [5] and Masato Minabe [2]

1 Department of Dental Hygiene, Kanagawa Dental University, Junior College, 82 Inaoka, Yokosuka 2388580, Kanagawa, Japan; yamamoto.yuko@kdu.ac.jp
2 Division of Periodontology, Department of Oral Interdisciplinary Medicine, Graduate School of Dentistry, Kanagawa Dental University, 82 Inaoka, Yokosuka 2388580, Kanagawa, Japan; t.hirata@kdu.ac.jp (T.H.); minabe@kdu.ac.jp (M.M.)
3 Department of Health and Nutrition, Faculty of Human Health, Kanazawa Gakuin University, 10 Sue-machi, Kanazawa 9201392, Ishikawa, Japan; t-takahasi@kanazawa-gu.ac.jp
4 Department of Disaster Medicine and Dental Sociology, Graduate School of Dentistry, Kanagawa Dental University, 82 Inaoka, Yokosuka 2388580, Kanagawa, Japan; fuchida@kdu.ac.jp
5 Nakajima Internal Medicine Clinic, 1-17 Yonegahamadori, Yokosuka 2380011, Kanagawa, Japan; toyoda@nakajima-naika.com (M.T.); nakajima@nakajima-naika.com (S.N.)
* Correspondence: morozumi@kdu.ac.jp

Abstract: Both periodontal disease and diabetes are common chronic inflammatory diseases. One of the major problems with type 2 diabetes is that unregulated blood glucose levels damage the vascular endothelium and cause complications. A bidirectional relationship between periodontal disease and diabetic complications has been reported previously. However, whether periodontal disease affects the presence of diabetic complications has not been clarified. Therefore, we examined the effect of the periodontal disease status on diabetic complications in patients with type 2 diabetes. Periodontal doctors examined the periodontal disease status of 104 type 2 diabetic patients who visited a private diabetes medical clinic once a month between 2016 and 2018. The subject's diabetic status was obtained from their medical records. Bayesian network analysis showed that bleeding on probing directly influenced the presence of diabetic retinopathy in type 2 diabetes patients. In addition, bleeding on probing was higher in the diabetic retinopathy group (n = 36) than in the group without diabetic retinopathy (n = 68, p = 0.006, Welch's t-test). Bleeding on probing represents gingival inflammation, which might affect the presence of diabetic retinopathy in type 2 diabetes patients who regularly visit diabetic clinics.

Keywords: periodontal disease; diabetes; diabetic retinopathy; bleeding on probing; probing pocket depth; fasting blood sugar

1. Introduction

Both periodontal disease and type 2 diabetes are known to be common chronic inflammatory diseases [1,2]. In addition, many studies have reported a bidirectional relationship between periodontal disease and type 2 diabetes [3–5]. Epidemiological studies show that diabetics with poor glycemic control have an increased risk of periodontal disease [6]. On the other hand, it has been reported that severe periodontitis adversely affects glycemic control in type 2 diabetic patients [7]. It has become clear that the treatment of periodontal disease and type 2 diabetes has an effect on the pathophysiology of both diseases. Further, it has been reported that hemoglobin A1c (HbA1c) levels are reduced when type 2 diabetic patients are treated for periodontal disease [8–10]. Additionally, it was reported that when blood glucose was controlled in type 2 diabetic patients, the bleeding on probing (BOP) value, which represents the inflammation state of periodontal disease, improved [11]. Both periodontal disease and type 2 diabetes have a high prevalence worldwide [12]; however, the mechanism underlying the bidirectional relationship between them remains unclear.

Type 2 diabetes is a disorder of dysregulated blood glucose homeostasis due to a decrease in insulin action [13]. One of the major problems with type 2 diabetes is that unregulated blood glucose levels damage the vascular endothelium and cause complications in diabetics [14]. Diabetes complications include cardiovascular disease, diabetic nephropathy, neuropathy, leg amputation, and diabetic retinopathy [15]. Diabetic retinopathy is one of the most common diabetic complications and, as it progresses, can cause blindness and poor quality of life [16]. Although diabetic retinopathy is a major cause of blindness in the working population, only 35–55% of patients with diabetes undergo regular ophthalmic evaluations. This is because the disease progresses gradually and the patient barely notices the progression of diabetic retinopathy [16]. Therefore, it is important to prevent the development of diabetic retinopathy in diabetic patients.

It has recently been shown that there is a correlation between the severity of periodontal disease and diabetic retinopathy and that many diabetic retinopathy patients have periodontal disease [17,18]. However, it remains unclear as to whether periodontal disease affects the presence of diabetic retinopathy. Commisso et al. reported that poor oral health care was observed in the diabetic population [19]. It is known that effective oral health behaviors, such as brushing teeth two or more times a day, improve the condition of periodontal disease [20]. However, the relationship between the toothbrushing habits of type 2 diabetic patients and the pathological condition of diabetes has not been fully clarified. Therefore, the purpose of this study was to clarify the effect of periodontal disease status on diabetic complications, including diabetic retinopathy, in type 2 diabetic patients who visit our hospital once a month for diabetes management. Furthermore, this study also aimed to examine the relationship between tooth brushing habits and the pathophysiology of diabetes in patients with type 2 diabetes.

2. Methods

2.1. Study Population

We recruited 104 (45 men and 59 women) diabetic patients who visited a private diabetes medical clinic in Yokosuka City (Nakajima Internal Medicine Clinic) every month between October 2016 and August 2018. Patients with type 1 diabetes, toothless patients, patients who did not visit the diabetic department monthly, and those who did not consent to the study were excluded. The protocol of the present study was approved by the Ethics Committee of Kanagawa Dental University in 2016 (approval number: 359) and was conducted in accordance with the Helsinki Declaration of 1975, as revised in 2013. The study was registered with the Clinical Trial Registry of the University Hospital Medical Information Network Clinical Trials Registry (ID: UMIN000024627). On implementation, all participants were given written and verbal explanations regarding the purposes and methods of the study, any potential risks, potential benefits, protection of personal information, and freedom of consent and withdrawal. Subsequently, all participants signed the informed consent form.

2.2. Medical Examination

Data regarding age, height, weight, duration of diabetes, presence of diabetic retinopathy, and the presence of diabetic nephropathy were collected from the subject's medical records. For each subject, the diagnosis of diabetic retinopathy was made by an ophthalmologist based on the Davis classification as follows: no diabetic retinopathy (NDR); simple diabetic retinopathy (SDR); pre-proliferative diabetic retinopathy (pre-PDR); and proliferative diabetic retinopathy (PDR) [21]. Peripheral blood samples were collected by a nurse who specializes in diabetes during the routine monthly medical consultations. HbA1c levels were measured by an HbA1c analyzer (ADAMS™ A1c HA-8180, ARKRAY Inc., Kyoto, Japan), and fasting blood sugar (FBS) levels were measured by a glucose analyzer (Glutest mint, SANWA KAGAKU KENKYUSHO Co., LTD., Aichi, Japan). The remaining peripheral blood was used to measure creatinine and triglyceride levels in a clinical laboratory (SRL, Inc., Tokyo, Japan).

2.3. Periodontal Examination

The periodontal disease status test was performed at the diabetic medical clinic on the day of the subject's visit by three trained periodontists. The probing pocket depth (PPD) and BOP were recorded with a manual probe (No.9550, YDM Corporation, Tokyo, Japan) at four points (mesial-buccal, mid-buccal, distal-buccal, and mid-lingual) for all teeth. Measurements of PPD and BOP were performed by three periodontists and then calibrated by a periodontist with the longest clinical experience (M.M.). Tooth mobility was measured for each tooth in the oral cavity. The Miller tooth mobility scale (0 degree, 1 degree, 2 degree, and 3 degree) was used to classify the degree of tooth mobility [22]. The presence of dental plaque on the surface adjacent to each tooth was determined by scratching the adjacent surface on the gingival margin with an explorer. Adherence of dental plaque to the adjacent surface even at one place led to the plaque adhesion on a surface that is adjacent to the tooth to be judged as "Yes". The number of times patients brushed their teeth per day and whether they underwent regular dental check-ups were confirmed by a questionnaire that was completed by the subjects.

2.4. Bayesian Network

A Bayesian network is a directed acyclic graph that is composed of a set of variables $\{X_1, X_2, \ldots, X_N\}$ and a set of directed edges between the variables [23]. Bayesian networks are very successful in probabilistic knowledge representation and reasoning. In Bayesian networks, the joint probability distribution function of all nodes can be calculated as follows:

$$P(X_1, X_2, \ldots, X_N) = \prod_{i=1}^{N} P(Xi \mid Pai) \quad (1)$$

where *Pai* is the set of random variables whose corresponding nodes are parent nodes of *Xi*.

A Bayesian network contains two elements: structure and parameters. Each arc begins at a parent node and ends at a child node. *Pa* (X) represents the parent nodes of node X. X_1 is the root node because it has no input arcs. Root nodes have prior probabilities. Each child node has conditional probabilities based on the combination of states of its parent nodes.

Although this study was a cross-sectional study, it was analyzed by a Bayesian network with reference to previous studies by Tsuruta et al. [24].

2.5. Statistical Analysis

All statistical analyses were performed using JMP version 12 (SAS Institute Japan, Tokyo, Japan) and R version 3.2.0 (The R Project for Statistical Computing, Vienna, Austria, 2013). Results are expressed as the mean and the standard error of the mean (SEM). Comparisons between the two groups were analyzed using Welch's *t*-test. Spearman's rank correlation was employed to analyze the statistical significance of the correlation between two variables. Causal effects between variables were calculated using Bayesian network analysis. *p*-Values less than 0.05 were considered statistically significant.

3. Results

3.1. Subject Characteristics

The characteristics of the subjects included in this study are shown in Table 1. The mean age of the subjects was 70.0 ± 1.22 years (range: 23–86 years). In terms of dental characteristics, the mean number of teeth was 21.4 ± 0.735, and the number of teeth tended to decrease with age. The average BOP was 27.3%, and 13.2% of subjects had an average ratio of a PPD of 4 mm or greater, with most subjects having periodontal disease. Thirty-eight subjects underwent supportive periodontal therapy at the dental clinic, and 66 did not. In terms of medical characteristics, the average duration of diabetes was 13.6 ± 1.02 years. The mean HbA1c was 7.15%, the mean FBS was 147 mg/dL, and the mean serum creatinine concentration was 1.08 mg/dL. In addition, 36 subjects had diabetic retinopathy, 30 had SDR, 4 had pre-PDR, and 2 had PDR. Twelve subjects had diabetic nephropathy and two subjects had diabetic neuropathy. Most of the subjects in this study had a history of diabetes for more than 10 years, and some had diabetic complications.

Table 1. Characteristics of the subjects in this study.

Total number	n = 104
Sex (n): Female/male	59/45
Age (year): Mean ± SEM	70.0 ± 1.22
Age (year): Minimum/maximum	23/86
Number of teeth: Mean ± SEM	21.4 ± 0.735
BOP (%)	27.3 ± 1.74
Ratio of PPD, 4 mm or greater (%)	13.2 ± 1.61
Percentage of teeth with more than 1 degree of movement (%)	9.90 ± 1.74
Plaque adhesion on a surface that is adjacent to the tooth (n): Yes/no	69/35
Brushing the teeth 2 or more times a day: Yes/no	65/39
SPT in the dental clinic: Yes/no	38/66
Duration of diabetes (years): Mean ± SEM	13.6 ± 1.02
BMI (%): Mean ± SEM	29.4 ± 0.467
FBS (mg/dL): Mean ± SEM	147 ± 4.95
HbA1c (%): Mean ± SEM	7.15 ± 0.0948
Serum creatinine (mg/dL)	1.08 ± 0.178
Diabetic nephropathy: Yes/no	12/92
Diabetic retinopathy: Yes/no	36/68
Diabetic retinopathy: PDR/total number	30/36
Diabetic retinopathy: pre-PDR/total number	4/36
Diabetic retinopathy: PDR/total number	2/36
Diabetic neuropathy: Yes/no	2/102
Serum LDL cholesterol (mg/dL): Mean ± SEM	113 ± 3.09
Serum HDL cholesterol (mg/dL): Mean ± SEM	57.3 ± 1.48
Serum triglyceride (mg/dL): Mean ± SEM	161 ± 1.48

BOP, Bleeding on probing; PPD, probing pocket depth; SPT, supportive periodontal therapy; BMI, body mass index; FBS, fasting blood sugar; HbA1c, hemoglobin A1c; NDR, no diabetic retinopathy; SDR, simple diabetic retinopathy; PDR, proliferative diabetic retinopathy; LDL, low-density lipoprotein; HDL, high-density lipoprotein; SEM, standard error of the mean.

3.2. Hemoglobin A1c in Type 2 Diabetic Patients with Adjacent Dental Plaque Attached to the Tooth Surface

The subjects were divided into a group with dental plaque attached to the adjacent tooth surface (n = 69) and a group without adjacent dental plaque attachment (n = 35). HbA1c was higher in the group with dental plaque attachment compared to the group without ($p < 0.05$, Welch's t-test, Table 2). No other differences were found between the two groups (Welch's t-test, Table 2).

Table 2. Characteristics of the groups with and without adjacent dental plaque attachment.

Variable	Adjacent Dental Plaque Attachment ($n = 69$)	No Adjacent Dental Plaque Attachment ($n = 35$)	p-Value *
Duration of diabetes (years)	14.3 ± 8.44	12.3 ± 13.4	0.4
BMI (%)	29.5 ± 4.69	29.1 ± 4.97	0.7
FBS (mg/dL)	154 ± 49.1	134 ± 51.2	0.06
HbA1c (%)	7.27 ± 1.01	6.90 ± 0.835	<0.05
Creatinine (mg/dL)	1.25 ± 2.21	0.735 ± 0.190	0.06
LDL cholesterol (mg/dL)	112 ± 32.5	113 ± 29.7	0.9
HDL cholesterol (mg/dL)	55.6 ± 14.1	60.5 ± 11.6	0.1
Triglyceride (mg/dL)	164 ± 88.4	156 ± 112	0.8

Data are presented as the mean ± standard error of the mean. BMI, body mass index; FBS, fasting blood sugar; HbA1c, hemoglobin A1c; Creatinine, serum creatinine; LDL, low-density lipoprotein; HDL, high-density lipoprotein; Triglyceride: serum triglyceride. * Welch's t-test. p-values < 0.05 are considered statistically significant.

3.3. Fasting Blood Sugar of Type 2 Diabetic Patients Who Brushed Their Teeth more than Twice a Day

The subjects were divided into two groups: those who brushed their teeth less than once per day ($n = 39$) and those who brushed their teeth two or more times per day ($n = 65$). The FBS in the group who brushed their teeth more than twice per day was lower than that in the group who brushed once a day or less ($p < 0.0001$, Welch's t-test, Table 3). No other differences were found between the two groups (Welch's t-test, Table 3).

Table 3. Characteristics of the groups who brushed their teeth <1 and ≥2 times per day.

Variable	Group Who Brushed Their Teeth ≥ 2 Times per Day ($n = 65$)	Group Who Brushed Their Teeth < 1 Time per Day ($n = 39$)	p-Value *
Duration of diabetes (years)	12.7 ± 10.7	15.1 ± 9.70	0.2
BMI (%)	28.9 ± 4.66	30.3 ± 4.88	0.2
FBS (mg/dL)	128 ± 31.4	179 ± 60.0	<0.0001
HbA1c (%)	7.00 ± 0.906	7.39 ± 1.03	0.05
Creatinine (mg/dL)	0.945 ± 1.56	1.31 ± 2.17	0.4
LDL cholesterol (mg/dL)	115 ± 32.0	108 ± 30.4	0.3
HDL cholesterol (mg/dL)	59.1 ± 13.8	54.2 ± 16.8	0.1
Triglyceride (mg/dL)	153 ± 93.2	173 ± 102	0.3

Data are presented as the mean ± standard error of the mean. BMI, body mass index; FBS, fasting blood sugar; HbA1c, hemoglobin A1c; Creatinine, serum creatinine; LDL, low-density lipoprotein; HDL, high-density lipoprotein; Triglyceride, serum triglyceride. * Welch's t-test. p-values < 0.05 are considered statistically significant.

3.4. Bleeding on Probing in Type 2 Diabetic Patients with Diabetic Retinopathy (1)

The subjects were divided into the diabetic retinopathy group ($n = 36$) and the non-diabetic retinopathy group ($n = 68$). The BOP was higher in the group with diabetic retinopathy than in the group without diabetic retinopathy ($p = 0.006$, Welch's t-test, Table 4). No other differences were found between the two groups (Welch's t-test, Table 4).

Table 4. Characteristics of the groups with and without diabetic retinopathy.

Variable	Diabetic Retinopathy ($n = 36$)	No Diabetic Retinopathy ($n = 68$)	p-Value *
Number of teeth	20.7 ± 8.50	21.7 ± 6.94	0.5
BOP (%)	34.1 ± 18.1	23.7 ± 16.6	0.006
Ratio of PPD, 4 mm or greater (%)	17.2 ± 19.0	11.1 ± 14.6	0.09
Proportion of teeth with more than 1 degree of movement (%)	12.0 ± 24.6	8.76 ± 12.7	0.5
Number of times the subjects brushed their teeth per day	1.53 ± 0.774	1.78 ± 0.666	0.1

Data are presented as the mean ± standard error of the mean. BOP, bleeding on probing; PPD, probing pocket depth. * Welch's t-test. p-values < 0.05 are considered statistically significant.

3.5. *Bleeding on Probing in Type 2 Diabetic Patients with Diabetic Retinopathy (2)*

Using Spearman's rank correlation, we found that the FBS positively correlated with the ratio of PPD of 4 mm or greater ($r_S = 0.29$, $p = 0.003$, $n = 104$) and BOP ($r_S = 0.21$, $p = 0.04$, $n = 104$) (Table 2). In contrast, FBS was not correlated with the percentage of teeth with more than 1 degree of movement ($r_S = -0.041$, $p = 0.7$, $n = 104$, Table 5) or the number of teeth ($r_S = 0.034$, $p = 0.7$, $n = 104$, Table 5).

Table 5. Correlations among fasting blood sugar, the PPD ratio (4 mm or greater), and BOP.

Variable	Fasting Blood Sugar (mg/dL)		
	r_S *	*p*-Value	*n*
Ratio of PPD 4 mm or greater (%)	0.29	0.0029	104
BOP (%)	0.21	0.037	104
Proportion of teeth with more than 1 degree of movement (%)	−0.041	0.68	104
Number of teeth	0.034	0.73	104

PPD, Probing pocket depth; BOP, bleeding on probing. * Spearman's rank correlation coefficient. *p*-values < 0.05 are considered statistically significant.

3.6. *Determination of Causal Effects Using Bayesian Network Analysis*

Bayesian network analysis showed that the presence of diabetic retinopathy was directly affected by BOP. In addition, the number of times patients brushed their teeth per day was directly affected by HbA1c and FBS.

4. Discussion

4.1. *Effect of Bleeding on Probing on Diabetic Retinopathy*

In this study, the subjects with diabetic retinopathy had a higher BOP compared to those without diabetic retinopathy (Table 4). Furthermore, the Bayesian network analysis showed that the presence of diabetic retinopathy was directly affected by the BOP (Figure 1). The BOP indicates the gingival inflammatory conditions caused by periodontal disease [25]. Accordingly, these results indicate that gingival inflammation in diabetic patients might have affected the development of diabetic retinopathy.

The involvement of reactive oxygen species (ROS) is considered to be a factor in which inflammation of the gingiva affected diabetic retinopathy [26–33]. *Porphyromonas gingivalis* (*P. gingivalis*) and *Fusobacterium nucleatum* (*F. nucleatum*) are the major periodontal bacteria that cause gingival inflammation [26,27]. It has been reported that diabetic model rats infected with *P. gingivalis* have increased maxillofacial oxidative stress and decreased gingival microvascular reactivity [28]. Tothova et al. reported that gingival inflammation caused by periodontitis leads to the production of ROS by neutrophils [29]. Furthermore, ROS production by neutrophils against *F. nucleatum* has been shown to be higher than that of *P. gingivalis* [30]. Overproduced ROS in the oral cavity can cause oxidative stress and oxidative damage to cells, proteins, and lipids throughout the body, which can lead to systemic disease [31]. Oxidative stress has been shown to reduce neuroretinal function [32]. In addition, oxidative stress has been found to be associated with the accelerated onset of diabetic retinopathy [33]. Therefore, ROS produced during inflammation of the gingiva in type 2 diabetic patients might induce oxidative stress and contribute to the development of diabetic retinopathy. Suppressing the production of ROS by treating periodontal disease might reduce the development of diabetic retinopathy in diabetic patients.

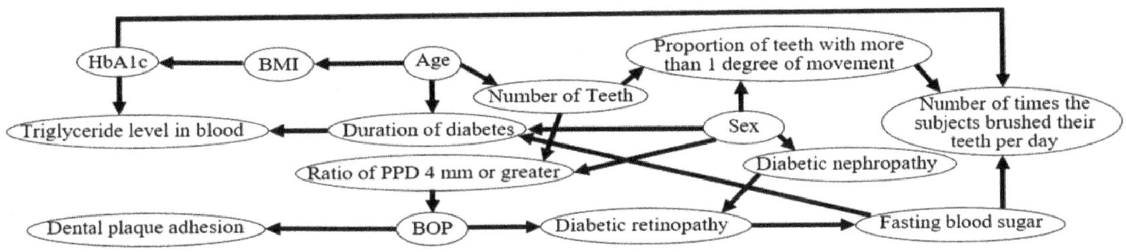

Figure 1. Bayesian network showing the causal effects among the following parameters: gender, age, number of teeth, bleeding on probing (BOP), ratio of probing pocket depth (PPD) of 4 mm or greater, proportion of teeth with more than 1 degree of movement, dental plaque adhesion, number of times the patients brushed their teeth per day, duration of diabetes, body mass index (BMI), fasting blood sugar, hemoglobin A1c (HbA1c), presence of diabetic retinopathy, presence of diabetic nephropathy, and triglyceride level in the blood. Causes and effects are indicated by arrowheads and lines, respectively.

Interleukin-17 (IL-17), which is secreted by IL-17-producing cells (T helper-17 cell: Th-17), causes inflammation and is involved in the development of chronic diseases such as autoimmune diseases [34]. IL-17 and Th-17 cells are present in human periodontal disease lesions and cause gingival inflammation [35]. Patients with a high BOP ratio have been found to have higher IL-17A concentrations in the saliva and gingival crevicular fluid compared with those without periodontal disease [36]. Furthermore, patients with periodontal disease have been found to have more Th-17 cells that produce IL-17 in the serum compared to healthy individuals [37]; in addition, the serum IL-17 concentration decreased due to a decrease in the BOP ratio in periodontal patients [38]. IL-17A has been reported to exacerbate diabetic retinopathy by impairing the function of Muller cells, which are the major glial cells in the retina [39]. Furthermore, IL-17A receptors have been found to be expressed in Muller glial cells, retinal endothelial cells, and photoreceptors [40]. Increased production of IL-17A in the periodontal lesions of patients with type 2 diabetes might have affected the development of diabetic retinopathy via the IL-17A receptor in the retina. Therefore, suppression of gingival inflammation with proper periodontal treatment might reduce IL-17 production in the gingiva and reduce the development of diabetic retinopathy in diabetic patients.

4.2. Relationship between Glycemic Control and Oral Hygiene Behavior

The Bayesian network analysis showed that the number of times patients brushed their teeth per day was directly affected by the HbA1c and FBS (Figure 1). In addition, HbA1c was higher in the group with dental plaque on the adjacent surfaces of the teeth compared to the group without adjacent dental plaque (Table 2). The FBS in subjects who brushed more than twice a day was lower than that of the subjects who brushed once a day or less (Table 3). It is well known that the amount of plaque on the tooth surface increases when the number of times toothbrushing is performed decreases [41]. Furthermore, HbA1c tended to be lower in the group who brushed more than twice a day than in the group who brushed once a day or less ($p = 0.05$, Table 3). From these findings, it is inferred that not only do FBS and HbA1c directly affect the number of times that diabetic patients brush their teeth per day, but also that oral hygiene habits and oral hygiene in diabetic patients are related to glycemic control.

Health literacy is the ability of an individual to obtain, understand, evaluate, and use health information to make decisions regarding the treatment of illnesses and overall health, and to maintain and improve the quality of life [42]. Sense of coherence (SOC) is a personality trait that allows individuals to adapt to and cope with stress to promote their health [43]. Recently, it has been reported that health literacy and SOC influence the pathophysiology of chronic diseases [42,44]. Patients with type 2 diabetes who have poor glycemic control have been shown to have poor health literacy [45]. Since SOC is indirectly involved in the glycemic control of patients with type 2 diabetes, it is necessary to increase SOC to improve glycemic control in such patients [46,47]. In addition, it has been reported that health literacy and SOC also affect oral hygiene behavior. Those who brush their teeth more than twice a day had a higher health literacy [48,49]. It has been reported that subjects who brush their teeth more than twice a day had higher SOC scores [49]. Inferring from these reports, the diabetic patients in this study with a higher health literacy and SOC would have been aware of not only blood glucose control, but also oral health improvement and behavior. Moreover, the ability to maintain and promote the health of diabetics would have been associated with glycemic control and oral hygiene habits. As a result, FBS and HbA1c would have had an effect on the number of times toothbrushing was performed per day, even in the Bayesian network analysis (Figure 1). Patients with type 2 diabetes who brush their teeth less often (per day) and have a large amount of plaque in the oral cavity might have poor glycemic control. Therefore, dentists and dental hygienists need to educate type 2 diabetics who are not interested in oral health in order to improve their health literacy and SOC, which might improve glycemic control in type 2 diabetics.

4.3. Relationship Between Periodontal Inflammation and Fasting Blood Sugar

In this study, there was a correlation between FBS and the ratio of both PPD of 4 mm or greater and BOP (Table 5). Similar to BOP, a PPD of 4 mm or greater indicates inflammation of the periodontal tissue [50]. Therefore, this relationship between periodontal inflammation and FBS in patients with type 2 diabetes was expected. There are many reports regarding the relationship between periodontal disease and FBS. Bleeding on probing (BOP) and PPD of 4 mm or greater were associated with fasting blood glucose [51]. For example, Joshipura et al. reported that the FBS of diabetic patients was reduced due to reduced periodontal pockets and improved BOP [52]. Further, Choi et al. reported that the FBS increased as the PPD increased [53]. Periodontal disease increases insulin resistance and raises blood sugar in diabetic patients [54]. Moreover, Colombo et al. reported that periodontal disease model rats had elevated plasma concentrations of tumor necrosis factor-α and increased insulin resistance [55]. The subjects in the present study might have also had high FBS levels due to periodontal inflammation causing insulin resistance. Treatment and education to reduce periodontal inflammation in dental clinics would help to control blood glucose levels in patients with type 2 diabetes.

4.4. Considerations

To the best of our knowledge, this study is the first to clarify the effect of periodontal disease on diabetic retinopathy in type 2 diabetic patients, as assessed by the diabetes department. However, this study has some limitations. First, we could not determine the smoking history of subjects because this was not described in the diabetes medical charts of the subjects. Second, we were unable to obtain data on the subjects' insulin injection status and medication status. As such, future studies will need to consider the association between these data and the effect of periodontal disease on diabetic retinopathy. Third, analysis of the Bayesian network revealed a causal relationship between multiple items. However, since the main purpose of this study was to clarify the effect of periodontal disease on diabetic complications, we considered only the causal relationship between the two diseases.

5. Conclusions

In conclusion, the BOP of subjects with diabetic retinopathy was higher than that of the subjects without diabetic retinopathy. Moreover, the gingival inflammation exhibited by BOP affected the presence of diabetic retinopathy in type 2 diabetics who regularly visit diabetic clinics. Controlling gingival inflammation by treating periodontal disease in dental clinics might suppress the development of diabetic retinopathy in patients with type 2 diabetes.

Author Contributions: T.M., Y.Y., and M.M. designed the study. T.H., Y.Y., T.M., M.M., M.T., and S.N. conducted the study. S.F. and T.T. performed the statistical analysis. Y.Y. and T.M. wrote the paper. M.M. and T.M. acquired the funding. All authors have read and agreed to the published version of the manuscript.

Acknowledgments: The authors thank the staff of the Nakajima Internal Medicine Clinic who cooperated with the data collection.

References

1. Doğan, Ş.B.; Ballı, U.; Dede, F.Ö.; Sertoğlu, E.; Tazegül, K. Chemerin as a novel crevicular fluid marker of patients with periodontitis and type 2 diabetes mellitus. *J. Periodontol.* **2016**, *87*, 923–933. [CrossRef] [PubMed]
2. Jourdain, M.L.; Velard, F.; Pierrard, L.; Sergheraert, J.; Gangloff, S.C.; Braux, J. Cationic antimicrobial peptides and periodontal physiopathology: A systematic review. *J. Periodontal Res.* **2019**, *54*, 589–600. [CrossRef] [PubMed]
3. Sanz, M.; Ceriello, A.; Buysschaert, M.; Chapple, I.; Demmer, R.T.; Graziani, F.; Herrera, D.; Jepsen, S.; Lione, L.; Madianos, P.; et al. Scientific evidence on the links between periodontal diseases and diabetes: Consensus report and guidelines of the joint workshop on periodontal diseases and diabetes by the International Diabetes Federation and the European Federation of Periodontology. *J. Clin. Periodontol.* **2018**, *45*, 138–149. [CrossRef] [PubMed]
4. Mohamed, H.G.; Idris, S.B.; Mustafa, M.; Ahmed, M.F.; Åstrøm, A.N.; Mustafa, K.; Ibrahim, S.O. Impact of chronic periodontitis on levels of glucoregulatory biomarkers in gingival crevicular fluid of adults with and without type 2 diabetes. *PLoS ONE* **2015**, *10*, e0127660. [CrossRef] [PubMed]
5. Casanova, L.; Hughes, F.J.; Preshaw, P.M. Diabetes and periodontal disease: A two-way relationship. *Br. Dent. J.* **2014**, *217*, 433–437. [CrossRef] [PubMed]
6. Mealey, B.L.; Ocampo, G.L. Diabetes mellitus and periodontal disease. *Periodontol. 2000* **2007**, *44*, 127–153. [CrossRef]
7. Taylor, G.W.; Burt, B.A.; Becker, M.P.; Genco, R.J.; Shlossman, M.; Knowler, W.C.; Pettitt, D.J. Severe periodontitis and risk for poor glycemic control in patients with non-insulin dependent diabetes mellitus. *J. Periodontol.* **1996**, *67*, 1085–1093. [CrossRef] [PubMed]
8. Madianos, P.N.; Koromantzos, P.A. An update of the evidence on the potential impact of periodontal therapy on diabetes outcomes. *J. Clin. Periodontol.* **2018**, *45*, 188–195. [CrossRef]
9. Darré, L.; Vergnes, J.N.; Gourdy, P.; Sixou, M. Efficacy of periodontal treatment on glycaemic control in diabetic patients: A meta-analysis of interventional studies. *Diabet. Metab.* **2008**, *34*, 497–506. [CrossRef]
10. Choi, S.E.; Sima, C.; Pandya, A. Impact of treating oral disease on preventing vascular diseases: A model-based cost-effectiveness analysis of periodontal treatment among patients with type 2 diabetes. *Diabet. Care* **2020**, *43*, 563–571. [CrossRef]
11. Katagiri, S.; Nitta, H.; Nagasawa, T.; Izumi, Y.; Kanazawa, M.; Matsuo, A.; Chiba, H.; Fukui, M.; Nakamura, N.; Oseko, F.; et al. Effect of glycemic control on periodontitis in type 2 diabetic patients with periodontal disease. *J. Diabet. Investig.* **2013**, *4*, 320–325. [CrossRef] [PubMed]
12. Sonnenschein, S.K.; Meyle, J. Local inflammatory reactions in patients with diabetes and periodontitis. *Periodontol. 2000* **2015**, *69*, 221–254. [CrossRef] [PubMed]
13. Merino, J.; Leong, A.; Liu, C.T.; Porneala, B.; Walford, G.A.; von Grotthuss, M.; Wang, T.J.; Flannick, J.; Dupuis, J.; Levy, D.; et al. Metabolomics insights into early type 2 diabetes pathogenesis and detection in individuals with normal fasting glucose. *Diabetologia* **2018**, *61*, 1315–1324. [CrossRef] [PubMed]
14. Forbes, J.M.; Cooper, M.E. Mechanisms of diabetic complications. *Physiol. Rev.* **2013**, *93*, 137–188. [CrossRef] [PubMed]
15. Deshpande, A.D.; Harris-Hayes, M.; Schootman, M. Epidemiology of diabetes and diabetes-related complications. *Phys. Ther.* **2008**, *88*, 1254–1264. [CrossRef]
16. Sinclair, S.H.; Schwartz, S.S. Diabetic retinopathy-an underdiagnosed and undertreated inflammatory, neuro-vascular complication of diabetes. *Front. Endocrinol. (Lausanne)* **2019**, *10*, 843. [CrossRef]
17. Veena, H.R.; Natesh, S.; Patil, S.R. Association between diabetic retinopathy and chronic periodontitis—A cross-sectional study. *Med. Sci.* **2018**, *6*, 104.
18. Song, S.J.; Lee, S.S.; Han, K.; Park, J.B. Periodontitis is associated with diabetic retinopathy in non-obese adults. *Endocrine* **2017**, *56*, 82–89. [CrossRef]
19. Commisso, L.; Monami, M.; Mannucci, E. Periodontal disease and oral hygiene habits in a type 2 diabetic population. *Int. J. Dent. Hyg.* **2011**, *9*, 68–73. [CrossRef]
20. Mizutani, S.; Ekuni, D.; Tomofuji, T.; Irie, K.; Azuma, T.; Iwasaki, Y.; Morita, M. Self-efficacy and progression of periodontal disease: A prospective cohort study. *J. Clin. Periodontol.* **2015**, *42*, 1083–1089. [CrossRef]
21. Tanaka, K.; Kawai, T.; Saisho, Y.; Meguro, S.; Harada, K.; Satoh, Y.; Kobayashi, K.; Mizushima, K.; Abe, T.; Itoh, H. Relationship between stage of diabetic retinopathy and pulse wave velocity in Japanese patients with type 2 diabetes. *J. Diabet. Res.* **2013**, *2013*, 193514. [CrossRef] [PubMed]

22. Miller, P.D. A classification of marginal tissue recession. *Int. J. Periodont. Restorat. Dent.* **1985**, *5*, 8–13.
23. Maglogiannis, I.; Zafiropoulos, E.; Platis, A.; Lambrinoudakis, C. Risk analysis of a patient monitoring system using Bayesian Network modeling. *J. Biomed. Inform.* **2006**, *39*, 637–647. [CrossRef] [PubMed]
24. Tsuruta, M.; Takahashi, T.; Tokunaga, M.; Iwasaki, M.; Kataoka, S.; Kakuta, S.; Soh, I.; Awano, S.; Hirata, H.; Kagawa, M.; et al. Relationships between pathologic subjective halitosis, olfactory reference syndrome, and social anxiety in young Japanese women. *BMC Psychol.* **2017**, *5*, 7. [CrossRef]
25. Killeen, A.C.; Harn, J.A.; Erickson, L.M.; Yu, F.; Reinhardt, R.A. Local minocycline effect on inflammation and clinical attachment during periodontal maintenance: Randomized clinical trial. *J. Periodont.* **2016**, *87*, 1149–1157. [CrossRef]
26. Huck, O.; Mulhall, H.; Rubin, G.; Kizelnik, Z.; Iyer, R.; Perpich, J.D.; Haque, N.; Cani, P.D.; de Vos, W.M.; Amar, S. Akkermansia muciniphila reduces *Porphyromonas gingivalis*-induced inflammation and periodontal bone destruction. *J. Clin. Periodont.* **2020**, *47*, 202–212. [CrossRef] [PubMed]
27. Yang, N.Y.; Zhang, Q.; Li, J.L.; Yang, S.H.; Shi, Q. Progression of periodontal inflammation in adolescents is associated with increased number of *Porphyromonas gingivalis*, *Prevotella intermedia*, *Tannerella forsythensis*, and *Fusobacterium nucleatum*. *Int. J. Paediatr. Dent.* **2014**, *24*, 226–233. [CrossRef] [PubMed]
28. Sugiyama, S.; Takahashi, S.S.; Tokutomi, F.A.; Yoshida, A.; Kobayashi, K.; Yoshino, F.; Wada-Takahashi, S.; Toyama, T.; Watanabe, K.; Hamada, N.; et al. Gingival vascular functions are altered in type 2 diabetes mellitus model and/or periodontitis model. *J. Clin. Biochem. Nutr.* **2012**, *51*, 108–113. [CrossRef]
29. Tóthová, L.; Celec, P. Oxidative stress and antioxidants in the diagnosis and therapy of periodontitis. *Front. Physiol.* **2017**, *8*, 1055. [CrossRef]
30. Wright, H.J.; Chapple, I.L.; Matthews, J.B.; Cooper, P.R. Fusobacterium nucleatum regulation of neutrophil transcription. *J. Periodont. Res.* **2011**, *46*, 1–12. [CrossRef] [PubMed]
31. Żukowski, P.; Maciejczyk, M.; Waszkiel, D. Sources of free radicals and oxidative stress in the oral cavity. *Arch. Oral Biol.* **2018**, *92*, 8–17. [CrossRef] [PubMed]
32. Suzumura, A.; Kaneko, H.; Funahashi, Y.; Takayama, K.; Nagaya, M.; Ito, S.; Okuno, T.; Hirakata, T.; Nonobe, N.; Kataoka, K.; et al. n-3 fatty acid and its metabolite 18-HEPE ameliorate retinal neuronal cell dysfunction by enhancing Müller BDNF in diabetic retinopathy. *Diabetes* **2020**, *69*, 724–735. [CrossRef] [PubMed]
33. Cecilia, O.M.; José Alberto, C.G.; José, N.P.; Ernesto Germán, C.M.; Ana Karen, L.C.; Luis Miguel, R.P.; Ricardo Raúl, R.R.; Adolfo Daniel, R.C. Oxidative stress as the main target in diabetic retinopathy pathophysiology. *J. Diabet. Res.* **2019**, *2019*, 8562408. [CrossRef] [PubMed]
34. Ren, S.; Hu, J.; Chen, Y.; Yuan, T.; Hu, H.; Li, S. Human umbilical cord derived mesenchymal stem cells promote interleukin-17 production from human peripheral blood mononuclear cells of healthy donors and systemic lupus erythematosus patients. *Clin. Exp. Immunol.* **2016**, *183*, 389–396. [CrossRef] [PubMed]
35. Cheng, W.C.; Hughes, F.J.; Taams, L.S. The presence, function and regulation of IL-17 and Th17 cells in periodontitis. *J. Clin. Periodont.* **2014**, *41*, 541–549. [CrossRef] [PubMed]
36. Apatzidou, D.A.; Iskas, A.; Konstantinidis, A.; Alghamdi, A.M.; Tumelty, M.; Lappin, D.F.; Nile, C.J. Clinical associations between acetylcholine levels and cholinesterase activity in saliva and gingival crevicular fluid and periodontal diseases. *J. Clin. Periodont.* **2018**, *45*, 1173–1183. [CrossRef]
37. Chen, X.T.; Chen, L.L.; Tan, J.Y.; Shi, D.H.; Ke, T.; Lei, L.H. Th17 and Th1 lymphocytes are correlated with chronic periodontitis. *Immunol. Investig.* **2016**, *45*, 243–254. [CrossRef]
38. Duarte, P.M.; da Rocha, M.; Sampaio, E.; Mestnik, M.J.; Feres, M.; Figueiredo, L.C.; Bastos, M.F.; Faveri, M. Serum levels of cytokines in subjects with generalized chronic and aggressive periodontitis before and after non-surgical periodontal therapy: A pilot study. *J. Periodont.* **2010**, *81*, 1056–1063. [CrossRef] [PubMed]
39. Qiu, A.W.; Liu, Q.H.; Wang, J.L. Blocking IL-17A alleviates diabetic retinopathy in rodents. *Cell Physiol. Biochem.* **2017**, *41*, 960–972. [CrossRef]
40. Sigurdardottir, S.; Zapadka, T.E.; Lindstrom, S.I.; Liu, H.; Taylor, B.E.; Lee, C.A.; Kern, T.S.; Taylor, P.R. Diabetes-mediated IL-17A enhances retinal inflammation, oxidative stress, and vascular permeability. *Cell Immunol.* **2019**, *341*, 103921. [CrossRef]
41. Kinane, D.F.; Zhang, P.; Benakanakere, M.; Singleton, J.; Biesbrock, A.; Nonnenmacher, C.; He, T. Experimental gingivitis, bacteremia and systemic biomarkers: A randomized clinical trial. *J. Periodont. Res.* **2015**, *50*, 864–869. [CrossRef] [PubMed]

42. Wang, W.; Zhang, Y.; Lin, B.; Mei, Y.; Ping, Z.; Zhang, Z. The urban-rural disparity in the status and risk factors of health literacy: A cross-sectional survey in Central China. *Int. J. Environ. Res. Public Health* **2020**, *17*, 3848. [CrossRef] [PubMed]
43. Tsiligianni, I.; Sifaki-Pistolla, D.; Gergianaki, I.; Kampouraki, M.; Papadokostakis, P.; Poulonirakis, I.; Gialamas, I.; Bempi, V.; Ierodiakonou, D. Associations of sense of coherence and self-efficacy with health status and disease severity in COPD. *NPJ Prim. Care Respir. Med.* **2020**, *30*, 27. [CrossRef] [PubMed]
44. Robat-Sarpooshi, D.; Mahdizadeh, M.; Alizadeh Siuki, H.; Haddadi, M.; Robatsarpooshi, H.; Peyman, N. The relationship between health literacy level and self-care behaviors in patients with diabetes. *Pat. Relat. Outcome Meas.* **2020**, *11*, 129–135. [CrossRef] [PubMed]
45. Saeed, H.; Saleem, Z.; Naeem, R.; Shahzadi, I.; Islam, M. Impact of health literacy on diabetes outcomes: A cross-sectional study from Lahore, Pakistan. *Public Health* **2018**, *156*, 8–14. [CrossRef] [PubMed]
46. Cohen, M.; Kanter, Y. Relation between sense of coherence and glycemic control in type 1 and type 2 diabetes. *Behav. Med.* **2004**, *29*, 175–183. [CrossRef]
47. Odajima, Y.; Sumi, N. Factors related to sense of coherence in adult patients with Type 2 diabetes. *Nagoya J. Med. Sci.* **2018**, *80*, 61–71.
48. Cepova, E.; Cicvakova, M.; Kolarcik, P.; Markovska, N.; Geckova, A.M. Associations of multidimensional health literacy with reported oral health promoting behaviour among Slovak adults: A cross-sectional study. *BMC Oral Health* **2018**, *18*, 44. [CrossRef]
49. Bernabé, E.; Kivimäki, M.; Tsakos, G.; Suominen-Taipale, A.L.; Nordblad, A.; Savolainen, J.; Uutela, A.; Sheiham, A.; Watt, R.G. The relationship among sense of coherence, socio-economic status, and oral health-related behaviours among Finnish dentate adults. *Eur. J. Oral. Sci.* **2009**, *117*, 413–418. [CrossRef]
50. Javed, F.; Al Amri, M.D.; Al-Kheraif, A.A.; Qadri, T.; Ahmed, A.; Ghanem, A.; Calvo-Guirado, J.L.; Romanos, G.E. Efficacy of non-surgical periodontal therapy with adjunct Nd:YAG laser therapy in the treatment of periodontal inflammation among patients with and without type 2 diabetes mellitus: A short-term pilot study. *J. Photochem. Photobiol. B* **2015**, *149*, 230–234. [CrossRef]
51. Jung, Y.S.; Shin, M.H.; Kweon, S.S.; Lee, Y.H.; Kim, O.J.; Kim, Y.J.; Chung, H.J.; Kim, O.S. Periodontal disease associated with blood glucose levels in urban Koreans aged 50 years and older: The Dong-gu study. *Gerodontology* **2015**, *32*, 267–273. [CrossRef] [PubMed]
52. Joshipura, K.J.; Muñoz-Torres, F.J.; Dye, B.A.; Leroux, B.G.; Ramírez-Vick, M.; Pérez, C.M. Longitudinal association between periodontitis and development of diabetes. *Diabet. Res. Clin. Pract.* **2018**, *141*, 284293. [CrossRef] [PubMed]
53. Choi, Y.H.; McKeown, R.E.; Mayer-Davis, E.J.; Liese, A.D.; Song, K.B.; Merchant, A.T. Association between periodontitis and impaired fasting glucose and diabetes. *Diabet. Care* **2011**, *34*, 381–386. [CrossRef] [PubMed]
54. Akutagawa, K.; Fujita, T.; Ouhara, K.; Takemura, T.; Tari, M.; Kajiya, M.; Matsuda, S.; Kuramitsu, S.; Mizuno, N.; Shiba, H.; et al. Glycyrrhizic acid suppresses inflammation and reduces the increased glucose levels induced by the combination of *Porphyromonas gulae* and ligature placement in diabetic model mice. *Int. Immunopharmacol.* **2019**, *68*, 30–38. [CrossRef] [PubMed]
55. Colombo, N.H.; Shirakashi, D.J.; Chiba, F.Y.; Coutinho, M.S.; Ervolino, E.; Garbin, C.A.; Machado, U.F.; Sumida, D.H. Periodontal disease decreases insulin sensitivity and insulin signaling. *J. Periodontol.* **2012**, *83*, 864–870. [CrossRef] [PubMed]

9

Importance of Virulence Factors for the Persistence of Oral Bacteria in the Inflamed Gingival Crevice and in the Pathogenesis of Periodontal Disease

Gunnar Dahlen *, Amina Basic and Johan Bylund

Department of Oral Microbiology and Immunology, Institute of Odontology, Sahlgrenska Academy, University of Gothenburg, SE-40530 Gothenburg, Sweden
* Correspondence: dahlen@odontologi.gu.se

Abstract: Periodontitis is a chronic inflammation that develops due to a destructive tissue response to prolonged inflammation and a disturbed homeostasis (dysbiosis) in the interplay between the microorganisms of the dental biofilm and the host. The infectious nature of the microbes associated with periodontitis is unclear, as is the role of specific bacterial species and virulence factors that interfere with the host defense and tissue repair. This review highlights the impact of classical virulence factors, such as exotoxins, endotoxins, fimbriae and capsule, but also aims to emphasize the often-neglected cascade of metabolic products (e.g., those generated by anaerobic and proteolytic metabolism) that are produced by the bacterial phenotypes that survive and thrive in deep, inflamed periodontal pockets. This metabolic activity of the microbes aggravates the inflammatory response from a low-grade physiologic (homeostatic) inflammation (i.e., gingivitis) into more destructive or tissue remodeling processes in periodontitis. That bacteria associated with periodontitis are linked with a number of systemic diseases of importance in clinical medicine is highlighted and exemplified with rheumatoid arthritis, The unclear significance of a number of potential "virulence factors" that contribute to the pathogenicity of specific bacterial species in the complex biofilm–host interaction clinically is discussed in this review.

Keywords: periodontal disease; host response; infection; inflammation; oral microbiota; virulence factors; metabolites

---

1. Introduction

Periodontal diseases affect the supporting tissues of teeth. The most common, gingivitis and periodontitis, are inflammatory diseases that are induced and maintained by the polymicrobial biofilm (dental plaque) that are formed on teeth in the absence of daily oral hygiene procedures. While gingivitis is a reversible inflammatory response without loss of bone support, periodontitis includes the destruction of the periodontal attachment and the alveolar bone. Peri-implantitis is the term used for a similar inflammatory reaction as periodontitis, but around dental implants, also here including the loss of bone support [1].

Periodontitis is the result of a complex interplay between microorganisms of the dental biofilm and the host. The role of specific microorganisms and their products in the disease initiation and propagation is still unclear [2,3]. The severity of the periodontal disease also depends on environmental (e.g., smoking) and host risk factors (for example genetic susceptibility) [4]. Lately, numerous studies have shown associations between periodontal disease and a number of systemic diseases, such as cardiovascular disease, diabetes mellitus, Alzheimer's disease, and rheumatoid arthritis [5]. This has intensified the research on the role of the microorganisms and their virulence factors in periodontitis. The purpose of this review is to high-light the complexity of the host-microbe relationship in periodontitis as well as the capacity of ordinary low virulent oral commensals to adapt and survive in the periodontal pocket, and to become infectious and contribute to systemic effects on the host.

2. The Role of Micro-organisms in Periodontitis—A Historical Perspective

The paradigm that dental plaque was the cause of gingivitis was established in the "gingivitis in man study" [6], where, in an experimental approach, a group of volunteers abstained from oral hygiene procedures resulting in plaque accumulation and gingivitis development. When oral hygiene procedures were reinstalled, the gingivitis was resolved within a week. The interpretation that followed was that the dental plaque induced the gingival inflammation and, if left untreated, this would inevitably lead to periodontitis [3]. Plaque was thought to cause periodontitis, and therefore plaque control became the cornerstone in the treatment of periodontal disease, and still is. Since the periodontitis distribution in the population was skewed, focus was next directed to specific bacteria, present in the dental biofilm of gingival/periodontal pockets and were more or less associated with periodontitis. Specific microorganisms, termed "putative periodontal pathogens", were hypothesized to be responsible for gingival tissue breakdown and the disease progression [7,8]. Even if Koch's postulate was found to be inadequate to apply to complex diseases like periodontitis, additional criteria for the elucidation of pathogens capable of causing periodontitis were suggested [9]. This bacteria-centered view of the disease led to the concept of an infectious nature of periodontitis, where treatment was aimed at eliminating putative pathogens e.g., with antibiotics [10].

It soon became clear that bacteria in the polymicrobial biofilm were necessary but not sufficient to explain why some individuals developed periodontitis while others did not, despite a similar composition of the subgingival microbiota. The existence of refractory cases that responded poorly to treatment and in which the disease continued to progress despite comprehensive periodontal treatment directed the focus towards the host and the inflammatory response—the disease susceptibility model [3,11,12]. This host-centered approach in search for high-risk groups and individuals discovered that diabetes patients or smokers were overrepresented among those with severe periodontitis [13,14]. The focus was on the host response and search for genetic grounds became intensive based on family pattern and twin studies of periodontitis [15,16]. The general epidemiological pattern, comprising of approximately 10–12% of the populations worldwide, irrespective of hygiene level and access to dental treatment, suffering from severe periodontitis with the risk of tooth loss [17] indicates that subgroups with genetic susceptibility for severe periodontitis exist in all populations. In a recent review it was concluded that up to one third of the variance of periodontitis is due to genetic factors [16]. The search for specific genes or gene polymorphism to explain the genetic role in periodontitis have so far been only moderately successful but the heritability of the disease is extremely complex and likely also influenced by epigenetic mechanisms [18,19].

While bacteria have a clear role in the periodontal disease aetiology, the relationship to other microorganisms, such as yeasts, is more uncertain [20]. Herpesviruses and Epstein-Barr virus, on the other hand, have been more strongly implicated in periodontitis and a link has also been suggested between periodontal herpesviruses and systemic diseases [21].

Nowadays periodontitis is described as an inflammatory disease induced and maintained by the polymicrobial biofilm formed on teeth, based on the polymicrobial synergy and dysbiosis hypothesis [22–24]. This hypothesis implies that the balance (homeostasis) between the microorganisms in the dental biofilm and the host response is disrupted due to fluctuations and burst of activity of the microorganisms or due to an imbalanced host response. This imbalanced condition in which the normal microbiome structure is disturbed is termed dysbiosis [24]. The magnitude of the inflammatory response is host related (susceptibility) and host related factors are responsible for the disease progression. The role of the classic, putative periodontal pathogens is still unclear and the infectious nature of the disease has been depreciated [23–25]. However, the enormous complexity and variability that takes place within the dental biofilm community and the similar complexity and variability in the inflammatory response is challenging. The role of the microorganisms in periodontitis is poorly understood and the many hypothesis launched are still hypotheses.

3. "Putative Periodontal Pathogens"

Aggregatibacter actinomycetemcomitans (previously *Actinobacillus actinomycetemcomitans*) was discovered to be closely related to localized forms of periodontal disease in young individuals. This discovery made it plausible that some microorganisms were more important for periodontal disease development than others and such microorganisms were termed "putative periodontal pathogens" [25,26]. Later, Socransky et al. [27] grouped three species (*Porphyromonas gingivalis, Tannerella forsythia* and *Treponema denticola*) to the so-called red complex, which was statistically strongly associated with periodontitis (Table 1). Another group including species such as *Prevotella intermedia, Fusobacterium nucleatum, Campylobacter rectus* and *Campylobacter gracilis* were associated with periodontitis to a milder degree and these were termed the orange complex [27]. Notably, most of these putative periodontopathogens are Gram-negative, strictly anaerobic species (except for *A. acinomyctemcomitans*), as well as proteolytic and thus well adapted to the inflamed periodontal pocket (Table 1). Occasional Gram-positive species, e.g., *Parvimonas micra* (formerly *Peptostreptococcus micros*) were included in the orange complex [27].

While some species, such as *A. actinomyctemcomitans* and *P. gingivalis,* are extremely well studied and described in several recent reviews, e.g., [28–30], phenotypical characterization of other bacterial species is more limited. Spirochetes are seriously underestimated, although they have been known to predominate the deep periodontal pocket from microscopic studies in the 1970s [31]. Studies using molecular biology methods have disclosed a number of unculturable *Treponema* genotypes, but their phenotypic characteristics are largely unknown [32,33].

It should also be noted that the concept of "species" is a man-made distinction and most species can be further specified into genotypic and/or phenotypic subtypes based on defined criteria. Clearly certain subtypes are more associated to oral infections than others, but unfortunately, the identification of bacterial species to a subtype level is rare in clinical oral microbiology studies. The best-known example of a specific bacterial subtype with implications for periodontal disease is the JP2 genotype of *A. actinomycetemcomitans,* which is a high virulent clone (high toxic clone) strongly associated with severe periodontal breakdown in young individuals of West African populations [34].

The list of "putative periodontal pathogens", or bacterial species associated to periodontitis, has gradually expanded and included 17 different species in a recent review [35]. Along with the use of more sensitive detection methods such as NGS (Next generation sequencing) the number periodontitis associated microorganisms have expanded further but their role in the pathogenesis of periodontitis remains elusive [36,37]. It is possible that certain microorganisms are more important for periodontal disease progression than others, but that can only be ruled out in prospective longitudinal studies over years without intervention, and very few such studies have been conducted [38].

Table 1. Important characteristics for eight "putative periodontal pathogens" as described by Socransky et al. (1998) in colored complexes (as indicated in the table by the red and orange color) associated with periodontitis. *A. actinomycetemcomitans* (serotype b) did not fit into any of the complexes and is colored grey in the table.

"Putative Periodontal Pathogens"	Gram Stain	Main Metabolic Trait	Motility	Proteolytic Activity	Carbohydrate Fermentation	Major end Products	Factors of Significance	Subtyping
Aggregatibacter actinomycetemcomitans	Gramneg	Facultative anaerobic	No	Weak	Glycolytic	Lactic acid, Succinic acid Acetic acid, Propionic acid	Leukotoxin Cytodescen-ding (Cdt) toxin	Serotypes a-e, Non-serotypable isolates are frequent Specific genotypes (JP2)
Porphyromonas gingivalis	Gramneg	Anaerobic	No	Strong	Asaccharolytic	NH_3 H_2S Phenylacetic acid Indole	Gingipains (RgpA and Kgp)	FimA genotypes: I-V Arg-specific RgpA: A-C Lys-specific Kgp: I and II Capsular subtypes: K1-K6
Tannerella forsythia	Gramneg	Anaerobic	No	Strong	Weak glycolytic	H_2S (weak) Acetic acid Propionic acid	Trypsin-like and PrtH proteases	Variations in the leucine-rich repeat BspA protein are existing but no subtyping is presented
Treponema denticola	Gramneg	Anaerobic	Strong	Strong	Weak glycolytic	H_2S (strong)	Spirochetes (spiral shaped)	Seven oral Treponema species identified but no subtyping is known Hundreds of spirochetal genotypes (OTU's) found
Prevotella intermedia/nigrescens	Gramneg	Anaerobic	No	Strong	Glycolytic	NH_3 H_2S Succinic acid Acetic	Indole	Capsule is produced but no subtyping is known
Fusobacterium nucleatum	Gramneg	Anaerobic	No	Strong	Glycolytic	NH_3 H2S (strong) Butyric acid	Fusiform Morphology (threadlike)	Three subspecies reported variation in the outer-membrane structure
Campylobacter rectus/gracilis	Gramneg	Microaerophilic	weak	Weak	Asaccharolytic	H_2S Succinic acid	Nd	not known
Parvimonas micra	Grampos	Anaerobic	No	Strong	Glycolytic	NH_3 H_2S (weak), Acetic acid	Nd	not known

4. Periodontitis—An Inflammatory Disease or an Infectious Disease?

Inflammation is a host tissue response to an assault commonly triggered by microorganisms (or other stimuli such as chemicals, radiation and trauma) and their products (metabolites, endotoxins) released from them. Clinically, inflammation often relates to some kind of pathology, but it is important to remember that inflammatory reactions are absolutely critical for our well-being and the process has evolved to provide rapid and early protection. We likely experience thousands of small clinically 'invisible' inflammatory reactions along the mucosal membranes every day as a result of various assaults involving microorganisms, without considering these inflammatory responses as infections (or even disease). These cases could not be considered pathologic and represent situations where the inflammatory response is physiologic and provide early protection from potentially dangerous events (see below).

There are many definitions of infection, most of them aimed at primary pathogens and specific infections, while it is more controversial to find a definition that fits to infections involving commensals [39]. In line with the "damage-response framework" [39], which can be applied to various oral infections, the term infection can be defined as "the process in which pathogenic organisms (ambionts) invade the tissues or organs of the body and cause injury (damage) followed by reactive phenomena" according to Dorland´s Medical Dictionary [40,41]. The critical issue here is invasion (further discussed below) and ordinary commensals are not part of any infection as long as they are colonizing (present) on the external side of the epithelial lining (barrier). That is a 'normal' condition. This means that in a state of commensalism and colonization (such as the subgingival dental plaque in health or gingivitis) a homeostatic balance between the microbiota and the host response (a homeostatic inflammation) is created, according to Lamont et al. [23]. This controlled immune-inflammatory state where the inflammatory response of the host causes no apparent damage should not be considered as pathological but rather as a normal response (a physiological inflammation). Thus, gingival inflammation as a response to the dental biofilm is a state of normality developed through the evolution and present in almost 100% of adults of all populations worldwide [24,42].

Infection occurs when the virulence, the number, and the exposed time supersede the local and general host's defense, which leads to a pathological reaction in the host's tissues [43]. Virulence is the relative ability of a microorganism to cause disease and consequently, virulence is a microbial property that can only be expressed in a susceptible host. Hence, virulence is not an independent microbial property, because it cannot be defined independently of a host [39]. In that perspective all bacteria in the dental biofilm may contribute to the host response and it is not meaningful to distinguish pathogenic microbes from non-pathogenic at that stage (gingivitis). The dental biofilm is the natural habit for these microorganisms and the change in microbial composition that occurs over time may just be a consequence of the changing environment brought about by the host (inflammatory) response. This implies that bacterial species that are better adapted to the changing environment (deeper pocket, anaerobiosis, mechanical retention, alkaline environment, and increased exudate flow with an abundance of serum proteins, complement factors, neutrophils, lysozyme) will thrive and thereby increasingly (or at least consistently) fuel the inflammatory response. This may occur without bacterial invasion and also without necessarily causing any apparent damage. Therefore, gingivitis is not defined as an infection.

In certain periodontal conditions aside from chronic periodontitis, the case for an infectious nature of the problem is strong, e.g., exacerbations and abscess formation due to trauma or blockage of drainage by, e.g., calculus, fillings, or prosthesis. Periodontal infections resemble other dentoalveolar infections regarding their microbial composition and progression [44]. They are endogenic polymicrobial, predominantly anaerobic infections that are characterized by a destroyed internal regulation in the biofilm community with increased activity and growth of bacteria (burst) originating from the dental biofilm. In addition, periodontal infections usually feature bacterial invasion which requires detachment from the plaque. One other condition where bacterial invasion is rather obvious is peri-implantitis which is an endogenic polymicrobial anaerobic infection where the bacteria originate from the biofilm on the implant surface and with a microbiota which resembles that of the periodontal pocket [45]. Due to the anatomical difference from teeth and lack of an intact epithelial barrier, bacterial invasion can be facilitated in peri-implantitis. Clinically visible pus formation and increased number of neutrophils found in biopsies support the view of peri-implantitis as an infectious process [46].

In these conditions mentioned above (periodontal infections), the infections are polymicrobial and although some bacterial species are more frequently found (and may even play an important role), it is not possible to exclude any of the microorganisms from taking part in the "infection" and to solely act as innocent bystanders [2]. Numerous studies have been performed to explain virulence mechanisms in vitro but in accordance with the above definition of virulence this cannot be fully evaluated for various microorganisms independently of a host. However, experimental infections in animals have clearly shown that mixed infections are more infectious than mono-infections, and have also emphasized the importance of anaerobes without the necessity to include "putative pathogens" in such infections [47].

In contrast to periodontal infections, chronic periodontitis is a pathological inflammatory disease, as a response to prolonged (months, years) exposure to, and not infected by a polymicrobial community in the gingival/periodontal pocket. The tissue responses involve alternating destructive phases and repair or healing phases, but with a net loss of attachment and bone. The microorganisms are necessary components but not sufficient to explain the tissue damage. In view of the "damage–response framework" as discussed earlier, both the host and microbes contribute to pathogenesis. As mentioned, the role of specific microorganisms and certain virulence mechanisms in triggering this pathologic inflammation remain unclear. Most factors that are commonly discussed in terms of "virulence factors" among the putative periodontal pathogens should rather be termed "survival factors" since they do not necessarily constitute factors for pathogenicity and damage but for the living, growth and survival of the bacteria in deep, inflamed periodontal pockets.

5. Factors that Promote Bacterial Colonization and Persistence

The oral microbiome in humans is distinctly different from that of other species. Similarly, the human oral microbiome is distinctly different from that of other body compartments, such as the skin, intestine, and vagina [48]. The oral microbiome comprises a highly diverse microbial population, involving more than 700 species [49]. Furthermore, within the oral microbiome, the dental biofilm has its own microbiome characterized by strong tooth surface adhering streptococci and Actinomyces [50]. Adhesion is essential for colonisation within the oral cavity, and it is regulated primarily by the host and host receptors on the mucosal surface and teeth. In fact, the host selectively, very early after birth, allows the microorganisms that best fit to the receptors of each individual and the specific environment of the oral cavity to colonize. The receptor interaction is mediated by microbial adhesins, which are surface structures such as fimbriae, capsule, lipopolysaccharides and others.

In the area of the gingival crevice, the microenvironment is different from other parts of the tooth surface, with the major nutrition probably coming from gingival crevicular fluid (GCF). Since GCF, in contrast to saliva, does not contain any sugars, the main source of nutrition for the microbiota in this niche are the proteins. Hence, the main metabolic pathway is proteolytic, thus favouring the proteolytic rather than the saccharolytic microorganisms. In addition, the GCF, which is a serum exudate, also contains a number of growth supporting factors such as vitamins (e.g., K-vitamin or menadione), hormones (e.g., oestrogen) and specific serum proteins/peptides (e.g., hemin) all favouring many of the fastidious Gram-negative anaerobes that adapt and grow concomitantly with gingival inflammation and deepening gingival pockets [24,50,51].

Gingival inflammation typically results in a deepening of the gingival pocket owing to swelling, oedema and resulting in increased flow of GCF. This has an impact on the type of colonizing and growing bacteria since it further provides nutritious advantages to proteolytic species. Furthermore, the lowering redox potential (Eh), which is arising from the swelling, favours the anaerobes. In contrast to the supragingival plaque, the adhesion of the microorganisms does not play a crucial role in the gingival pocket and motile bacteria (*Treponema, Campylobacter, Selenomonas* spp.) are able to establish themselves by mechanical retention [50]. The GCF contains humoral defence factors (antibodies, complement, antimicrobial peptides) as well as inflammatory cells such as neutrophils and monocytes. This selects for bacteria that can escape phagocytosis and killing by producing anti-phagocytic capsules (*P. gingivalis*) or leukotoxins (*A. actinomycetemcomitans*), or that simply are proteolytic enough to degrade most proteins, including humoral antimicrobial factors such as immunoglobulins (IgG), complement factors, or antimicrobial host defence peptides [52]. The exudate also contains lysozyme, an enzyme directed towards the peptidoglycan of the bacterial cell wall, which is protected by the outer membrane of Gram-negative microorganisms (Gram-positives lack such outer membrane). Consequently, Gram-negatives appear to have a higher survival rate in the inflamed gingival pocket. Inevitably, inflamed gingival pockets contain a microbiota dominated by Gram-negative, anaerobic, proteolytic, and motile bacteria as they are favoured by and adapted to the changing pocket environment (Table 1). This character of the subgingival plaque microbiota has been repeatedly shown in numerous studies for decades using microscopic-, culture- and molecular biology methods [8,53–56]. The composition of the subgingival microbiota can thus convincingly be explained as a result of a changing ecology involving only commensals (essentially non-pathogenic microorganisms) that are adapting to the new environment [8].

6. Factors Promoting Gingival Inflammation

6.1. Bacterial Metabolites as Pro-Inflammatory and/or Cytotoxic Agents

The products of bacterial metabolic processes, the metabolites, can be used by the bacteria for the construction of new macromolecules, but may also remain by-products with cytotoxic potential and take part in the host-microbe interplay. In a combined metagenome/metatranscriptome analysis that compared active and non-progressing sites in periodontitis patients it was confirmed that proteolysis is associated with progressing periodontal sites [57]. Such bacterial metabolism results in the formation of various compounds, some of which are suggested to participate in the pathogenesis of periodontitis [58].

Bacterial hydrogen sulfide (H_2S) is formed predominantly by degradation of the amino acid L-cysteine or the peptide glutathione by various bacterial species that are associated with periodontitis [59]. H_2S is also formed from sulfate by sulfate reducing bacteria. It is a volatile sulfur compound that has been shown to induce the secretion of the pro-inflammatory cytokines IL-1β and IL-18 in monocytes in vitro through the formation of the NLRP3 inflammasome (Figure 1) [59]. These and other pro-inflammatory cytokines are necessary to sustain or even strengthen the inflammatory reactions in the gingiva. Furthermore, H_2S can induce apoptosis in human gingival fibroblasts [60] and split disulfide bonds in host proteins. These mechanisms, that in different ways trigger inflammatory reactions, are proposed to contribute to the disruption of homeostasis between host cells and bacteria, and to participate in the development of disease. In support of this notion, the sulfur compound metabolic processes have been shown to be enhanced in periodontitis progressing sites [57]. Other volatile sulfur compounds, such as methyl mercaptan, dimethyl disulfide, and dimethyl sulfide, are formed from the degradation of L-methionine among other metabolic pathways, and have similarly been suggested to participate in the host-microbiome crosstalk during the induction and progression of periodontal disease [61].

Additional products of the catabolism of L-cysteine and L-methionine are, together with H_2S and methyl mercaptan, ammonia and pyruvate. Ammonia (NH_3), a product of numerous metabolic processes that take place in the periodontal pocket including the transformation of arginine or lysine [62], is suggested to, apart from its effects on pH, also affect neutrophil function [63]. Apart from ammonia, the degradation of arginine can also, result in the by-product and amino acid citrulline [62]. Pyruvate can be degraded into acetic acid or formic acid for energy production [64].

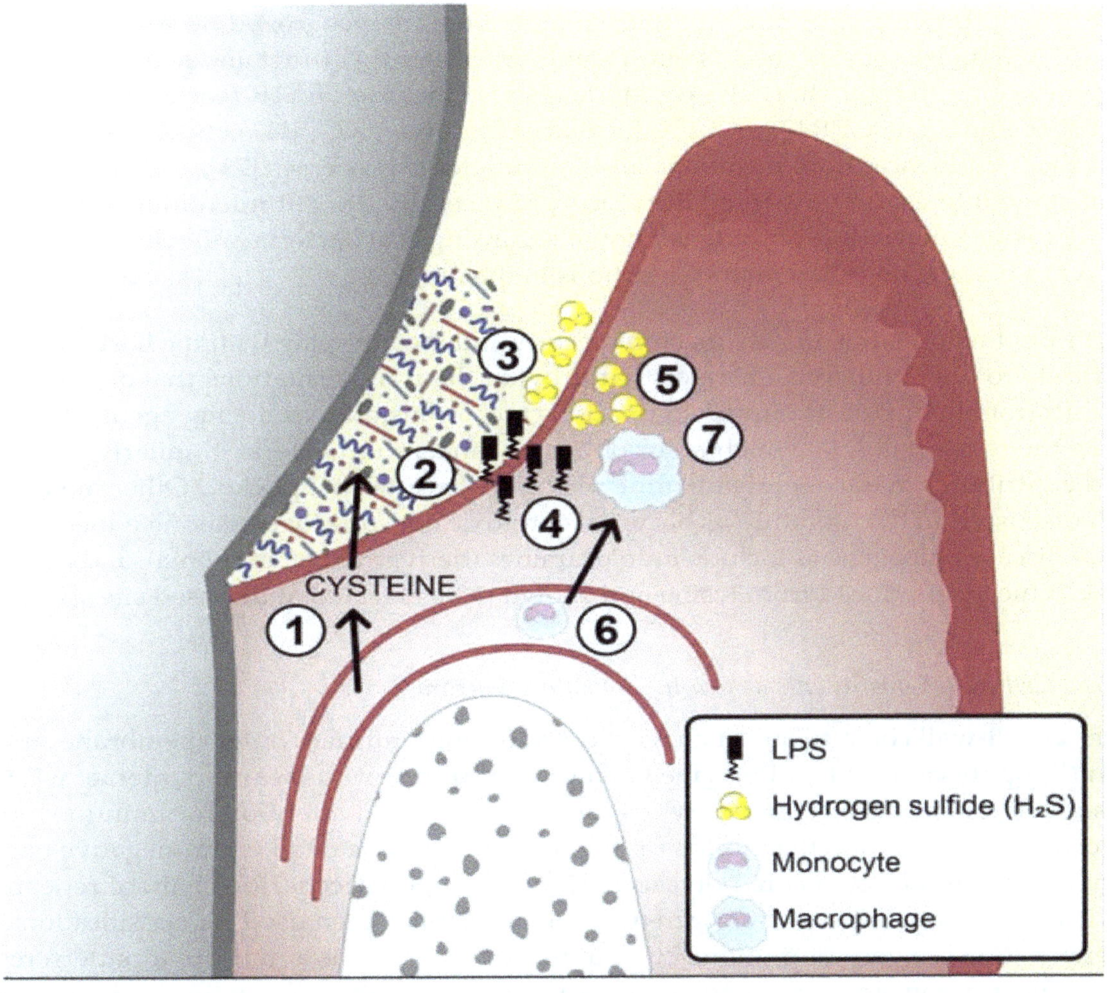

Figure 1. A schematic figure of an inflamed gingival pocket with subgingival plaque (biofilm) and the two signals that lead to the production and secretion of IL-1ß and IL-18 from monocytes/macrophages as reprinted from Basic et al. [59]. The numbers in the figure indicates the following: 1. Serum exudate from blood vessels containing serum proteins, peptides and amino acids including cysteine. 2. The exudate (gingival crevicular fluid, GCF) continues through the thin pocket epithelium (junctional epithelium) into the subgingival pocket. 3. The subgingival plaque, containing numerous, mainly Gram-negative, anaerobic bacteria with proteolytic capacity, degrade proteins, peptides and amino acids including cysteine. 4. Growing Gram-negative anaerobes release lipopolysaccharides (LPS) that penetrate the junctional epithelium into gingival connective tissues. 5. Growing Gram-negative anaerobes (*Fusobacterium* spp. *P. gingivalis*, *Treponema* spp., and others) produce metabolites e.g., hydrogen sulfide (H_2S). 6. The inflammatory lesion attracts monocytes that migrate into the connective tissue and differentiate to macrophages. 7. The effect of LPS and H_2S on macrophages and the subsequent production of the pro-inflammatory cytokines IL-1β and IL-18.

Various carboxylic acids, i.e., acetic acid, butyric acid, formic acid, isobutyric acid, isovaleric acid, lactic acid, propionic acid, phenylacetic acid, succinic acid, and valeric acid are by-products of the deamination of amino acids to generate energy. The presence of many of these have been found to be elevated at inflamed and diseased periodontal sites [65–68]. Comparably to other metabolites, also these mainly short-chain fatty acids have been suggested to act as potent and modifying factors in periodontitis. Butyric acid (Table 1) has for instance been shown to be capable of inducing apoptosis and autophagic cell death in gingival epithelial cells [69], to induce apoptosis in inflamed fibroblasts [70], to induce ROS production, and to impair the cell growth of gingival fibroblasts [71]. These effects stimulate inflammation and are thus, thought to contribute to initiation and the prolongation of periodontitis [66]. Interestingly, many of these metabolites are recognized by specific free fatty acid receptors (FFAR) on leukocytes such as neutrophils and potently attract and activate these cells [72]. This receptor group all bind short-chain fatty acids and include FFA1R (earlier known as GPR40), FFA2R (earlier known as GPR43) and FFA3R (earlier known as GPR41). Such recognition of free fatty acids likely influences both metabolic and immunologic processes [73], and although there has been quite some interest on how free fatty acids produced by the gut microbiota affect health and disease [74], to our knowledge, nothing is known regarding oral bacteria and whether free fatty acid production has bearing on inflammatory reactions in the gingiva.

Apart from the formation of new macromolecules and the interplay with the host, the metabolites also contribute to environmental changes that provide the transformations that are needed for the bacterial shift from homeostasis. Sulfur compounds are, for instance, reducing agents that contribute to lowering the redox potential which favor obligately anaerobic bacteria. Similarly, ammonia is an advocated contributor to the slightly alkaline pH of the periodontal pocket. Other metabolites that have been discussed in the literature as bacterial cytotoxic end-products playing a mediating role in periodontal disease pathogenesis include indole, amines (derivatives of ammonia), and the polyamine cadaverine, which is produced from lysine and shown to be elevated at diseased sites [75].

6.2. *Bacterial Cell-Wall Constituents as Pro-inflammatory Factors*

Bacterial cell-wall constituents such as short and long fimbriae, outer membrane vesicles and endotoxin (lipopolysaccharide; LPS) have been proposed in various ways to interact with (or even to cause subversion of) the inflammatory response [76,77]. Most attention for immune modulation has been directed toward LPS that builds up the outer membrane of all Gram-negative bacteria and consists of a Lipid A moiety, a core polysaccharide, and a polysaccharide chain of repeating sugar subunits. The latter is an important antigen (O-antigen) that has been used for classification of several enteric genera. LPS is a very immunoreactive molecule and seen as a molecular pattern recognized by potential host organisms—genome-encoded receptors capable of reacting to LPS are found in organisms ranging from plants to mammals [78]. In humans, LPS is sensed primarily by toll-like receptor (TLR) 4, which is expressed by immune cells, but also by a wide variety of other cell types. When bound by LPS, TLR4 activates the pro-inflammatory transcription factor NF-κB that enters the nucleus and initiates gene transcription (Figure 2).

This is a pivotal event that regulates the production of multiple pro-inflammatory cytokines [78]. The broad pro-inflammatory response triggered by NF-κB makes LPS a primary candidate for immune-modulation of gingival inflammation. Since all Gram-negative bacteria release LPS, they may all be involved in triggering/sustaining periodontal inflammation. However, the potency of LPS to trigger inflammation varies among different bacteria, and although this has been studied extensively for *P. gingivalis* [79], less is known about the bioactivity of LPS from other Gram-negatives residing in inflamed gingival pockets.

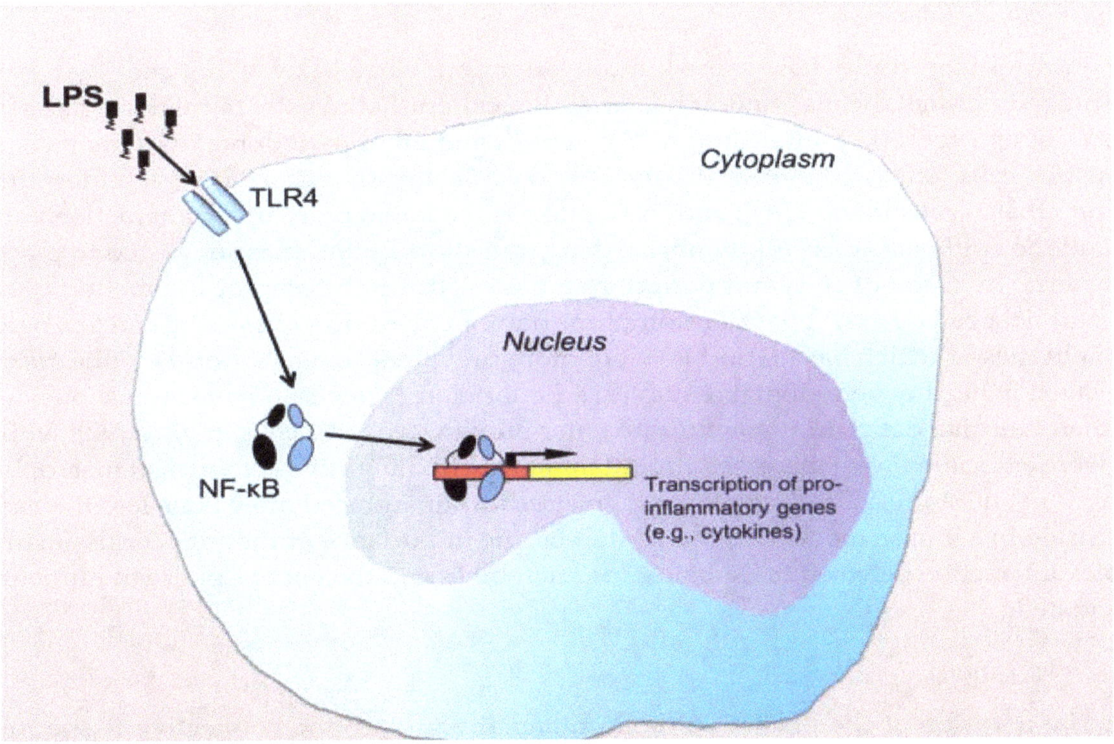

Figure 2. LPS from Gram-negative bacteria bind and activate TLR4 which leads to the activation and translocation from the cytoplasm of the transcription factor NF-κB. Inside the nucleus, NF-κB initiates the transcription of a wide variety of pro-inflammatory genes, e.g., those encoding for pro-inflammatory cytokines.

7. Invasion and Factors that Promote Tissue Degradation

As mentioned above, bacterial invasion is a key process in order to define infections by commensal bacteria, and although invasion seems well established for, e.g., peri-implantitis, it is less clear if it occurs and if it is of importance for chronic periodontitis. How bacteria penetrate through the epithelium and reach the gingival connective tissues is also unclear [80,81], but the pathways commonly discussed [81,82] are: the intercellular route, the intracellular route and by trauma.

7.1. The Intercellular Route

An intercellular route is suggested to take place primarily by motile species, e.g., spirochetes [82]. The junctional epithelium is non-keratinized and thin (4–5 cells thick), and in a state of inflammation, the cells are not tightly joined in order to facilitate gingival exudate and migration of neutrophils and monocytes through the gingival barrier. It is hypothesized that this intercellular passage also allows motile bacteria such as *Treponema* and *Campylobacter* species to penetrate the barrier. *Treponema* spp. and *P. gingivalis* produce specific gingipains that can degrade epithelial junctional proteins (E-cadherin and occludin), and this impairs the junction-related structures [83,84].

Invasion is more likely to take place if the epithelial barrier (junctional epithelium) is disrupted in the case of ulceration. In acute necrotizing ulcerative gingivitis (ANUG) spirochetes are shown to invade the underlying connective tissue by motility [85]. A similar situation is also seen in peri-implantitis where the epithelium fails to cover the connective tissues of the apical part of the peri-implant pocket [46,86]. The periodontal abscess is another example of invasion into the tissues by bacterial growth, and the abscess can sometimes even lead to fistula formation. Invasion in these examples is due to bacterial multiplication and expansion, and it is associated with heavy neutrophil attraction and suppuration, and sometimes symptoms characteristic of an acute infection.

7.2. *The Intracellular Route*

The intracellular route has gained more attention since it was noticed that viable and non-keratinized epithelial cells contain bacteria. Buccal epithelial cells regularly contain bacterial cells, mainly streptococci [87]. Interestingly, *P. gingivalis* and other periodontal bacteria have also been shown in such cells [88]. *T. forsythia, Prevotella intermedia* and *C. rectus* have been identified inside crevicular epithelial cells in vivo [89], and this uptake is mediated by receptor interaction between the bacteria and the epithelial cells [90]. Fimbriae (long and short fimbriae) is suggested to play a crucial role in bacterial invasion of cells and periodontal tissues through receptor interaction between the fimbriae and host cells [76]. *P. gingivalis* long fimbriae can be divided based on the *fimA* gene into 6 different subtypes of which *fimA* II and IV were more prevalent in periodontitis while *fimA* type I is more prevalent in healthy periodontal tissues [91]. Fimbriated *P. gingivalis* have been shown to be more efficient than fimbriae-deficient *P. gingivalis* to enter human dendritic cells in vitro [92], while Type II fimbriae were associated with increased proinflammatory and invasive activities in macrophages [76]. Interestingly, in one study a Type-1 fimbriae *P. gingivalis* strain induced more bone loss than a Type-II *P. gingivalis* strain in a mouse model [93]. Nevertheless, the importance of fimbriae for tissue invasion in the complex interaction between the subgingival microbiota and the host response in humans remains to be elucidated.

7.3. *Invasion by Trauma*

Bacterial invasion of the pocket epithelium and the underlying connective tissue in gingival biopsies from patients with periodontitis has been reported using various methods [81]. These studies clearly show presence of various periodontitis associated bacteria intracellularly in epithelial cells as well as in the connective tissue, but without explaining whether they have passed the barrier actively or accidentally by trauma (e.g., while taking the biopsies). Bacteria are commonly pushed into the connective tissues during manipulations and hygienic procedures (tooth brushing, flossing, tooth picks) and chewing. Dental hygienists or dentists, during cleaning and treatment procedures (depuration, scaling, ultrasonication, probing, periodontal surgery and tooth extractions), frequently cause the spread of microorganisms into the blood stream. Bacteremia during dental procedures is thus a well-known phenomenon, and poor oral hygiene, with an abundance of plaque and inflammation, increases the likelihood of bacterial spread out in the tissues. It is likely that most people have bacteremia daily without any (severe) consequences but it is also possible that bacteria can survive within the periodontal tissues and not being immediately eliminated by the host defense.

7.4. *Tissue Degrading Factors*

Tissue degrading or histolytic enzymes produced by bacteria were previously thought to be directly responsible for periodontal tissue breakdown [94], comparably to similar enzymes of pathogenic tissue invading bacteria such as *Clostridium histolyticum, Staphylococcus aureus* and *Streptococcus pyogenes* (Group A streptococci) [94]. Hyaluronidase ("spreading factor"), chondroitin sulphatase, and beta-glucuronidase produced by various oral bacteria such as streptococci, peptostreptococci, and corynebacteria (diphteroids) were thought to facilitate the spread of infections by degrading tissue components. Similarly, various bacterial proteases including collagenases were thought to play a major role by degrading tissue constituents in infections involving anaerobic proteolytic bacteria [94]. It was tempting to argue that collagenases and gingipains (previously termed "trypsin-like") produced by several *Porphyromonas* species (e.g., *P. gingivalis* and *P. gulae*) degrading almost any protein in vitro also had a role in periodontal pathology. Although, realizing that host defense cells, e.g., neutrophils and macrophages, also produce similar enzymes, the possibility that bacterial enzymes contribute to tissue degradation has been diminished.

8. Factors for Evasion of Host Defence

The host reacts extensively to the microbial challenge by employing the inflammatory reaction and assembling defense factors such as neutrophils, complement factors, and antibodies in the exudate and gingival pocket [95]. Microorganisms with the capacity to evade such host factors will increase their survival rate. As mentioned above, proteolytic enzymes may split or degrade the host's defense molecules such as immunoglobulins and complement [96], but there are also more sophisticated mechanisms for the evasion of host defense.

8.1. Exotoxins

Toxins that destroy leukocytes, leukotoxins, are well-known virulence factors found in several pathogenic bacteria such as the PV-leucocidin in *Staphylococcus aureus* [97] and *Fusobacterium necrophorum* [98]. This explains the invasive and abscess-promoting character of these pathogens. Therefore, the leukotoxin-producing microorganism, *A. actinomycetemcomitans*, among the periodontal bacteria, has been extensively studied due to this particular factor [99,100]. The importance of leukotoxin in *A. actinomycetemcomitans* was emphasized when discovering the high toxic JP2 clone, which produces highly elevated levels of leukotoxin. Interestingly, Höglund et al. [101] correctly predicted that children of a Ghanaian cohort harboring *A. actinomycetemcomitans* and the high-toxic clone (JP2) in particular, at periodontal sites, had significantly more periodontal breakdown after 2 years compared with baseline, indicating a specific impact of the JP2 clone on the disease progression. The leukotoxin explains the specific ability of this bacterium to survive or escape the host's defense (neutrophils present in the gingival pockets), but it does not explain the periodontal breakdown that is associated with this bacterium in aggressive forms of periodontitis in children and adolescents [102]. The fact that the toxin is both membrane-associated and secreted may be important since (at least) the secreted form would likely create a local niche free from viable neutrophils, which would benefit all bacteria present at this site.

8.2. Capsule Formation

The formation of an anti-phagocytic capsule is a well-known virulence strategy of many pathogenic microorganisms. *Streptococcus pneumoniae* and *Haemophilus influence* are exclusively dependent on capsule formation and vaccination of children towards their capsular antigens is today a reality [103,104]. Capsules are produced by many Gram-negative anaerobic rods, e.g., *Bacteroides, Prevotella,* and *Porphyromonas* [105,106]. The capsule is produced to escape phagocytosis and thereby intracellular killing by neutrophils and macrophages. The inability of the host's defense to kill capsulated bacteria may result in spread of infections and to complications such as sepsis [107]. Six capsular serotypes have been identified among periodontal *P. gingivalis* isolates (Table 1). Two capsular types, K1 and K6, seem to include isolates with a lower adhesion capacity to human leukocytes in vitro than the other capsular types [105,108]. However, in vivo evidence supporting that any of the capsular types would be more associated with periodontitis than others are lacking.

9. Systemic Implications of Periodontal Bacteria

Bacteraemia and focal infections from the oral cavity have been associated with teeth and oral conditions for more than hundred years [109]. Formerly, the total extraction of all teeth was a common way to avoid future problems and full dentures was the only option for adults, and still is in many countries in the world. Incomplete endodontic treatment was thought to be the major cause of focal infections and apical periodontitis is still a suspected (by the medical profession) major point of entry for oral bacteria into the blood stream and further to various organs of the body. Today, the systemic effects from marginal periodontitis is considered to be much more important [109]. Not only bacteria as such but also products from subgingival bacteria (e.g., metabolites and endotoxins), and inflammatory mediators produced locally in the periodontal tissues, are being linked to the chronic inflammation seen in a number of systemic diseases such as atherosclerosis, diabetes, preterm birth, rheumatoid arthritis and Alzheimer's disease [5,110]. Especially, the association between periodontitis and putative periodontal pathogens to Alzheimer's disease has been in focus during the last decade and *P. gingivalis* LPS and outer-membrane vesicles have been suggested to be accumulated in brain tissues of patients with Alzheimer's disease [77,111]. Most studies linking periodontitis to systemic diseases are association studies and it is less clear what (if any) unique contribution periodontitis might have that would not be found for other chronic inflammatory diseases in the body (e.g., in the gut).

However, one disease where the connection to periodontitis appears more solid than a mere association between the two diseases, is rheumatoid arthritis (RA), a widespread systemic inflammatory disease that is mainly manifested as peripheral polyarthritis (i.e., inflammation of peripheral joints) and that affects up to 1% of the global population [112]. RA is a heterogeneous disease but the majority of cases feature auto-antibodies directed towards citrullinated epitopes, so-called anti-citrullinated protein antibodies (ACPAs). Citrullination is a biochemical post-translational modification where arginine residues of peptides and proteins are converted into citrulline residues. In general, protein citrullination is of great physiological importance and endogenous citrullination is ascertained by a family of human enzymes known as peptidylarginine deiminases (PADs), some of which are primarily located immune cells, such as neutrophils. PAD-mediated citrullination of arginine residues may create neo-epitopes that could give rise to the development of ACPAs and one major research questions in RA deal with how, when, and where tolerance is broken to allow for the generation of ACPAs.

A. acinomycetemcomitans has been shown to trigger dysregulated citrullination of proteins, a process mediated by the activation and release of endogenous neutrophil PAD by the actions of the bacterial leukotoxin [113]. Although the pore-forming leukotoxin of *A. actinomycetemcomitans* is exclusive among oral bacteria, pore formation is by no means a unique feature of bacterial toxins in general. Additionally, *P. gingivalis* has been implicated as a potentially even more interesting link between periodontitis and RA when it was found that it expresses a bacterial PAD, typically referred to as PPAD, to distinguish it from the human isoforms [114]. PPAD seems to be rather uniquely expressed by *P. gingivalis* among the bacteria that interact with humans and it has the ability to create citrullinated neo-epitopes that are recognized by ACPAs from RA patients. Interestingly, *P. gingivalis* appears especially fit to do this, since the PPAD is specific for C-terminal arginine residues and such peptides are typically generated by the gingipains. Thus, these two *P. gingivalis* enzymes (PPAD and gingipains) appear to work in concert, in a way that maximize the levels of citrullinated epitopes which might thereby break tolerance and facilitate the generation of ACPAs [112].

10. Conclusions

Inflammation in the gingiva (gingivitis) is a normal host tissue response (a physiological inflammation) triggered by ordinary commensal microorganisms and the products (metabolites, endotoxins) released from them during growth. Periodontitis is a pathological inflammatory disease, as a response to years of prolonged exposure to a polymicrobial community in the gingival/periodontal pocket, involving tissue responses with alternating destructive (damage) and healing (repair) phases, but with a net loss of attachment and bone. The infectious nature of the microbes, and to what extent specific bacterial species, with specific virulence factors capable of interference with host defense and tissue repair, play in disease onset and progression, are still unclear. Most of the factors that used to be discussed in terms of virulence (proteases, LPS, invasive ability, fimbriae, capsule, leukotoxin) among microorganisms commonly associated with periodontitis should rather be termed survival factors, since they do not necessarily constitute factors for pathogenicity and damage but for the living, growth, and survival of the bacteria in deep, inflamed periodontal pockets. One exception is the leukotoxin produced by *A. actinomycetemcomitans* (and the JP2 genotype where clinical evidence support a causative role in disease progression) [101] and although the mechanism whereby the leukotoxin leads to tissue damage is still not known, this bacterial species best fulfils the designation of a putative periodontal pathogen in the human oral microbiota.

Author Contributions: G.D., A.B. and J.B. reviewed the literature and wrote the review.

Acknowledgments: (Figure 1 is published in an Open Access journal and is distributed under the terms of the Creative Commons Attribution ver. 4.0 International License *https://creativecommons.org/licenses/by/4.0/*, which is hereby acknowledged.

References

1. Hashim, D.; Cionca, N.; Combescure, C.; Mombelli, A. The diagnosis of peri-implantitis: A systematic review on the predictive value of bleeding on probing. *Clin. Oral Implants Res.* **2018**, *29* (Suppl. S16), 276–293. [CrossRef]
2. Teles, R.; Teles, F.; Frias-Lopez, J.; Paster, B.; Haffajee, A. Lessons learned and unlearned in periodontal microbiology. *Periodontology 2000* **2013**, *62*, 95–162. [CrossRef] [PubMed]
3. Baelum, V.; Lopez, R. Periodontal disease epidemiology—Learned and unlearned? *Periodontology 2000* **2013**, *62*, 37–58. [CrossRef] [PubMed]
4. Kinane, D.F.; Stathopoulou, P.G.; Papapanou, P.N. Periodontal diseases. *Nat. Rev. Dis. Primers* **2017**, *3*, 17038. [CrossRef]
5. Bui, F.Q.; Almeida-da-Silva, C.L.C.; Huynh, B.; Trinh, A.; Liu, J.; Woodward, J.; Asadi, H.; Ojcius, D.M. Association between periodontal pathogens and systemic disease. *Biomed. J.* **2019**, *42*, 27–35. [CrossRef] [PubMed]
6. Loe, H.; Theilade, E.; Jensen, S.B. Experimental gingivitis in man. *J. Periodontal.* **1965**, *36*, 177–187. [CrossRef] [PubMed]
7. Socransky, S.S.; Haffajee, A.D. Evidence of bacterial etiology: A historical perspective. *Periodontology 2000* **1994**, *5*, 7–25. [CrossRef] [PubMed]
8. Socransky, S.S.; Haffajee, A.D. Periodontal microbial ecology. *Periodontology 2000* **2005**, *38*, 135–187. [CrossRef] [PubMed]
9. Socransky, S.S. Criteria for the infectious agents in dental caries and periodontal disease. *J. Clin. Periodontal.* **1979**, *6*, 16–21. [CrossRef] [PubMed]
10. Loesche, W.J. The therapeutic use of antimicrobial agents in patients with periodontal disease. *Scand. J. Infect. Dis. Suppl.* **1985**, *46*, 106–114. [PubMed]
11. Page, R.C.; Kornman, K.S. The pathogenesis of human periodontitis: An introduction. *Periodontology 2000* **1997**, *14*, 9–11. [CrossRef] [PubMed]
12. Meyle, J.; Chapple, I. Molecular aspects of the pathogenesis of periodontitis. *Periodontology 2000* **2015**, *69*, 7–17. [CrossRef] [PubMed]
13. Haber, J.; Wattles, J.; Crowley, M.; Mandell, R.; Joshipura, K.; Kent, R.L. Evidence for cigarette smoking as a major risk factor for periodontitis. *J. Periodontal.* **1993**, *64*, 16–23. [CrossRef] [PubMed]
14. Emrich, L.J.; Shlossman, M.; Genco, R.J. Periodontal disease in non-insulin-dependent diabetes mellitus. *J. Periodontal.* **1991**, *62*, 123–131. [CrossRef] [PubMed]
15. Loos, B.G.; Papantonopoulos, G.; Jepsen, S.; Laine, M.L. What is the contribution of genetics to periodontal risk? *Dent. Clin.* **2015**, *59*, 761–780. [CrossRef]
16. Nibali, L.; Bayliss-Chapman, J.; Almofareh, S.A.; Zhou, Y.; Divaris, K.; Vieira, A.R. What Is the heritability of periodontitis? A systematic review. *J. Dent. Res.* **2019**, *98*, 632–641. [CrossRef]
17. Kassebaum, N.J.; Bernabe, E.; Dahiya, M.; Bhandari, B.; Murray, C.J.; Marcenes, W. Global burden of severe periodontitis in 1990–2010: A systematic review and meta-regression. *J. Dent. Res.* **2014**, *93*, 1045–1053. [CrossRef]
18. Larsson, L. Current concepts of epigenetics and its role in periodontitis. *Curr. Oral Health Rep.* **2017**, *4*, 286–293. [CrossRef]
19. Luo, Y.; Peng, X.; Duan, D.; Liu, C.; Xu, X.; Zhou, X. Epigenetic regulations in the pathogenesis of periodontitis. *Curr. Stem Cell Res. Ther.* **2018**, *13*, 144–150. [CrossRef]
20. De-La-Torre, J.; Quindos, G.; Marcos-Arias, C.; Marichalar-Mendia, X.; Gainza, M.L.; Eraso, E.; Acha-Sagredo, A.; Aguirre-Urizar, J.M. Oral Candida colonization in patients with chronic periodontitis. Is there any relationship? *Rev. Iberoam. Micol.* **2018**, *35*, 134–139. [CrossRef]

21. Slots, J. Periodontitis: Facts, fallacies and the future. *Periodontology 2000* **2017**, *75*, 7–23. [CrossRef] [PubMed]
22. Rosier, B.T.; Marsh, P.D.; Mira, A. Resilience of the oral microbiota in health: Mechanisms that prevent dysbiosis. *J. Dent. Res.* **2018**, *97*, 371–380. [CrossRef] [PubMed]
23. Lamont, R.J.; Koo, H.; Hajishengallis, G. The oral microbiota: Dynamic communities and host interactions. *Nat. Rev. Microbiol.* **2018**, *16*, 745–759. [CrossRef] [PubMed]
24. Kilian, M.; Chapple, I.L.; Hannig, M.; Marsh, P.D.; Meuric, V.; Pedersen, A.M.; Tonetti, M.S.; Wade, W.G.; Zaura, E. The oral microbiome—An update for oral healthcare professionals. *Br. Dent. J.* **2016**, *221*, 657–666. [CrossRef] [PubMed]
25. Lopez, R.; Hujoel, P.; Belibasakis, G.N. On putative periodontal pathogens: An epidemiological perspective. *Virulence* **2015**, *6*, 249–257. [CrossRef] [PubMed]
26. Dahlen, G.; Manji, F.; Baelum, V.; Fejerskov, O. Putative periodontopathogens in "diseased" and "non-diseased" persons exhibiting poor oral hygiene. *J. Clin. Periodontal.* **1992**, *19*, 35–42. [CrossRef]
27. Socransky, S.S.; Haffajee, A.D.; Cugini, M.A.; Smith, C.; Kent, R.L., Jr. Microbial complexes in subgingival plaque. *J. Clin. Periodontal.* **1998**, *25*, 134–144. [CrossRef]
28. Lamont, R.J.; Jenkinson, H.F. Life below the gum line: Pathogenic mechanisms of *Porphyromonas gingivalis*. *Microbiol. Mol. Biol. Rev.* **1998**, *62*, 1244–1263.
29. Holt, S.C.; Ebersole, J.L. Porphyromonas gingivalis, *Treponema denticola*, and *Tannerella forsythia*: The "red complex", a prototype polybacterial pathogenic consortium in periodontitis. *Periodontology 2000* **2005**, *38*, 72–122. [CrossRef]
30. Fine, D.H.; Patil, A.G.; Velusamy, S.K. *Aggregatibacter actinomycetemcomitans* (Aa) under the radar: Myths and misunderstandings of Aa and its role in aggressive periodontitis. *Front. Immunol.* **2019**, *10*, 728. [CrossRef]
31. Listgarten, M.A.; Hellden, L. Relative distribution of bacteria at clinically healthy and periodontally diseased sites in humans. *J. Clin. Periodontal.* **1978**, *5*, 115–132. [CrossRef] [PubMed]
32. Huo, Y.B.; Chan, Y.; Lacap-Bugler, D.C.; Mo, S.; Woo, P.C.Y.; Leung, W.K.; Watt, R.M. Multilocus sequence analysis of phylogroup 1 and 2 oral treponeme strains. *Appl. Environ. Microbiol.* **2017**, *83*, e02499-16. [CrossRef] [PubMed]
33. You, M.; Mo, S.; Leung, W.K.; Watt, R.M. Comparative analysis of oral treponemes associated with periodontal health and disease. *BMC Infect. Dis.* **2013**, *13*, 174. [CrossRef] [PubMed]
34. Haubek, D.; Ennibi, O.K.; Poulsen, K.; Vaeth, M.; Poulsen, S.; Kilian, M. Risk of aggressive periodontitis in adolescent carriers of the JP2 clone of *Aggregatibacter* (*Actinobacillus*) *actinomycetemcomitans* in Morocco: A prospective longitudinal cohort study. *Lancet* **2008**, *371*, 237–242. [CrossRef]
35. Perez-Chaparro, P.J.; Goncalves, C.; Figueiredo, L.C.; Faveri, M.; Lobao, E.; Tamashiro, N.; Duarte, P.; Feres, M. Newly identified pathogens associated with periodontitis: A systematic review. *J. Dent. Res.* **2014**, *93*, 846–858. [CrossRef] [PubMed]
36. Wade, W.G. Has the use of molecular methods for the characterization of the human oral microbiome changed our understanding of the role of bacteria in the pathogenesis of periodontal disease? *J. Clin. Periodontal.* **2011**, *38* (Suppl. S11), 7–16. [CrossRef] [PubMed]
37. Curtis, M.A. Periodontal microbiology—The lid's off the box again. *J. Dent. Res.* **2014**, *93*, 840–842. [CrossRef]
38. Charalampakis, G.; Dahlen, G.; Carlen, A.; Leonhardt, A. Bacterial markers vs. clinical markers to predict progression of chronic periodontitis: A 2-yr prospective observational study. *Eur. J. Oral Sci.* **2013**, *121*, 394–402. [CrossRef]
39. Casadevall, A.; Pirofski, L.A. Virulence factors and their mechanisms of action: The view from a damage-response framework. *J. Water Health* **2009**, *7* (Suppl. S1), S2–S18. [CrossRef]
40. Isenberg, H.D. Pathogenicity and virulence: Another view. *Clin. Microbiol. Rev.* **1988**, *1*, 40–53. [CrossRef]
41. Anonymous. *Dorland´s Medical Dictionary*; Saunders: Philadelphia, PA, USA, 2007.
42. Manji, F.; Dahlen, G.; Fejerskov, O. Caries and periodontitis: Contesting the conventional wisdom on their aetiology. *Caries Res.* **2018**, *52*, 548–564. [CrossRef] [PubMed]
43. Dahlen, G. Microbiology and treatment of dental abscesses and periodontal-endodontic lesions. *Periodontology 2000* **2002**, *28*, 206–239. [CrossRef] [PubMed]
44. Lewis, M.A.; MacFarlane, T.W.; McGowan, D.A. Quantitative bacteriology of acute dento-alveolar abscesses. *J. Med. Microbiol.* **1986**, *21*, 101–104. [CrossRef] [PubMed]
45. Charalampakis, G.; Belibasakis, G.N. Microbiome of peri-implant infections: Lessons from conventional, molecular and metagenomic analyses. *Virulence* **2015**, *6*, 183–187. [CrossRef] [PubMed]

46. Berglundh, T.; Gislason, O.; Lekholm, U.; Sennerby, L.; Lindhe, J. Histopathological observations of human periimplantitis lesions. *J. Clin. Periodontal.* **2004**, *31*, 341–347. [CrossRef] [PubMed]
47. Dahlen, G.; Fabricius, L.; Holm, S.E.; Moller, A. Interactions within a collection of eight bacterial strains isolated from a monkey dental root canal. *Oral Microbiol. Immunol.* **1987**, *2*, 164–170. [CrossRef] [PubMed]
48. Project, C.H.M. Structure, function and diversity of the healthy human microbiome. *Nature* **2012**, *486*, 207–214. [CrossRef]
49. Verma, D.; Garg, P.K.; Dubey, A.K. Insights into the human oral microbiome. *Arch. Microbiol.* **2018**, *200*, 525–540. [CrossRef] [PubMed]
50. Marsh, P.; Lewis, M.; Williams, D.; Marsh, P.; Martin, M.; Lewis, M.; Williams, D. *Oral Microbiology*, 5th ed.; Churchill Livingstone: Edingburgh, UK, 2009.
51. Carlsson, J. Growth and nutrition as ecological factors. In *Oral Bacterial Ecology. The Molecular Basis*; Kuramitsu, H.K., Ellen, R.P., Eds.; Horizon Scientific Press: Norfolk, UK, 2000; pp. 68–130.
52. Devine, D.A.; Cosseau, C. Host defense peptides in the oral cavity. *Adv. Appl. Microbiol.* **2008**, *63*, 281–322. [CrossRef] [PubMed]
53. Theilade, E.; Wright, W.H.; Jensen, S.B.; Loe, H. Experimental gingivitis in man. II. A longitudinal clinical and bacteriological investigation. *J. Periodontal Res.* **1966**, *1*, 1–13. [CrossRef] [PubMed]
54. Moore, L.V.; Moore, W.E.; Cato, E.P.; Smibert, R.M.; Burmeister, J.A.; Best, A.M.; Ranney, R.R. Bacteriology of human gingivitis. *J. Dent. Res.* **1987**, *66*, 989–995. [CrossRef] [PubMed]
55. Slots, J. Subgingival microflora and periodontal disease. *J. Clin. Periodontal.* **1979**, *6*, 351–382. [CrossRef] [PubMed]
56. Griffen, A.L.; Beall, C.J.; Campbell, J.H.; Firestone, N.D.; Kumar, P.S.; Yang, Z.K.; Podar, M.; Leys, E.J. Distinct and complex bacterial profiles in human periodontitis and health revealed by 16S pyrosequencing. *ISME J.* **2012**, *6*, 1176–1185. [CrossRef] [PubMed]
57. Yost, S.; Duran-Pinedo, A.E.; Teles, R.; Krishnan, K.; Frias-Lopez, J. Functional signatures of oral dysbiosis during periodontitis progression revealed by microbial metatranscriptome analysis. *Genome Med.* **2015**, *7*, 27. [CrossRef]
58. Takahashi, N. Oral microbiome metabolism: From "who are they?" to "what are they doing?". *J. Dent. Res.* **2015**, *94*, 1628–1637. [CrossRef]
59. Basic, A.; Alizadehgharib, S.; Dahlen, G.; Dahlgren, U. Hydrogen sulfide exposure induces NLRP3 inflammasome-dependent IL-1beta and IL-18 secretion in human mononuclear leukocytes in vitro. *Clin. Exp. Dent. Res.* **2017**, *3*, 115–120. [CrossRef]
60. Zhang, J.H.; Dong, Z.; Chu, L. Hydrogen sulfide induces apoptosis in human periodontium cells. *J. Periodontal Res.* **2010**, *45*, 71–78. [CrossRef]
61. Nakano, Y.; Yoshimura, M.; Koga, T. Methyl mercaptan production by periodontal bacteria. *Int. Dent. J.* **2002**, *52* (Suppl. S3), 217–220. [CrossRef]
62. Uematsu, H.; Sato, N.; Djais, A.; Hoshino, E. Degradation of arginine by *Slackia exigua* ATCC 700122 and *Cryptobacterium curtum* ATCC 700683. *Oral Microbiol. Immunol.* **2006**, *21*, 381–384. [CrossRef]
63. Niederman, R.; Brunkhorst, B.; Smith, S.; Weinreb, R.N.; Ryder, M.I. Ammonia as a potential mediator of adult human periodontal infection: Inhibition of neutrophil function. *Arch. Oral Biol.* **1990**, *35*, S205–S209. [CrossRef]
64. Uematsu, H.; Sato, N.; Hossain, M.Z.; Ikeda, T.; Hoshino, E. Degradation of arginine and other amino acids by butyrate-producing asaccharolytic anaerobic gram-positive rods in periodontal pockets. *Arch. Oral Biol.* **2003**, *48*, 423–429. [CrossRef]
65. Niederman, R.; Zhang, J.; Kashket, S. Short-chain carboxylic-acid-stimulated, PMN-mediated gingival inflammation. *Crit. Rev. Oral Biol. Med.* **1997**, *8*, 269–290. [CrossRef] [PubMed]
66. Niederman, R.; Buyle-Bodin, Y.; Lu, B.Y.; Robinson, P.; Naleway, C. Short-chain carboxylic acid concentration in human gingival crevicular fluid. *J. Dent. Res.* **1997**, *76*, 575–579. [CrossRef] [PubMed]
67. Qiqiang, L.; Huanxin, M.; Xuejun, G. Longitudinal study of volatile fatty acids in the gingival crevicular fluid of patients with periodontitis before and after nonsurgical therapy. *J. Periodontal Res.* **2012**, *47*, 740–749. [CrossRef] [PubMed]
68. Lu, R.; Meng, H.; Gao, X.; Xu, L.; Feng, X. Effect of non-surgical periodontal treatment on short chain fatty acid levels in gingival crevicular fluid of patients with generalized aggressive periodontitis. *J. Periodontal Res.* **2014**, *49*, 574–583. [CrossRef] [PubMed]

69. Tsuda, H.; Ochiai, K.; Suzuki, N.; Otsuka, K. Butyrate, a bacterial metabolite, induces apoptosis and autophagic cell death in gingival epithelial cells. *J. Periodontal Res.* **2010**, *45*, 626–634. [CrossRef] [PubMed]
70. Kurita-Ochiai, T.; Seto, S.; Suzuki, N.; Yamamoto, M.; Otsuka, K.; Abe, K.; Ochiai, K. Butyric acid induces apoptosis in inflamed fibroblasts. *J. Dent. Res.* **2008**, *87*, 51–55. [CrossRef]
71. Chang, M.C.; Tsai, Y.L.; Chen, Y.W.; Chan, C.P.; Huang, C.F.; Lan, W.C.; Lin, C.C.; Lan, W.H.; Jeng, J.H. Butyrate induces reactive oxygen species production and affects cell cycle progression in human gingival fibroblasts. *J. Periodontal Res.* **2013**, *48*, 66–73. [CrossRef]
72. Bjorkman, L.; Martensson, J.; Winther, M.; Gabl, M.; Holdfeldt, A.; Uhrbom, M.; Bylund, J.; Hojgaard Hansen, A.; Pandey, S.K.; Ulven, T.; et al. The Neutrophil response induced by an agonist for free fatty acid receptor 2 (GPR43) is primed by tumor necrosis factor alpha and by Receptor UNCOUPLING from the cytoskeleton but attenuated by tissue recruitment. *Mol. Cell Biol.* **2016**, *36*, 2583–2595. [CrossRef]
73. Alvarez-Curto, E.; Milligan, G. Metabolism meets immunity: The role of free fatty acid receptors in the immune system. *Biochem. Pharmacol.* **2016**, *114*, 3–13. [CrossRef]
74. Maslowski, K.M.; Vieira, A.T.; Ng, A.; Kranich, J.; Sierro, F.; Yu, D.; Schilter, H.C.; Rolph, M.S.; Mackay, F.; Artis, D.; et al. Regulation of inflammatory responses by gut microbiota and chemoattractant receptor GPR43. *Nature* **2009**, *461*, 1282–1286. [CrossRef] [PubMed]
75. Barnes, V.M.; Teles, R.; Trivedi, H.M.; Devizio, W.; Xu, T.; Mitchell, M.W.; Milburn, M.V.; Guo, L. Acceleration of purine degradation by periodontal diseases. *J. Dent. Res.* **2009**, *88*, 851–855. [CrossRef] [PubMed]
76. Enersen, M.; Nakano, K.; Amano, A. Porphyromonas gingivalis fimbriae. *J. Oral Microbiol.* **2013**, *5*, 20265. [CrossRef] [PubMed]
77. Singhrao, S.K.; Olsen, I. Are *Porphyromonas gingivalis* outer membrane vesicles microbullets for sporadic Alzheimer's disease manifestation? *J. Alzheimers Dis. Rep.* **2018**, *2*, 219–228. [CrossRef] [PubMed]
78. Neyen, C.; Lemaitre, B. Sensing gram-negative bacteria: A phylogenetic perspective. *Curr. Opin. Immunol.* **2016**, *38*, 8–17. [CrossRef] [PubMed]
79. Paramonov, N.; Aduse-Opoku, J.; Hashim, A.; Rangarajan, M.; Curtis, M.A. Identification of the linkage between A-polysaccharide and the core in the A-lipopolysaccharide of *Porphyromonas gingivalis* W50. *J. Bacteriol.* **2015**, *197*, 1735–1746. [CrossRef]
80. Tribble, G.D.; Lamont, R.J. Bacterial invasion of epithelial cells and spreading in periodontal tissue. *Periodontology 2000* **2010**, *52*, 68–83. [CrossRef]
81. Ji, S.; Choi, Y.S.; Choi, Y. Bacterial invasion and persistence: Critical events in the pathogenesis of periodontitis? *J. Periodontal Res.* **2015**, *50*, 570–585. [CrossRef]
82. Lux, R.; Miller, J.N.; Park, N.H.; Shi, W. Motility and chemotaxis in tissue penetration of oral epithelial cell layers by Treponema denticola. *Infect. Immun.* **2001**, *69*, 6276–6283. [CrossRef]
83. Katz, J.; Yang, Q.B.; Zhang, P.; Potempa, J.; Travis, J.; Michalek, S.M.; Balkovetz, D.F. Hydrolysis of epithelial junctional proteins by *Porphyromonas gingivalis* gingipains. *Infect. Immun.* **2002**, *70*, 2512–2518. [CrossRef]
84. Listgarten, M.A. Electron microscopic observations on the bacterial flora of acute necrotizing *Ulcerative gingivitis*. *J. Periodontal.* **1965**, *36*, 328–339. [CrossRef] [PubMed]
85. Listgarten, M.A.; Socransky, S.S. Ultrastructural characteristics of a spirochete in the lesion of acute necrotizing *Ulcerative gingivostomatitis* (Vincent's infection). *Arch. Oral Biol.* **1964**, *9*, 95–96. [CrossRef]
86. Berglundh, T.; Zitzmann, N.U.; Donati, M. Are peri-implantitis lesions different from periodontitis lesions? *J. Clin. Periodontol.* **2011**, *38* (Suppl. S11), 188–202. [CrossRef]
87. Rudney, J.D.; Chen, R.; Zhang, G. Streptococci dominate the diverse flora within buccal cells. *J. Dent. Res.* **2005**, *84*, 1165–1171. [CrossRef] [PubMed]
88. Rudney, J.D.; Chen, R.; Sedgewick, G.J. *Actinobacillus actinomycetemcomitans*, *Porphyromonas gingivalis*, and *Tannerella forsythensis* are components of a polymicrobial intracellular flora within human buccal cells. *J. Dent. Res.* **2005**, *84*, 59–63. [CrossRef] [PubMed]
89. Dibart, S.; Skobe, Z.; Snapp, K.R.; Socransky, S.S.; Smith, C.M.; Kent, R. Identification of bacterial species on or in crevicular epithelial cells from healthy and periodontally diseased patients using DNA-DNA hybridization. *Oral Microbiol. Immunol.* **1998**, *13*, 30–35. [CrossRef] [PubMed]
90. Madianos, P.N.; Papapanou, P.N.; Nannmark, U.; Dahlen, G.; Sandros, J. Porphyromonas gingivalis FDC381 multiplies and persists within human oral epithelial cells in vitro. *Infect. Immun.* **1996**, *64*, 660–664.

91. Amano, A.; Kuboniwa, M.; Nakagawa, I.; Akiyama, S.; Morisaki, I.; Hamada, S. Prevalence of specific genotypes of *Porphyromonas gingivalis* fimA and periodontal health status. *J. Dent. Res.* **2000**, *79*, 1664–1668. [CrossRef]
92. Jotwani, R.; Cutler, C.W. Fimbriated *Porphyromonas gingivalis* is more efficient than fimbria-deficient *P. gingivalis* in entering human dendritic cells in vitro and induces an inflammatory Th1 effector response. *Infect. Immun.* **2004**, *72*, 1725–1732. [CrossRef]
93. Wang, M.; Liang, S.; Hosur, K.B.; Domon, H.; Yoshimura, F.; Amano, A.; Hajishengallis, G. Differential virulence and innate immune interactions of Type I and II fimbrial genotypes of *Porphyromonas gingivalis*. *Oral Microbiol. Immunol.* **2009**, *24*, 478–484. [CrossRef]
94. Burnett, G.W.; Scherp, H.W. *Oral Microbiology and Infectious Disease*, 3rd ed.; The William & Wilkins Company: Baltimore, MD, USA, 1968; p. 982.
95. Attstrom, R.; Schroeder, H.E. Effect of experimental neutropenia on initial gingivitis in dogs. *Scand. J. Dent. Res.* **1979**, *87*, 7–23. [CrossRef] [PubMed]
96. Sundqvist, G.; Carlsson, J.; Herrmann, B.; Tarnvik, A. Degradation of human immunoglobulins G and M and complement factors C3 and C5 by black-pigmented bacteroides. *J. Med. Microbiol.* **1985**, *19*, 85–94. [CrossRef] [PubMed]
97. Lina, G.; Piemont, Y.; Godail-Gamot, F.; Bes, M.; Peter, M.O.; Gauduchon, V.; Vandenesch, F.; Etienne, J. Involvement of Panton-Valentine leukocidin-producing *Staphylococcus aureus* in primary skin infections and pneumonia. *Clin. Infect. Dis.* **1999**, *29*, 1128–1132. [CrossRef]
98. Tadepalli, S.; Stewart, G.C.; Nagaraja, T.G.; Narayanan, S.K. Human *Fusobacterium necrophorum* strains have a leukotoxin gene and exhibit leukotoxic activity. *J. Med. Microbiol.* **2008**, *57*, 225–231. [CrossRef]
99. Kachlany, S.C. Aggregatibacter actinomycetemcomitans leukotoxin: From threat to therapy. *J. Dent. Res.* **2010**, *89*, 561–570. [CrossRef] [PubMed]
100. Johansson, A. *Aggregatibacter actinomycetemcomitans* leukotoxin: A powerful tool with capacity to cause imbalance in the host inflammatory response. *Toxins* **2011**, *3*, 242–259. [CrossRef] [PubMed]
101. Hoglund Aberg, C.; Kwamin, F.; Claesson, R.; Dahlen, G.; Johansson, A.; Haubek, D. Progression of attachment loss is strongly associated with presence of the JP2 genotype of *Aggregatibacter actinomycetemcomitans*: A prospective cohort study of a young adolescent population. *J. Clin. Periodontal.* **2014**, *41*, 232–241. [CrossRef]
102. Aberg, C.H.; Kelk, P.; Johansson, A. *Aggregatibacter actinomycetemcomitans*: Virulence of its leukotoxin and association with aggressive periodontitis. *Virulence* **2015**, *6*, 188–195. [CrossRef]
103. Fortanier, A.C.; Venekamp, R.P.; Boonacker, C.W.; Hak, E.; Schilder, A.G.; Sanders, E.A.; Damoiseaux, R.A. Pneumococcal conjugate vaccines for preventing acute otitis media in children. *Cochrane Database Syst. Rev.* **2019**, *5*, Cd001480. [CrossRef]
104. Wang, S.; Tafalla, M.; Hanssens, L.; Dolhain, J. A review of *Haemophilus influenzae* disease in Europe from 2000–2014: Challenges, successes and the contribution of hexavalent combination vaccines. *Expert Rev. Vaccines* **2017**, *16*, 1095–1105. [CrossRef]
105. Laine, M.L.; van Winkelhoff, A.J. Virulence of six capsular serotypes of *Porphyromonas gingivalis* in a mouse model. *Oral Microbiol. Immunol.* **1998**, *13*, 322–325. [CrossRef] [PubMed]
106. Gharbia, S.E.; Haapasalo, M.; Shah, H.N.; Kotiranta, A.; Lounatmaa, K.; Pearce, M.A.; Devine, D.A. Characterization of *Prevotella intermedia* and *Prevotella nigrescens* isolates from periodontic and endodontic infections. *J. Periodontal.* **1994**, *65*, 56–61. [CrossRef] [PubMed]
107. Singh, A.; Wyant, T.; Anaya-Bergman, C.; Aduse-Opoku, J.; Brunner, J.; Laine, M.L.; Curtis, M.A.; Lewis, J.P. The capsule of *Porphyromonas gingivalis* leads to a reduction in the host inflammatory response, evasion of phagocytosis, and increase in virulence. *Infect. Immun.* **2011**, *79*, 4533–4542. [CrossRef] [PubMed]
108. Yoshino, T.; Laine, M.L.; van Winkelhoff, A.J.; Dahlen, G. Genotype variation and capsular serotypes of *Porphyromonas gingivalis* from chronic periodontitis and periodontal abscesses. *FEMS Microbiol. Lett.* **2007**, *270*, 75–81. [CrossRef] [PubMed]
109. Slots, J. Focal infection of periodontal origin. *Periodontology 2000* **2019**, *79*, 233–235. [CrossRef] [PubMed]
110. Jepsen, S.; Caton, J.G.; Albandar, J.M.; Bissada, N.F.; Bouchard, P.; Cortellini, P.; Demirel, K.; de Sanctis, M.; Ercoli, C.; Fan, J.; et al. Periodontal manifestations of systemic diseases and developmental and acquired conditions: Consensus report of workgroup 3 of the 2017 world workshop on the classification of periodontal and peri-implant diseases and conditions. *J. Periodontal.* **2018**, *89* (Suppl. S1), S237–S248. [CrossRef] [PubMed]

111. Chen, C.K.; Wu, Y.T.; Chang, Y.C. Association between chronic periodontitis and the risk of Alzheimer's disease: A retrospective, population-based, matched-cohort study. *Alzheimers Res. Ther.* **2017**, *9*, 56. [CrossRef]
112. Potempa, J.; Mydel, P.; Koziel, J. The case for periodontitis in the pathogenesis of rheumatoid arthritis. *Nat. Rev. Rheumatol.* **2017**, *13*, 606–620. [CrossRef]
113. Konig, M.F.; Abusleme, L.; Reinholdt, J.; Palmer, R.J.; Teles, R.P.; Sampson, K.; Rosen, A.; Nigrovic, P.A.; Sokolove, J.; Giles, J.T.; et al. *Aggregatibacter actinomycetemcomitans*-induced hypercitrullination links periodontal infection to autoimmunity in rheumatoid arthritis. *Sci. Transl. Med.* **2016**, *8*, 369ra176. [CrossRef]
114. McGraw, W.T.; Potempa, J.; Farley, D.; Travis, J. Purification, characterization, and sequence analysis of a potential virulence factor from *Porphyromonas gingivalis*, peptidylarginine deiminase. *Infect. Immun.* **1999**, *67*, 3248–3256.

10

Optimal Examination Sites for Periodontal Disease Evaluation: Applying the Item Response Theory Graded Response Model

Yoshiaki Nomura [1], Toshiya Morozumi [2,*], Mitsuo Fukuda [3], Nobuhiro Hanada [1], Erika Kakuta [4], Hiroaki Kobayashi [5], Masato Minabe [2], Toshiaki Nakamura [6], Yohei Nakayama [7], Fusanori Nishimura [8], Kazuyuki Noguchi [6], Yukihiro Numabe [9], Yorimasa Ogata [7], Atsushi Saito [10], Soh Sato [11], Satoshi Sekino [9], Naoyuki Sugano [12], Tsutomu Sugaya [13], Fumihiko Suzuki [14], Keiso Takahashi [15], Hideki Takai [7], Shogo Takashiba [16], Makoto Umeda [17], Hiromasa Yoshie [18], Atsutoshi Yoshimura [19], Nobuo Yoshinari [20] and Taneaki Nakagawa [21]

1 Department of Translational Research, Tsurumi University School of Dental Medicine, Yokohama 230-8501, Japan; nomura-y@tsurumi-u.ac.jp (Y.N.); hanada-n@tsurumi-u.ac.jp (N.H.)

2 Division of Periodontology, Department of Oral Interdisciplinary Medicine, Graduate School of Dentistry, Kanagawa Dental University, Yokosuka 238-8580, Japan; minabe@kdu.ac.jp

3 Department of Periodontology, School of Dentistry, Aichi Gakuin University, Nagoya 464-8650, Japan; fukuda-m@dpc.agu.ac.jp

4 Department of Oral Microbiology, Tsurumi University School of Dental Medicine, Yokohama 230-8501, Japan; kakuta-erika@tsurumi-u.ac.jp

5 Department of Periodontology, Graduate School of Medical and Dental Sciences, Tokyo Medical and Dental University, Tokyo 113-8510, Japan; h-kobayashi.peri@tmd.ac.jp

6 Department of Periodontology, Kagoshima University Graduate School of Medical and Dental Sciences, Kagoshima 890-8544, Japan; toshi-n@dent.kagoshima-u.ac.jp (T.N.); kazuperi@dent.kagoshima-u.ac.jp (K.N.)

7 Department of Periodontology, Nihon University School of Dentistry at Matsudo, Matsudo 271-8587, Japan; nakayama.youhei@nihon-u.ac.jp (Y.N.); ogata.yorimasa@nihon-u.ac.jp (Y.O.); takai.hideki@nihon-u.ac.jp (H.T.)

8 Section of Periodontology, Division of Oral Rehabilitation, Faculty of Dental Science, Kyushu University, Fukuoka 819-0395, Japan; fusanori@dent.kyushu-u.ac.jp

9 Department of Periodontology, School of Life Dentistry at Tokyo, The Nippon Dental University, Tokyo 102-8159, Japan; numabe-y@tky.ndu.ac.jp (Y.N.); sekino-s@tky.ndu.ac.jp (S.S.)

10 Department of Periodontology, Tokyo Dental College, Tokyo 101-0061, Japan; atsaito@tdc.ac.jp

11 Department of Periodontology, School of life Dentistry at Niigata, The Nippon Dental University, Niigata 951-8580, Japan; s-sato@ngt.ndu.ac.jp

12 Department of Periodontology, Nihon University School of Dentistry, Tokyo 101-8310, Japan; sugano.naoyuki@nihon-u.ac.jp

13 Division of Periodontology and Endodontology, Department of Oral Health Science, Hokkaido University Graduate School of Dental Medicine, Sapporo 060-8586, Japan; sugaya@den.hokudai.ac.jp

14 Division of Dental Anesthesiology, Department of Oral Surgery, Ohu University School of Dentistry, Koriyama 963-8611, Japan; f-suzuki@den.ohu-u.ac.jp

15 Division of Periodontics, Department of Conservative Dentistry, Ohu University School of Dentistry, Koriyama 963-8611, Japan; ke-takahashi@den.ohu-u.ac.jp

16 Department of Pathophysiology-Periodontal Science, Okayama University Graduate School of Medicine, Dentistry and Pharmaceutical Sciences, Okayama 700-8525, Japan; stakashi@okayama-u.ac.jp

17 Department of Periodontology, Osaka Dental University, Hirakata 573-1121, Japan; umeda-m@cc.osaka-dent.ac.jp

18 Division of Periodontology, Department of Oral Biological Science, Niigata University Graduate School of Medical and Dental Sciences, Niigata 951-8514, Japan; yoshie119@galaxy.ocn.ne.jp

19 Department of Periodontology and Endodontology, Nagasaki University Graduate School of Biomedical Sciences, Nagasaki 852-8588, Japan; ayoshi@nagasaki-u.ac.jp

20 Department of Periodontology, School of Dentistry, Matsumoto Dental University, Shiojiri 399-0781, Japan; nobuo.yoshinari@mdu.ac.jp

[21] Department of Dentistry and Oral Surgery, School of Medicine, Keio University, Tokyo 60-8582, Japan; tane@z6.keio.jp
* Correspondence: morozumi@kdu.ac.jp

Abstract: Periodontal examination data have a complex structure. For epidemiological studies, mass screenings, and public health use, a simple index that represents the periodontal condition is necessary. Periodontal indices for partial examination of selected teeth have been developed. However, the selected teeth vary between indices, and a justification for the selection of examination teeth has not been presented. We applied a graded response model based on the item response theory to select optimal examination teeth and sites that represent periodontal conditions. Data were obtained from 254 patients who participated in a multicenter follow-up study. Baseline data were obtained from initial follow-up. Optimal examination sites were selected using item information calculated by graded response modeling. Twelve sites—maxillary 2nd premolar (palatal-medial), 1st premolar (palatal-distal), canine (palatal-medial), lateral incisor (palatal-central), central incisor (palatal-distal) and mandibular 1st premolar (lingual, medial)—were selected. Mean values for clinical attachment level, probing pocket depth, and bleeding on probing by full mouth examinations were used for objective variables. Measuring the clinical parameters of these sites can predict the results of full mouth examination. For calculating the periodontal index by partial oral examination, a justification for the selection of examination sites is essential. This study presents an evidence-based partial examination methodology and its modeling.

Keywords: periodontitis; epidemiological index; item response theory; oral examination; diagnosis; bleeding on probing

---

1. Introduction

Periodontal examination should be carried out precisely for the evaluation of periodontal diseases, especially their clinical parameters. Improvement in or progression of periodontitis should be monitored at the site-level along with periodontal treatment [1]. One of the important characteristics of periodontal disease is the localization of infectious processes at specific sites, which eventually leads to tissue destruction [2]. Therefore, the accumulated data obtained during periodontal examination is copious and structurally complex [1]. Each of the 28 teeth has six examination sites for measuring parameters such as bleeding on probing (BOP), periodontal pocket probing depth (PD), and clinical attachment level (CAL). These measurements are evaluated several times throughout the course of periodontal disease treatment. Representative summary statistics include the mean value of CAL and PD, maximum value of CAL and PD, and percentage of sites with BOP (BOP%). Conventionally, summary statistics have been used in several clinical trials for the patient-level evaluation of clinical parameters [3]. However, aggregating summary statistics like the mean value or maximum value can lead to the loss of information [4]. Full-mouth protocols are proven to be the most effective [5]. When time and labor are limited, a simplified index may be necessary to represent the periodontal condition.

Several periodontal indices have been developed for epidemiological surveys and periodontal disease screening: Periodontal disease index (PDI) [6,7], Periodontal Index (PI) [8], Community periodontal index (CPI or CPITN) [8,9], Gingival bone count [10], PMA index [11], Gingival index [12]. They are based on a partial-examination method in which the target teeth for examination vary between the indices. A justification for the selection of these target teeth is not always clear. However, the developers of epidemiological indices may notice that there are several teeth or examination sites within the oral cavity that represent periodontal conditions at an individual level.

In many educational and psychological studies, a latent variable is often used as the outcome variable. These variables cannot be measured directly and are estimated by their response to the observational items. Item response theory (IRT) modeling is an important methodology commonly used for the development of tests to measure the ability by total score of test consisted of items with weighted scores [13]. Through the application of IRT, we can examine each item's reliability and whether it contributes to an overall construct [14,15]. Total score correspond to the sum of the values of periodontal examinations. Items correspond to the values of periodontal examinations. Therefore, IRT is applicable for the indexes used in dental search.

IRT can be applied to the clinical parameters of periodontal disease. The progress of periodontal disease at an individual level corresponds to ability. Susceptibility to the progress of PD, CAL, and BOP corresponds to item difficulty. Discrimination parameter corresponds to the predictability of each site to represent all examination sites or teeth. Previous studies have shown that IRT can efficiently characterize dental caries susceptibility [16,17]. IRT graded response modeling has also been applied in the evaluation of existing measures in several clinical areas, such as those related to swallowing and communication disorders [18,19]. Furthermore, by using IRT models with clinical diagnoses from electronic health records, a constellation of high-risk patients could be identified [20]. Therefore, by applying the IRT model to periodontal data, evidence-based target sites or teeth can be selected to represent and reflect the periodontal conditions of all sites or teeth in the oral cavity.

This study aimed to identify the most reliable subset of teeth able to represent a full-mouth periodontal diagnosis.

2. Materials and Methods

2.1. Study Design

2.1.1. Setting

This study was part of a clinical research project by the Japanese Society of Periodontology, in cooperation with 17 facilities (one clinic and 16 university hospitals) in Japan for the diagnosis of periodontitis [1,21,22]. Two-hundred-fifty-four patients with chronic periodontitis were chosen between February 2009 and February 2012 for this study, who had completed their active treatment regulated by the Japanese health insurance system. All 254 patients who registered the study were analyzed.

2.1.2. Diagnosis

Each patient was diagnosed according to the guideline at the time (Guidelines of the American Academy of Periodontology) [23]. One examiner from each institute (T.M., M.F., H.K., M.M., T.N., Y.N., K.N., S.S., N.S., S.S., T.S., F.S., H.T., H.Y., A.Y., N.Y. and T.N.) was chosen to carry out the oral examinations. Each examiner was a periodontist licensed by the Japanese Society of Periodontology.

Intra- and inter-examiner calibration session were conducted at the beginning and middle of the study period. Diagnosis of periodontitis was based on the proposed criteria by the Center for Disease Control and Prevention (CDC) in partnership with the American Academy of Periodontology (AAP) [24].

2.1.3. Patients

Each patient was $\geq$ 30 years of age, possessed at least 20 teeth, was systemically healthy, and had not been administered immunosuppressive or anti-inflammatory drugs or systemic antibiotics within 3 months before the initiation of the investigation.

2.2. *Research Data*

In this study, we analyzed CAL, PD, BOP, plaque index (PlI), and tooth mobility. CAL was measured at six sites for all of the remaining teeth (mesiobuccal, buccal, distobuccal, mesiolingual, lingual, and distolingual). The data of CAL were categorized as < 4, 4–5, and > 5 mm.

2.3. *Statistical Analysis*

2.3.1. IRT Modeling

Based on the IRT model for ordinal polytomous data, we applied a Graded Response Model [25–29]. Item difficulty, item discrimination, item information for the examined sites, and ability of the subjects were calculated [30–34]. The R software with the ltm package was used to perform the IRT analysis [27]. To reduce the total number of examination sites, sites with small item information were removed from the IRT model. This procedure were based on a step-by-step analysis. Using the data for CAL, a model was constructed for all examination sites (Model 1). Next, out of all 168 examination sites, 28 sites representing the highest information for each tooth (sum of left and right side) were selected. An IRT model was constructed using these 28 sites (Model 2). Out of these 28 sites, 12 sites in six teeth were selected for depicting a higher information (Model 3). Finally, the data from the right and left side were categorized as follows: at least one site with >5 mm CAL; at least one site with 4–5 mm CAL; or both sites with <4 mm CAL. Even though there may be optimal examination sites for each clinical parameter, the examination of numerous sites for each clinical parameter may be a laborious procedure for an epidemiological examiner or clinician. IRT models for BOP and PD were constructed in the same manner as for CAL.

2.3.2. Model Evaluation

For the scatterplot, regression analysis was carried out. Generalized linear models were applied. For optimal link functions, models were evaluated using Akaike's information criteria [35]. Receiver operating characteristic (ROC) curve was used to analyze sensitivities and specificities. The cutoff points were determined as the minimum difference between specificity and sensitivity [36,37]. The mean CAL of all examination sites and community periodontal index (CPI) were used as reference. Diagnostic criteria by the CDC-AAP [24] was used. Statistical Package for the Social Sciences version 24.0 (IBM, Tokyo, Japan) was used to perform the analyses.

To compare the model to other studies, Sensitivity, relative bias (Severity) relative bias (Extent) were calculated [38–40].

2.4. *Ethical Approval*

The study was conducted in compliance with the principles outlined in the Helsinki Declaration. Informed written consent was obtained from each subject, and the protocol was approved by the Institutional Review Board of each participating institution. The ethics committee members' names and reference numbers are listed in Appendix A.

3. Results

3.1. *Descriptive Statistics of the Subjects Participated in this Study*

Descriptive statistics of periodontal clinical parameters were the 3.1 mm for mean of CAL, 2.5 mm for mean of PD, 15.0% for BOP%, and 0.3 for PlI.

3.2. *Optimal Site Selection by IRT Modeling*

The final model for CAL (Model 4) is shown in Table 1, accompanied with models for the remaining clinical parameters. Item information and item response curves of Model 4 are shown in Figure S1.

Using these steps, 168 examination sites were narrowed down to six variables located at 12 sites (same sites on the right and left side). The results of each step from Model 1 to 4 are shown in Table S1. A quick reference for the calculation of ability by Model 4 is presented in Appendix B.

Table 1. Final model (Model 4) for the clinical attachment level.

		Maxilla					Mandibular	AIC	BIC
		2nd Premolar	1st Premolar	Canine	Lateral Incisor	Central Incisor	1st Premolar		
		Palatal	Palatal	Palatal	Palatal	Palatal	Lingual		
		Medial	Distal	Medial	Central	Distal	Medial		
CAL	Extrmt1	0.28	0.45	0.65	1.13	0.75	0.53	1796.06	1859.73
	Extrmt2	1.28	1.24	1.31	1.59	1.38	1.57		
	Discrimination	3.07	3.42	4.51	4.83	3.16	2.03		
	Item information	5.47	5.92	7.97	7.93	5.02	3.27		
PD	Extrmt1	0.72	0.88	0.96	1.35	1.01	1.03	1198.73	1262.41
	Extrmt2	1.46	1.48	1.39	1.79	1.45	1.63		
	Discrimination	3.89	3.38	4.89	4.63	3.90	3.39		
	Item information	6.82	5.37	7.87	7.41	5.94	5.40		
BOP	Extrmt1	1.30	1.22	1.56	1.45	1.63	1.95	686.60	729.04
	Discrimination	3.70	7.71	2.93	16.96	2.48	2.09		
	Item information	3.70	7.62	2.93	16.65	2.48	2.09		
PlI	Extrmt1	0.38	0.47	0.35	0.27	0.47	0.82	1965.74	2029.41
	Extrmt2	1.85	1.70	1.65	1.81	1.96	2.03		
	Discrimination	2.78	3.85	3.86	2.66	2.14	2.19		
	Item information	5.25	7.44	7.50	5.03	3.85	3.76		
Tooth Mobility	Extrmt1	0.87	0.77	1.22	0.69	0.72	1.19	1445.90	1509.57
	Extrmt2	1.90	1.85	2.21	1.79	1.99	2.56		
	Discrimination	2.41	2.53	2.98	3.81	3.23	2.07		
	Item information	4.06	4.39	5.28	7.24	6.11	3.62		

Extrmt: extremity parameters; CAL: clinical attachment level; PD: probing depth; BOP: bleeding on probing; PlI: plaque index. For CAL, it shows the cutoff to discriminate CAL < 4 mm, CAL 4–5 mm, and CAL > 5 mm. Extrmt1 discriminates CAL < 4 mm and (CAL 4–5 mm and CAL > 5 mm), and Extrmt 2 discriminates (CAL < 4 mm and CAL 4–5 mm) and CAL > 5 mm. Discrimination: This parameter shows the height of item characteristic curves. For the item response theory (IRT) analysis, CAL and PD were categorized as at least one site with >6 mm, at least one site with 4–6 mm, or both sites with <4 mm on the left or right side. IRT analysis was carried out using a graded response model. AIC: Akaike's information criterion; BIC: Bayesian information criterion; both are fitness indices, in which small values are more suitable for a model fit.

3.3. *Model Evaluation*

3.3.1. Evaluation of Selected Sites

In clinical practice, the mean values of all examination sites are often used as summary statistics. The selected 12 sites were evaluated using a scatter plot by plotting the mean values of each clinical parameter against the mean values of the selected 12 sites. The results are shown in Figure 1. For each clinical parameter, adequate co-relations were obtained.

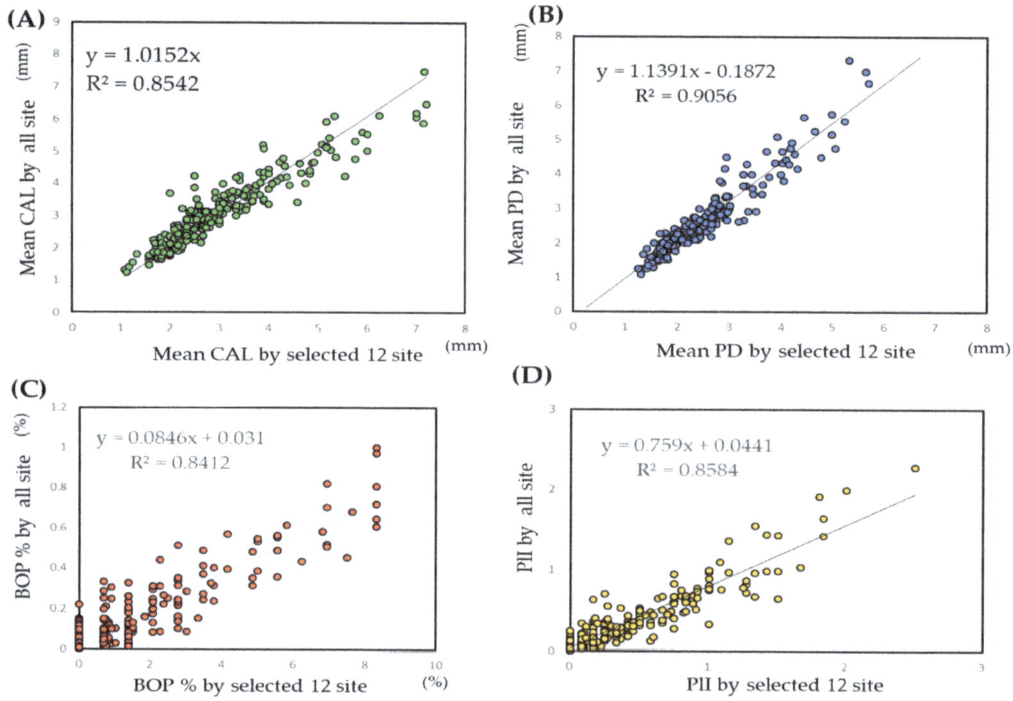

Figure 1. Scatter plot of the mean values of clinical parameters against the mean values of the selected 12 sites. (**A**) CAL: clinical attachment level. (**B**) PD: probing depth. (**C**) BOP: bleeding on probing. (**D**) PlI: plaque index. The selected 12 sites were the same sites that are listed in the Figure 1 legend.

3.3.2. Model Evaluation

The models were evaluated using two methods: correlation between predictive values and observed values and ROC curve analysis. Ability calculated by IRT analysis indicates the predictive value of the sample. The scatter plot of the ability calculated using Model 4 against the mean values of CAL is illustrated in Figure 2. A scatter plot of all 168 examination sites (Model 1) is also presented as a reference. As the plot appears to be a curve, the generalized linear model was applied. The coefficient and intercept were statistically significant. The scatter plot of the result of the generalized linear model against the models for other clinical parameters is shown in Table S2.

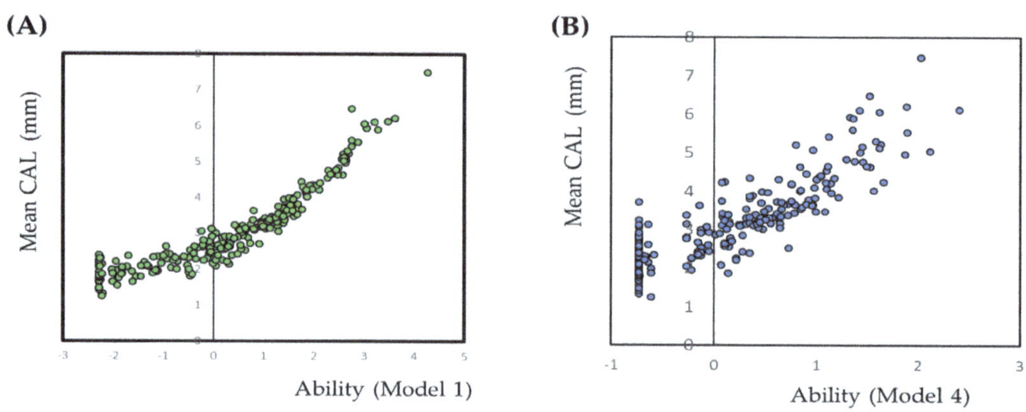

Figure 2. Scatter plot of the mean value of the clinical attachment level against the ability calculated by item response theory. Abilities are calculated using a graded response model under the item response theory approach. Abilities are calculated for all the 168 examined sites (**A**) and the selected six variables at the 12 sites (**B**). Ability means sum of the weighted scores of each items. In this case, ability indicate the sum of the weighted scores of positive for periodontal examination.

The data from the same location site are combined with at least one site with >6 mm, at least one site with 4–6 mm, or both sites <4 mm.

The plot appears to be a curve. Therefore, the generalized linear model is applied for the relationship.

The selected sites were maxillary 2nd premolar (palatal-distal), maxillary 1st premolar (palatal-medial), maxillary Canine (palatal-distal), maxillary lateral incisor (palatal-central), maxillary central incisor (palatal-medial), and mandibular 1st premolar (lingual-medial).

Based on the ROC analysis, sensitivity, specificity, likelihood, and area under ROC curve (AUR) are presented in Table 2. The results of the models for other clinical parameters are also shown in Table 2. For the mean value of CAL >3 mm, sensitivity and specificity were 0.832 and 0.852, respectively, and for >5 mm, they were 0.895 and 0.911, respectively. The ROC curve of each clinical parameter and various cutoff points are presented in Figure S2.

Table 2. Sensitivity, specificity, and area under the receiver operating characteristic curve for the six variables.

		Cutoff Point	Sensitivity	Specificity	AUR
	>3 mm	−0.190	0.832	0.852	0.922
	>3.5 mm	0.193	0.865	0.878	0.939
Mean CAL	>4 mm	0.546	0.891	0.885	0.960
	>4.5 mm	1.033	0.929	0.929	0.978
	>5 mm	1.082	0.895	0.911	0.977
	>3 mm	0.703	0.897	0.912	0.974
	>3.5 mm	0.891	0.926	0.930	0.983
Mean PD	>4 mm	1.202	0.947	0.949	0.985
	>4.5 mm	1.391	1.000	0.971	0.989
	>5 mm	1.548	1.000	0.984	0.992
	>2.5%	−0.097	0.453	0.913	0.671
	>5%	−0.097	0.388	0.939	0.698
BOP	>10%	−0.097	0.571	0.886	0.755
	>20%	−0.097	0.687	0.834	0.804
	>25%	−0.097	0.765	0.813	0.847
	>10	−0.141	0.849	0.829	0.890
	>20	0.313	0.838	0.839	0.915
PlI	>30	0.540	0.824	0.822	0.915
	>40	0.695	0.831	0.776	0.924
	>50	0.710	0.825	0.838	0.912

CAL: clinical attachment level; PD: probing depth; BOP: bleeding on probing; PlI: plaque index; AUR: area under receiver operating characteristic curve. Cutoff points are set in abilities calculated using graded response theory. Graded response theory is one of the models of item response theory.

3.4. *Application of the CAL Model for Diagnosis of Periodontal Disease*

The cutoff point, sensitivity, specificity, and AUR for the diagnosis of periodontal disease by the CDC-AAP are presented in Table 3. ROC curves are shown in Figure S3. For moderate periodontitis, the simple mean CAL of all examination sites is most useful, followed by the mean CAL of optimal examination sites. For severe periodontitis, the CPI is most useful. Simple mean CAL were not obtained similar AUR for CPI.

Table 3. Receiver operating characteristic analysis for the selected optimal examination sites for the diagnosis of periodontal disease.

Diagnosis	Moderate Periodontitis				Severe Periodontitis			
	Cutoff	Sensitivity	Specificity	AUR	Cutoff	Sensitivity	Specificity	AUR
CAL mean (12 sites)	2.20	0.82	0.88	0.91	2.65	0.75	0.72	0.85
CAL mean (All sites)	2.21	0.91	0.92	0.96	3.04	0.78	0.78	0.88
CAL ability (6 value)	−0.72	0.71	0.88	0.82	−0.47	0.86	0.62	0.83
CAL ability (12 sites)	−0.79	0.79	0.79	0.87	0.05	0.81	0.81	0.87
CPI	2	0.84	0.92	0.88	4	0.81	0.94	0.91

CPI: community periodontal index; CAL: clinical attachment level.

3.5. Prediction of Conventional Periodontal Indices by the CAL Model

The model was applied to conventionally use summary statistics, i.e., mean value of CAL, PD, and BOP%. Clinically useful cutoff points were set for each index. The results are presented in Table 4. The best predictors were the mean values of the clinical parameters by the mean values of the 12 selected sites (e.g., mean CAL by the mean CAL of the 12 sites). For obtaining the mean values of PD and BOP%, we were able to obtain higher values of the AUR compared to the CPI by calculating the simple mean CAL of the 12 selected sites. Ability of CAL, weighted CAL, could obtain higher AUR. All ROC curves are shown in Figure S4. By measuring the CAL, all other clinical parameters can be predicted.

3.6. Model Evaluation by Prevalence, Severity, and Extent

The prevalence, relative bias for severity and extent of model 4 were 62%, −0.0035, and −0.017, respectively.

Table 4. Receiver operating characteristic curve analysis of the selected optimal examination sites for the mean values of pocket probing depth, clinical attachment level, and bleeding on probing.

	Cutoff	Sensitivity	Specificity	AUR	Cutoff	Sensitivity	Specificity	AUR	Cutoff	Sensitivity	Specificity	AUR
Mean CAL	**Mean CAL > 3.5 mm**				**Mean CAL > 4 mm**				**Mean CAL > 4.5 mm**			
CAL mean (12 sites)	3.04	0.92	0.90	0.96	3.52	0.91	0.91	0.98	3.95	0.93	0.94	0.99
CAL ability (6 values)	0.16	0.89	0.88	0.95	0.55	0.89	0.88	0.96	1.03	0.93	0.93	0.98
CAL ability (12 site)	0.35	0.89	0.90	0.96	0.69	0.93	0.93	0.97	0.90	0.93	0.93	0.99
CPI	4	0.72	0.77	0.77	2	0.96	0.36	0.81	4	0.86	0.69	0.78
Mean PD	Mean PD > 3.5 mm				Mean PD > 4 mm				Mean PD > 5 mm			
CAL mean (12 sites)	3.90	0.08	0.11	0.96	4.13	0.95	0.92	0.97	5.04	1.00	0.96	0.99
CAL ability (6 values)	4.03	0.89	0.91	0.97	0.99	0.89	0.89	0.96	1.44	1.00	0.96	0.99
CAL ability (12 sites)	0.70	0.85	0.87	0.95	0.89	0.89	0.89	0.96	1.20	1.00	0.93	0.98
CPI	4	1.00	0.71	0.85	4	1.00	0.68	0.84	4	1.00	0.65	0.82
PD mean (12 sites)	0.68	0.89	0.86	0.95	3.78	1.00	0.95	0.99	4.46	1.00	0.97	0.99
BOP	BOP > 10%				BOP > 20%				BOP > 30%			
CAL mean (12 sites)	2.65	0.64	0.65	0.71	2.96	0.76	0.75	0.83	3.26	0.82	0.80	0.89
CAL ability (6 values)	−0.26	0.65	0.62	0.69	0.12	0.74	0.77	0.80	0.46	0.77	0.82	0.86
CAL ability (12 sites)	0.03	0.63	0.66	0.67	0.31	0.74	0.75	0.80	0.60	0.75	0.85	0.85
CPI	4	0.59	0.79	0.72	4	0.75	0.76	0.80	4	0.84	0.72	0.81
BOP% mean (12 sites)	0.73	0.84	0.87	0.91	1.97	0.81	0.94	0.95	2.18	0.91	0.92	0.97

CAL: clinical attachment level; PD: probing depth; BOP: bleeding on probing; AUR: area under receiver operating characteristic curve; CPI: community periodontal index.

4. Discussion

Public health applications of periodontal examination such as epidemiological surveys, mass screenings, and community diagnosis, simplified indices that represent an indivisible disease status are indispensable. For this purpose, several indices have been developed [6–12]. Developed by the World Health Organization, the CPI has been utilized in epidemiological surveys not just for community diagnosis but also for the screening of periodontal disease. Originally, the index was calculated through the examination of eight teeth [41]. It has currently been revised to include the examination of all teeth [42]; however, the original method of examining just eight teeth is also still applied. According to Japan's Survey of Dental Diseases, national oral health surveys, which are conducted every six years, still use the original CPI examination method. However, we were unable to find any justification for the tooth-selection methodology or periodontal indices used in these surveys [43].

Several methods that do not require oral examinations for the screening of periodontal disease have been proposed [36,44–48]. These include questionnaires [49,50] and biochemical analysis of the saliva [47] or gingival crevicular fluid [51]. However, the sensitivity and specificity of questionnaires used for periodontitis screening is not high enough, and using biochemical analyses requires a special measuring device. Therefore, oral examinations are still widely used for periodontal disease screenings.

In comparison to the CPI, our model was superior in predicting clinical parameters and almost equivalent in diagnosing moderate periodontitis. Further, partial examination using the CPI requires the examination of 60 sites; our model requires the examination of only 6–12 sites. Furthermore, the examination sites presented by our model are more representative of the periodontal conditions in an oral cavity. As shown in Table 4, the partial examination of these sites represents the mean value of each examined index by the mean value of all examination sites in the oral cavity. By simply measuring the CAL, all other clinical parameters can be predicted. The model presented in this study was derived using the IRT approach. The IRT model is very useful for the selection of items that have high information. However, IRT models can only process dichotomous variables or ordinal scale; they are unable to process contentious variables. At this stage, a loss of information can occur. Therefore, the simple mean of 12 selected sites is more suitable for calculating some of the predictions presented in this study.

When the 12 selected sites are compared with other partial examination protocol, sampling sites are predominantly small. Sampling sites of other protocols were 84 [38,39,52,53], 60 [54], and 56 [38,39,52]. Partial examination protocol by high number of examination site can detect small number of deep CAL or PD. The sensitivity indicate to detect subject with at least one site of CAL > 4 mm. The sensitivity by 84 examination site was 92% [52], by 56 site was 66% [52] and by 28 site was 57% [52]. The sensitivity by the 12 site in this study was 62%. In addition, relative bias of severity of the 12 sites, which estimate the difference of mean value of CAL between full mouth examination, was −0.0035. This value protocols by 84 site were 0.009 [52], −0.046 [38] and −0.01 [53]. The 12 sites based on statistical model may equal, in other partial examination protocol, more than 5 times higher numbers of examination sites.

In this study, the teeth selected for examination included premolars and anterior teeth; the molars were excluded. The molar is a double-rooted tooth with complex anatomical root morphology, including root length, furcation area, and divergence of root and root trunk. Cervical enamel projections and enamel pearls also occur commonly in molars and are considered to be risk factors for periodontal disease; however, their occurrence varies among different individuals [55]. Additionally, molars have to withstand high occlusal forces, which can contribute to periodontal tissue destruction. Therefore, we excluded molars from representing oral examination sites in our analysis.

The periodontal disease index is used for assessing the periodontal status in epidemiological surveys; six target teeth (maxillary right 1stmolar, maxillary left central incisor, maxillary left 1st premolar, mandibular left 1st molar, mandibular left 1st molar, and mandibular right 1st premolar) are scored for the assessment of the disease. However, a sufficient justification for the selection of these teeth has not been provided [6]. For the index, evidence is indispensable.

In this study, optimal sites were selected based in the item information through the models presented in Table S1, and Table 1. Twelve sites: maxillary 2nd premolar (palatal-medial), 1st premolar (palatal-distal), 3 canine (palatal-medial), lateral incisor (palatal-central), central incisor (palatal-distal) and mandibular 1st premolar (lingual-medial) selected in this study were based on statistical modeling and represented the periodontal conditions. a full mouth examination is a best method; however, as time and labor are limited, partial examination may be applicable. Partial examination of these sites may be useful tool for epidemiological studies, mass screenings, and public health use.

There are several limitations in this study. The study population was consisted of the patients who experienced active periodontal treatment. The wider population is necessary to confirm the robustness of the model presented in this study. However, several partial-mouth assessments were not based on the statistical modeling. The strength of the model presented in this study was based on the IRT model, and weights for the site were calculated to improve the predictive values.

5. Conclusions

For calculating the periodontal index by partial oral examination, a justification for the selection of examination sites is necessary. This study presents an evidence-based partial examination method and its modeling. The 12 sites presented in this study almost equal to other partial examination protocol, which have more than 5 times the number of sampling sites.

Author Contributions: Conceptualization, Y.N. (Yoshiaki Nomura) and T.M.; methodology, Y.N. (Yoshiaki Nomura); software, Y.N. (Yoshiaki Nomura); validation, E.K. and N.H.; formal analysis, Y.N. (Yoshiaki Nomura); investigation, T.M., M.F., H.K., M.M., T.N. (Taneaki Nakagawa), Y.N. (Yukihiro Numabe), F.N., K.N., Y.N. (Yohei Nakayama), Y.O., A.S., S.S. (Soh Sato), N.S., S.S. (Satoshi Sekino), T.S., F.S., K.T., H.T., M.U., H.Y., A.Y., N.Y. and T.N. (Toshiaki Nakamura); data curation, S.T.; writing—original draft preparation, Y.N. (Yoshiaki Nomura); writing—review and editing, Y.N. (Yoshiaki Nomura) and T.M.; visualization, Y.N. (Yoshiaki Nomura); supervision, T.M. and H.Y.; project administration, T.M., T.N. (Taneaki Nakagawa) and H.Y.; funding acquisition, T.N. (Taneaki Nakagawa) and H.Y. All authors have read and agreed to the published version of the manuscript.

Acknowledgments: The authors thank Toshihide Noguchi, Masamitsu Kawanami, Koichi Ito, Yuichi Izumi, Yoshitaka Hara, Osamu Fujise, Yuzo Abe, Tomoo Kono, Asako Makino-Oi, and Chie Fukaya, for their advice and useful comments.

Appendix A

List of ethical committees and their approval numbers.

Institution	Name of the Ethics Committee	Reference Number
Niigata University	The regional ethical committee of the Faculty of Dentistry, Niigata University	20-R17-08-06
Keio University	Keio University School of Medicine, Ethics Committee	20080096
Hokkaido University	Institutional Review Board for Clinical Research of Hokkaido University Hospital	008-0113
Ohu University	Ohu University Research Ethics Committee	52

Institution	Name of the Ethics Committee	Reference Number
School of life Dentistry at Niigata, The Nippon Dental University	The Ethical Review Committee of The Nippon Dental University School of Life Dentistry at Niigata	151
Tokyo Dental College	Ethics Committee of Tokyo Dental College	208
Bunkyo-Dori Dental Clinic	The regional ethical committee of the Faculty of Dentistry, Niigata University	20-R17-08-06
Nihon University School of Dentistry at Matsudo	Ethics Committee in Nihon University School of Dentistry at Matsudo	EC 08-014
Tokyo Medical and Dental University	Dental Research Ethics Committee of Tokyo Medical and Dental University	660
Nihon University School of Dentistry	Ethical Committee of Nihon University School of Dentistry	EP08D016
School of Life Dentistry at Tokyo, The Nippon Dental University	The Institutional Review Board of Nippon Dental University.	2-1-22
Matsumoto Dental University	The Ethics Committee of Matsumoto Dental University	0090
Aichi Gakuin University	Ethics Committee: Aichi Gakuin University, School of Dentistry	158
Osaka Dental University	the Ethics Committee of Osaka Dental University	80712
Kyushu University	Ethical Committee of Kyushu University Faculty of Dental Science	20-11
Nagasaki University	The Ethics Committee, Nagasaki University Graduate School of Biomedical Sciences	0846-2
Kagoshima University	Ethical Committee of Kagoshima University Medical and Dental Hospital.	20-58

Appendix B

Quick reference for the calculation of ability by Model 4.

Maxilla					Mandibular	Ability
5	4	3	2	1	4	
Palatal	Palatal	Palatal	Palatal	Palatal	Lingual	
Medial	Distal	Medial	Central	Distal	Medial	
1	1	1	1	1	1	−0.932
1	1	1	1	1	2	−0.442
1	1	1	1	2	1	−0.223
1	1	1	1	2	2	0.052
1	1	1	1	3	2	0.159
1	1	1	2	1	1	0.16
1	1	2	1	1	1	−0.013
1	1	2	1	1	2	0.21
1	1	2	1	2	1	0.321

Maxilla					Mandibular	Ability
5	4	3	2	1	4	
Palatal	Palatal	Palatal	Palatal	Palatal	Lingual	
Medial	Distal	Medial	Central	Distal	Medial	
1	1	3	1	1	1	0.108
1	1	3	3	2	2	1.315
1	2	1	1	1	1	−0.506
1	2	1	1	1	2	−0.156
1	2	1	1	1	3	−0.066
1	2	1	1	2	1	0.009
1	2	2	1	1	3	0.434
1	2	2	1	2	2	0.575
1	2	2	1	3	1	0.566
1	2	2	2	2	1	0.828
1	3	1	1	2	2	0.293
1	3	2	2	2	1	0.887
2	1	1	1	1	1	−0.306
2	1	1	1	1	2	−0.008
2	1	1	1	2	1	0.135
2	1	1	2	2	1	0.65
2	1	2	1	1	1	0.28
2	1	2	1	1	3	0.522
2	1	2	2	2	3	1.038
2	1	2	3	3	2	1.334
2	1	3	1	1	1	0.468
2	1	3	1	3	1	0.887
2	2	1	1	1	1	−0.053
2	2	1	1	1	2	0.176
2	2	1	1	1	3	0.262
2	2	1	1	2	2	0.449
2	2	1	1	2	3	0.53
2	2	1	2	1	1	0.542
2	2	2	1	1	1	0.411
2	2	2	1	1	2	0.549
2	2	2	1	2	2	0.727
2	2	2	1	3	2	0.847
2	2	2	2	2	2	1.027
2	2	2	2	3	3	1.228
2	2	2	3	2	1	1.121
2	2	3	1	1	1	0.613

Maxilla					Mandibular	Ability
5	4	3	2	1	4	
Palatal	Palatal	Palatal	Palatal	Palatal	Lingual	
Medial	Distal	Medial	Central	Distal	Medial	
2	2	3	2	2	2	1.229
2	2	3	2	2	3	1.31
2	2	3	2	3	2	1.373
2	3	1	1	1	1	0.023
2	3	1	1	1	3	0.339
2	3	2	1	2	1	0.68
2	3	2	1	2	2	0.785
2	3	2	1	3	3	0.991
2	3	2	2	2	2	1.083
2	3	2	2	3	2	1.213
2	3	3	1	2	3	1.081
2	3	3	1	3	1	1.048
2	3	3	2	1	1	1.097
2	3	3	2	2	3	1.38
2	3	3	3	2	3	1.701
3	1	1	1	2	3	0.61
3	1	1	1	3	2	0.663
3	1	3	3	3	3	1.979
3	2	1	1	1	2	0.393
3	2	2	1	2	1	0.773
3	2	2	1	2	2	0.868
3	2	2	1	3	2	0.995
3	2	2	2	3	1	1.209
3	2	2	3	3	3	1.684
3	2	3	2	1	1	1.181
3	2	3	2	3	2	1.521
3	2	3	3	3	1	1.801
3	2	3	3	3	3	2.042
3	3	1	1	1	2	0.468
3	3	2	1	2	2	0.927
3	3	2	2	1	3	1.185
3	3	2	2	2	1	1.137
3	3	2	2	3	3	1.442
3	3	2	3	2	2	1.475
3	3	2	3	3	2	1.664
3	3	3	1	2	3	1.243
3	3	3	1	3	1	1.222

Maxilla					Mandibular	Ability
5	4	3	2	1	4	
Palatal	Palatal	Palatal	Palatal	Palatal	Lingual	
Medial	Distal	Medial	Central	Distal	Medial	
3	3	3	2	1	3	1.439
3	3	3	2	2	1	1.362
3	3	3	2	2	3	1.53
3	3	3	3	2	3	1.9
3	3	3	3	3	2	2.012
3	3	3	3	3	3	2.228

1: CAL <4mm; 2: CAL = 4–6mm; 3: CAL >6mm.

References

1. Nomura, Y.; Morozumi, T.; Nakagawa, T.; Sugaya, T.; Kawanami, M.; Suzuki, F.; Takahashi, K.; Abe, Y.; Sato, S.; Makino-Oi, A.; et al. Site-level progression of periodontal disease during a follow-up period. *PLoS ONE* **2017**, *12*, e0188670. [CrossRef] [PubMed]
2. Socransky, S.S.; Haffajee, A.D. The nature of periodontal diseases. *Ann. Periodontol.* **1997**, *2*, 3–10. [CrossRef] [PubMed]
3. Sharma, P.; Cockwell, P.; Dietrich, T.; Ferro, C.; Ives, N.; Chapple, I.L.C. Influence of successful periodontal intervention in renal disease (INSPIRED): Study protocol for a randomized controlled pilot clinical trial. *Trials* **2017**, *18*, 535. [CrossRef] [PubMed]
4. Cho, Y.; Kim, H.Y. Analysis of periodontal data using mixed effects models. *J. Periodontal. Implant. Sci.* **2015**, *45*, 2–7. [CrossRef] [PubMed]
5. Botelho, J.; Machado, V.; Proença, L.; Mendes, J.J. The 2018 periodontitis case definition improves accuracy performance of full-mouth partial diagnostic protocols. *Sci. Rep.* **2020**, *10*, 7093. [CrossRef] [PubMed]
6. Ramfjord, S.P. The Periodontal Disease Index (PDI). *J. Periodontol.* **1967**, *38*, S602–S610. [CrossRef]
7. Wang, W.J.; Liu, C.Y.; Liu, D.Z.; Lee, C.J. Survey of periodontal disease among workers in Tianjin using Ramfjord's Periodontal Disease Index (PDI). *Community Dent. Oral Epidemiol.* **1987**, *15*, 98–99. [CrossRef] [PubMed]
8. Cutress, T.W.; Hunter, P.B.; Hoskins, D.I. Comparison of the Periodontal Index (PI) and Community Periodontal Index of Treatment Needs (CPITN). *Community Dent. Oral Epidemiol.* **1986**, *14*, 39–42. [CrossRef]
9. Ainamo, J.; Barmes, D.; Beagrie, G.; Cutress, T.; Martin, J.; Infirri, S.J. Development of the World Health Organization (WHO) community periodontal index of treatment needs (CPITN). *Int. Dent. J.* **1982**, *32*, 281–291.
10. Dunning, J.M.; Leach, L.B. Gingival-bone count: A method for epidemiological study of periodontal disease. *J. Dent. Res.* **1960**, *39*, 506–513. [CrossRef]
11. Massler, M. The P-M-A index for the assessment of gingivitis. *J. Periodontol.* **1967**, *38*, S592–S601. [CrossRef] [PubMed]
12. Löe, H. The Gingival Index, the Plaque Index and the Retention Index Systems. *J. Periodontol.* **1967**, *38*, S610–S616. [CrossRef]
13. Edelen, M.O.; Reeve, B.B. Applying item response theory (IRT) modeling to questionnaire development; evaluation; and refinement. *Qual. Life Res.* **2007**, *16*, 5–18. [CrossRef] [PubMed]
14. Thomas, M.L. Advances in applications of item response theory to clinical assessment. *Psychol. Assess.* **2019**, *12*, 1442–1455. [CrossRef]
15. Reise, S.P.; Waller, N.G. Item response theory and clinical measurement. *Annu. Rev. Clin. Psychol.* **2009**, *5*, 27–48. [CrossRef]
16. Nomura, Y.; Otsuka, R.; Wint, W.Y.; Okada, A.; Hasegawa, R.; Hanada, N. Tooth-Level Analysis of Dental Caries in Primary Dentition in Myanmar Children. *Int. J. Environ. Res. Public Health* **2020**, *17*, 7613. [CrossRef]

17. Nomura, Y.; Maung, K.; Khine, E.M.K.; Sint, K.M.; Lin, M.P.; Myint, M.K.W.; Aung, T.; Sogabe, K.; Otsuka, R.; Okada, A.; et al. Prevalence of dental caries in 5- and 6-year-old Myanmar children. *Int. J. Dent.* **2019**, *2019*, 5948379. [CrossRef]
18. Donovan, N.J.; Rosenbek, J.C.; Ketterson, T.U.; Velozo, C.A. Adding meaning to measurement: Initial rasch analysis of the ASHA FACS social communication subtest. *Aphasiology* **2006**, *20*, 362–373. [CrossRef]
19. Cordier, R.; Joosten, A.; Clavé, P.; Schindler, A.; Bülow, M.; Demir, N.; Arslan, S.S.; Speyer, R. Evaluating the psychometric properties of the eating assessment tool (EAT-10) using rasch analysis. *Dysphagia* **2017**, *32*, 250–260. [CrossRef]
20. Prenovost, K.M.; Fihn, S.D.; Maciejewski, M.L.; Nelson, K.; Vijan, S.; Rosland, A.M. Using item response theory with health system data to identify latent groups of patients with multiple health conditions. *PLoS ONE* **2018**, *13*, e0206915. [CrossRef]
21. Morozumi, T.; Nakagawa, T.; Nomura, Y.; Sugaya, T.; Kawanami, M.; Suzuki, F.; Takahashi, K.; Abe, Y.; Sato, S.; Makino-Oi, A.; et al. Salivary pathogen and serum antibody to assess the progression of chronic periodontitis: A 24-mo prospective multicenter cohort study. *J. Periodontal. Res.* **2016**, *51*, 768–778. [CrossRef] [PubMed]
22. Kakuta, E.; Nomura, Y.; Morozumi, T.; Nakagawa, T.; Nakamura, T.; Noguchi, K.; Yoshimura, A.; Hara, Y.; Fujise, O.; Nishimura, F.; et al. Assessing the progression of chronic periodontitis using subgingival pathogen levels: A 24-month prospective multicenter cohort study. *BMC Oral Health* **2017**, *17*, 46. [CrossRef] [PubMed]
23. Krebs, K.A.; Clem, D.S., 3rd. American Academy of Periodontology, Guidelines for the management of patients with periodontal diseases. *J. Periodontol.* **2006**, *77*, 1607–1611. [CrossRef] [PubMed]
24. Eke, P.I.; Page, R.C.; Wei, L.; Evans, G.T.; Genco, R.J. Update of the case definitions for population-based surveillance of periodontitis. *J. Periodontol.* **2012**, *83*, 1449–1454. [CrossRef]
25. Yang, R.; Donaldson, G.W.; Edelman, L.S.; Cloyes, K.G.; Sanders, N.A.; Pepper, G.A. Fear of older adult falling questionnaire for caregivers (FOAFQ-CG): Evidence from content validity and item-response theory graded-response modelling. *J. Adv. Nurs.* **2020**, *76*, 2768–2780. [CrossRef]
26. Khazaal, Y.; Breivik, K.; Billieux, J.; Zullino, D.; Thorens, G.; Achab, S.; Gmel, G.; Chatton, A. Game addiction scale assessment through a nationally representative sample of young adult men: Item response heory graded-response modeling. *J. Med. Internet Res.* **2018**, *20*, e10058. [CrossRef]
27. Rizopoulos, D. An R package for latent variable modelling and item response theory analyses. *J. Stat. Softw.* **2006**, *17*, 1–25. [CrossRef]
28. Molenaar, D.; Dolan, C.V.; Boeck, P.D. The Heteroscedastic graded response model with a skewed latent trait: Testing statistical and substantive hypotheses related to skewed item category functions. *Psychometrika* **2012**, *77*, 455–478. [CrossRef]
29. Kang, H.A.; Su, Y.H.; Chang, H.H. A note on monotonicity of item response functions for ordered polytomous item response theory models. *Br. J. Math. Stat. Psychol.* **2018**, *71*, 523–535. [CrossRef]
30. Nomura, Y.; Okada, A.; Kakuta, E.; Otsuka, R.; Saito, H.; Maekawa, H.; Daikoku, H.; Hanada, N.; Sato, T. Workforce and Contents of Home Dental Care in Japanese Insurance System. *Int. J. Dent.* **2020**, *2020*, 7316796. [CrossRef]
31. Nomura, Y.; Kakuta, E.; Okada, A.; Yamamoto, Y.; Tomonari, H.; Hosoya, N.; Hanada, N.; Yoshida, N.; Takei, N. Prioritization of the Skills to Be Mastered for the Daily Jobs of Japanese Dental Hygienists. *Int. J. Dent.* **2020**, *2020*, 4297646. [CrossRef] [PubMed]
32. Nomura, Y.; Kakuta, E.; Okada, A.; Otsuka, R.; Shimada, M.; Tomizawa, Y.; Taguchi, C.; Arikawa, K.; Daikoku, H.; Sato, T.; et al. Effects of self-assessed chewing ability, tooth loss and serum albumin on mortality in 80-year-old individuals: A 20-year follow-up study. *BMC Oral Health.* **2020**, *20*, 122. [CrossRef] [PubMed]
33. Nomura, Y.; Tsutsumi, I.; Nagasaki, M.; Tsuda, H.; Koga, F.; Kashima, N.; Uraguchi, M.; Okada, A.; Kakuta, E.; Hanada, N. Supplied Food Consistency and Oral Functions of Institutionalized Elderly. *Int. J. Dent.* **2020**, *2020*, 3463056. [CrossRef] [PubMed]
34. Nomura, Y.; Matsuyama, T.; Fukai, K.; Okada, A.; Ida, M.; Yamauchi, N.; Hanamura, H.; Yabuki, Y.; Watanabe, K.; Sugawara, M.; et al. PRECEDE-PROCEED model based questionnaire and saliva tests for oral health checkup in adult. *J. Oral Sci.* **2019**, *61*, 544–548. [CrossRef] [PubMed]
35. Zheng, B.; Agresti, A. Summarizing the predictive power of a generalized linear model. *Stat. Med.* **2000**, *19*, 1771–1781. [CrossRef]

36. Nomura, Y.; Okada, A.; Kakuta, E.; Gunji, T.; Kajiura, S.; Hanada, N. A new screening method for periodontitis: An alternative to the community periodontal index. *BMC Oral Health* **2016**, *16*, 64. [CrossRef]
37. Kudo, C.; Naruishi, K.; Maeda, H.; Abiko, Y.; Hino, T.; Iwata, M.; Mitsuhashi, C.; Murakami, S.; Nagasawa, T.; Nagata, T.; et al. Assessment of use of plasma/serum IgG test to screen for periodontitis. *J. Dent. Res.* **2012**, *91*, 1190–1195. [CrossRef]
38. Kingman, A.; Susin, C.; Albandar, J.M. Effect of partial recording protocols on severity estimates of periodontal disease. *J. Clin. Periodontol.* **2008**, *35*, 659–667. [CrossRef]
39. Susin, C.; Kingman, A.; Albandar, J.M. Effect of partial recording protocols on estimates of prevalence of periodontal disease. *J. Periodontol.* **2005**, *76*, 262–267. [CrossRef]
40. Tran, D.T.; Gay, I.; Du, X.L.; Fu, Y.; Bebermeyer, R.D.; Neumann, A.S.; Streckfus, C.; Chan, W.; Walji, M.F. Assessing periodontitis in populations: A systematic review of the validity of partial-mouth examination protocols. *J. Clin. Periodontol.* **2013**, *40*, 1064–1071. [CrossRef]
41. World Health Organization. *Oral Health Surveys Basic Methods*, 4th ed.; World Health Organization: Geneva, Switzerland, 1997; p. 39.
42. World Health Organization. *Oral Health Surveys Basic Methods*, 5th ed.; World Health Organization: Geneva, Switzerland, 2013; pp. 47–49.
43. Ministry of Health, Labour and Welfare Japan. Survey of Dental Diseases. Available online: https://www.mhlw.go.jp/toukei/list/62-28.html (accessed on 1 September 2020).
44. Okada, A.; Nomura, Y.; Sogabe, K.; Oku, H.; Gillbreath, S.A.; Hino, F.; Hayashi, H.; Yoshino, H.; Utsunomiya, H.; Suzuki, K.; et al. Comparison of salivary hemoglobin measurements for periodontitis screening. *J. Oral Sci.* **2017**, *59*, 63–69. [CrossRef] [PubMed]
45. Kakuta, E.; Nomura, Y.; Naono, Y.; Koresawa, K.; Shimizu, K.; Hanada, N. Correlation between health-care costs and salivary tests. *Int. Dent. J.* **2013**, *63*, 249–253. [CrossRef] [PubMed]
46. Nomura, Y.; Shimada, Y.; Hanada, N.; Numabe, Y.; Kamoi, K.; Sato, T.; Gomi, K.; Arai, T.; Inagaki, K.; Fukuda, M.; et al. Salivary biomarkers for predicting the progression of chronic periodontitis. *Arch. Oral Biol.* **2012**, *57*, 413–420. [CrossRef] [PubMed]
47. Nomura, Y.; Okada, A.; Tamaki, Y.; Miura, H. Salivary Levels of Hemoglobin for Screening Periodontal Disease: A Systematic Review. *Int. J. Dent.* **2018**, *2018*, 2541204. [CrossRef]
48. Nomura, Y.; Tamaki, Y.; Tanaka, T.; Arakawa, H.; Tsurumoto, A.; Kirimura, K.; Sato, T.; Hanada, N.; Kamoi, K. Screening of periodontitis with salivary enzyme tests. *J. Oral Sci.* **2006**, *48*, 177–183. [CrossRef]
49. Chatzopoulos, G.S.; Tsalikis, L.; Konstantinidis, A.; Kotsakis, G.A. A two-domain self-report measure of periodontal disease has good accuracy for periodontitis screening in dental school outpatients. *J. Periodontol.* **2016**, *87*, 1165–1173. [CrossRef]
50. Wright, N.M.; Cheng, B.; Tafreshi, S.N.; Lamster, I.B. A simple self-report health assessment questionnaire to identify oral diseases. *Int. Dent. J.* **2018**, *68*, 428–432. [CrossRef]
51. Preianò, M.; Savino, R.; Villella, C.; Pelaia, C.; Terracciano, R. Gingival crevicular fluid peptidome profiling in healthy and in periodontal diseases. *Int. J. Mol. Sci.* **2020**, *21*, 5270. [CrossRef]
52. Kingman, A.; Albandar, J.M. Methodological aspects of epidemiological studies of periodontal diseases. *Periodontology* **2002**, *29*, 11–30. [CrossRef]
53. Vettore, M.V.; de Lamarca, G.A.; Leao, A.T.; Sheiham, A.; do Leal, M.C. Partial recording protocols for periodontal disease assessment in epidemiological surveys. *Cademos Saude Publica* **2007**, *23*, 33–42. [CrossRef]
54. Benigeri, M.; Brodeur, J.M.; Payette, M.; Charbonneau, A.; Ismail, A.I. Community periodontal index of treatment needs and prevalence of periodontal conditions. *J. Clin. Periodontol.* **2000**, *27*, 308–312. [CrossRef] [PubMed]
55. Newman, M.G.; Takei, H.H.; Klokkevod, P.R.; Carranza, F.A. Clinical risk assessment. In *Carranza's Clinical Periodontology*; Elsevier Saunders: Philadelphia, PA, USA, 2012; pp. 370–372.

11

TREM-1 is Upregulated in Experimental Periodontitis and its Blockade Inhibits IL-17A and RANKL Expression and Suppresses Bone Loss

Nagihan Bostanci [1,2,*], Toshiharu Abe [3], Georgios N. Belibasakis [1,2] and George Hajishengallis [3]

1 Division of Oral Diseases, Department of Dental Medicine, Karolinska Institutet, 14104 Huddinge, Sweden; george.belibasakis@ki.se
2 Center of Dental Medicine, University of Zürich, 8032 Zürich, Switzerland
3 Department of Basic and Translational Sciences, School of Dental Medicine, University of Pennsylvania, Philadelphia, PA 19104, USA; toshiharu@ikeshita-abeshika.com (T.A.); geoh@upenn.edu (G.H.)
* Correspondence: nagihan.bostanci@ki.se

Abstract: Aim: Triggering receptor expressed on myeloid cells-1 (TREM-1) is a modifier of local and systemic inflammation. There is clinical evidence implicating TREM-1 in the pathogenesis of periodontitis. However, a cause-and-effect relationship has yet to be demonstrated, as is the underlying mechanism. The aim of this study was to elucidate the role of TREM-1 using the murine ligature-induced periodontitis model. Methods: A synthetic antagonistic LP17 peptide or sham control was microinjected locally into the palatal gingiva of the ligated molar teeth. Results: Mice treated with the LP17 inhibitor developed significantly less bone loss as compared to sham-treated mice, although there were no differences in total bacterial load on the ligatures. To elucidate the impact of LP17 on the host response, we analyzed the expression of a number of immune-modulating genes. The LP17 peptide altered the expression of 27/92 genes ≥ two-fold, but only interleukin (IL)-17A was significantly downregulated (4.9-fold). Importantly, LP17 also significantly downregulated the receptor activator of nuclear factor kappa-B-ligand (RANKL) to osteoprotegerin (OPG) ratio that drives osteoclastic bone resorption in periodontitis. Conclusion: Our findings show for the first time that TREM-1 regulates the IL-17A-RANKL/OPG axis and bone loss in experimental periodontitis, and its therapeutic blockade may pave the way to a novel treatment for human periodontitis.

Keywords: TREM-1; periodontal disease; intervention; inflammation; LP17; IL-17; RANKL; OPG

1. Introduction

Periodontitis entails the destruction of the tooth-supporting (periodontal) tissues, as an outcome of their inflammatory response to the juxtaposed microbial biofilm forming on the tooth surface [1,2]. Although oral bacteria are essential for initiation of the disease, the resulting inflammation is what causes collateral damage to the tissues, which may eventually lead to tooth loss. The inflammatory mediators that lead to alveolar bone destruction form an intricate network [3,4], in which the receptor activator of NF-κB ligand (RANKL)/osteoprotegerin (OPG) system plays a crucial role as a terminal regulator of the resulting osteoclastogenesis and bone resorption [5,6]. Recently discovered host molecules, acting between the microbial challenge and the RANKL/OPG system, may lead to better understanding of the pathogenesis of periodontal disease and offer novel targets for therapeutic intervention.

Triggering receptor expressed on myeloid cells 1 (TREM-1), a member of the immunoglobulin superfamily, has been defined as a modifier of local and systemic inflammation, especially in response to bacterial infections [7–9]. Bacterial infection can upregulate the membrane-bound and soluble forms of TREM-1, which in turn amplifies inflammation. This is a particularly crucial response associated with systemic sepsis [10,11]. Blockade of TREM-1 engagement by either soluble forms of TREM-1 or synthetic peptides thereof reduces hyper-inflammatory responses and morbidity [12]. In a TREM-1 knock-out mouse model of viral or parasitic infection, it was demonstrated that the lack of TREM-1 signaling mitigated the severity of inflammation and disease (as compared to the wild-type mice) without, however, affecting pathogen clearance [13]. The study by Weber et al. [13] suggested that TREM-1 regulates inflammation, and that its therapeutic targeting may be beneficial in infection-driven inflammatory diseases without compromising pathogen clearance.

There is also correlative evidence to suggest that TREM-1 might modify periodontal inflammation. Specifically, the presence or expression of TREM-1 is increased in saliva, serum [14,15], gingival crevicular fluid [16–18], and gingival tissues [19] of patients with periodontitis as compared to individuals with periodontal health. TREM-1 levels also positively correlate with the levels of putative periodontal pathogens present in subgingival biofilms or lysed gingival tissue [16,19]. In this respect, multispecies biofilms [19] or *Porphyromonas gingivalis* alone induce TREM-1 gene expression in monocytes [20], whereas sub-antimicrobial doses of doxycycline can abolish this upregulatory effect [21].

The studies discussed above collectively suggest that TREM-1 expression is upregulated in periodontitis as a result of microbial stimulation. However, there are as-yet no interventional studies in preclinical models to conclusively demonstrate TREM-1 involvement in periodontitis. Hence, this in vivo study in a validated model of murine ligature-induced periodontitis [22] was designed to investigate the effect of local TREM-1 inhibition on the induction of experimental periodontitis, as well as on the expression of inflammation- and osteoclastogenesis-associated molecules in the gingival tissue. Our results described below implicate for the first time TREM-1 in the pathogenesis of periodontitis in a preclinical model and suggest a novel therapeutic approach for the treatment of this oral inflammatory disease.

2. Materials and Methods

2.1. Ligature-Induced Periodontitis Model in Mice

The well-established ligature-induced periodontitis model in specific pathogen-free C57BL/6 mice was used as described earlier [22]. All animal procedures were performed according to protocols approved by the Institutional Animal Care and Use Committee of the University of Pennsylvania, and adequate measures were taken to minimize pain or discomfort. To induce experimental periodontitis, a 5-0 silk ligature was tied around the maxillary left second molar for up to 8 days (n = 4–5 mice/group). The unligated contralateral molar in each mouse was used as baseline control (unligated control). A synthetic peptide derived from the extracellular domain of TREM-1 (LP17; LQVTDSGLYRCVIYHPP, Pepscan, Lelystad, Netherlands) was used as described earlier [7]. The LP17 blocking peptide is considered as a competitive antagonist of membrane-bound TREM-1 for its natural ligand, therefore acting as a decoy receptor for TREM signaling [23]. For the intervention experiments performed in this study, 5 μg of LP17 peptide or PBS were injected into the palatal gingiva of the ligated second maxillary molar 1 days before placing the ligature and every day thereafter until the day before sacrifice (day 5).

The measurements on the alveolar bone height were done on defleshed maxillae under a Nikon SMZ800 microscope (Nikon Instruments, Melville, NY, USA), and images of the maxillae were captured using a Nikon Digital Sight DS-U3 camera controller. The distance between the cemento-enamel junction (CEJ) and alveolar bone crest (ABC) was measured at six predetermined points on the ligated molar and adjacent regions using NIS Elements software (Nikon Instruments, Melville, NY, USA) [22]. To calculate bone loss, the six-site total CEJ–ABC distance for the ligated side of each mouse was subtracted from the six-site total CEJ–ABC distance of the contralateral unligated side. The results are presented in millimeters, and negative values indicate bone loss relative to the unligated control.

2.2. *Bacterial Counts on Silk Sutures*

The ligated silk sutures obtained from LP17-treated or PBS-treated mice at day 5 were collected (n = 5 mice/group). These were suspended individually in sterile PBS, and adherent bacteria were disassociated from the sutures via high-speed vortexing for 2 min. Serial dilutions of the samples were plated onto blood agar plates (BD Difco Laboratories, Detroit, MI, USA), and the plates were incubated anaerobically at 37 °C for 7 days. Results are reported as the mean number of colony forming units (CFUs) per millimeter length of silk suture ± the standard error of the mean (SEM). Anaerobic CFUs were preferred over aerobic ones because of the stronger etiological association of anaerobic organisms with periodontitis.

2.3. *Antimicrobial Effects of the Synthetic Peptides in Vitro*

A 6-species oral biofilm model was used to investigate the potential antimicrobial effects of LP17. The biofilm consisted of *Actinomyces oris* OMZ 745, *Veillonella dispar* OMZ 493 (ATCC 17748T), *Fusobacterium nucleatum* OMZ 598 (KP-F2), *Streptococcus mutans* OMZ 918 (UA159), *Streptococcus oralis* OMZ 607 (SK 248), and *Candida albicans* OMZ 110. In brief, biofilms were grown according to the standard protocol in 24-well cell culture plates on sintered hydroxyapatite (HA) discs, which were pre-conditioned for 4 h with pooled human saliva, for pellicle formation. Throughout the following experimentation period, the biofilms were grown in the presence of LP17 or 0.9% NaCl (sham control). After 5 days of biofilm growth under anaerobic conditions, the HA discs were vortexed vigorously for 1 min in 1 mL of 0.9% NaCl and then sonicated (Branson Sonic Power Company, Danbury, CT, USA) for 5 s to harvest the adherent biofilms. Then, to determine the total CFUs, the bacterial suspensions were serially diluted in 0.9% NaCl and 50 μL aliquots were plated on agar plates supplemented with 5% whole human blood at 37 °C for 72 h.

2.4. *Quantitative TaqMan Real-Time PCR and TaqMan Array Analysis*

The TaqMan Array 96-well Mouse Immune Response kit (Applied Biosystems) was used to assess the expression of 92 predetermined genes mediating the immune response and four endogenous control genes including *GAPDH, HPRT, GUSB and 18S RNA*. For this analysis, gingival tissues were collected at day 5 (n = 3 mice/group). Total RNA was extracted from these tissues by Qiagen Fibrous Tissue Extraction kit. According to the manufacturer's protocol, cDNA was mixed with 2× TaqMan Universal Master Mix and H_2O to a total volume of 2160 μL. Subsequently, 20 μL of the mixture was placed into each well of the PCR array. The three steps of the cycling program were 95 °C for 10 min for 1 cycle, then 95 °C for 15 s, and 60 °C for 1 min for 40 cycles, using a Step One Plus Real-Time PCR System (Applied Biosystems). In addition, the transcription levels of TREM-1, interleukin (IL)-1β, RANKL, OPG, COX-2, and IL-6 were assessed by individual TaqMan Gene Expression Assays (Applied Biosytems). For TaqMan qPCR analysis, mouse ACTB (β-actin) was used as an endogenous control.

2.5. *Statistical Analysis*

All statistical analyses were performed using Prism v.6.0 software (GraphPad Software, La Jolla, CA, USA). One-way ANOVA was used to determine differences between three or more groups, whereas an unpaired, two-tailed Student t test was used to determine the statistical significance of differences between two groups. Differences were considered significant at $p < 0.05$.

3. Results

3.1. *Local Tissue Kinetics of TREM-1 Expression in Ligature-Induced Periodontitis*

Using the ligature-induced murine periodontitis model, we first investigated the regulation of TREM-1 expression in the gingival tissue. TREM-1 gene expression was significantly upregulated at the ligated sites in a time-dependent manner, peaking at day 8 compared to the unligated control sites forming the baseline (Figure 1A). Compared to the unligated control sites, TREM-1 mRNA levels in the ligated sites were approximately 16-fold and 17-fold higher at day 5 and day 8, respectively ($p < 0.01$). Since TREM-1 activation is involved in the upregulation of a number of key proinflammatory cytokines [20], including IL-1β, which is crucial in periodontal pathogenesis, IL-1β gene expression levels were also assessed. A similar expression pattern was observed for IL-1β. In particular, compared to the baseline control, IL-1β gene expression at ligated sites was approximately 13-fold, 21-fold, and 27-fold higher at days 3, 5, and 8, respectively ($p < 0.01$) (Figure 1B).

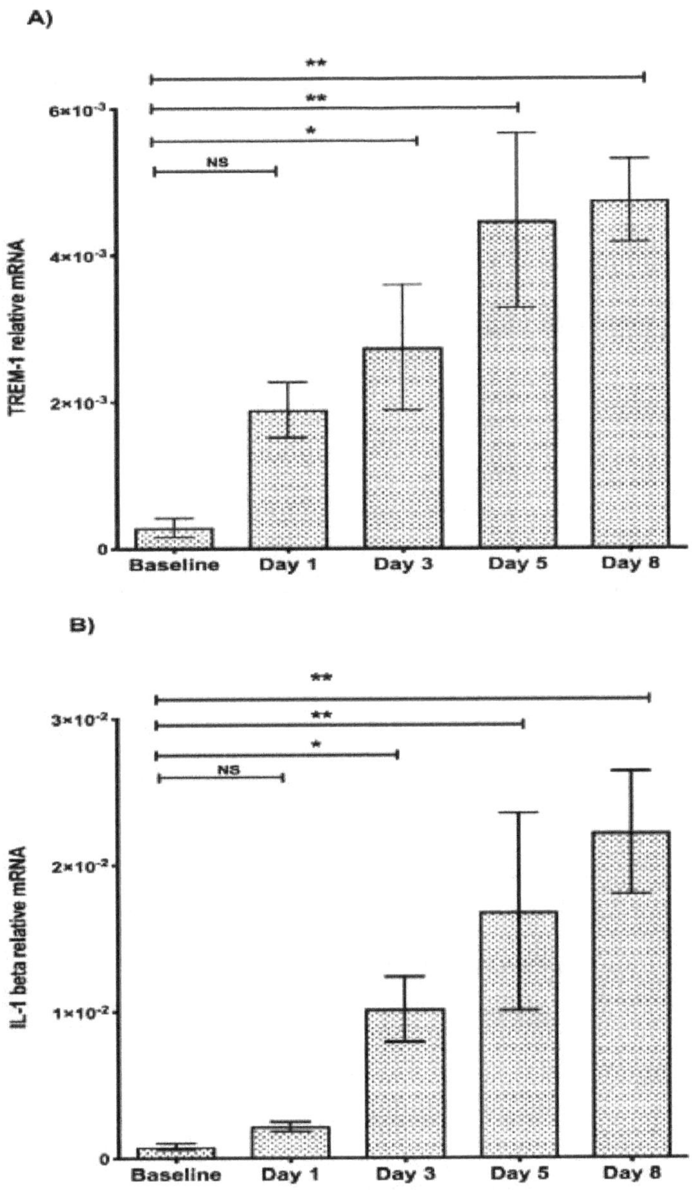

Figure 1. Kinetics of gingival tissue expression of TREM-1 and IL-1 beta in ligature-induced periodontitis. TREM-1 mRNA **(A)** and IL-1 beta mRNA **(B)** levels were examined in unligated control gingiva and ligature-induced periodontitis gingival tissues at 1 to 8 days. The gene expression levels were detected by TaqMan real-time qPCR and calibrated against the expression of housekeeping gene *β-actin*. Results are means ± SEM (n = 4 mice/group). * $p < 0.05$ and ** $p < 0.01$ between the indicated groups.

3.2. Role of TREM-1 in Alveolar Bone Loss

The kinetics of TREM-1 gene expression followed a pattern similar to those of ligature-induced bone loss seen in our previous publication [22]. To determine whether there was a cause-and-effect relationship between gingival TREM-1 expression and alveolar bone loss, we subjected groups of mice to ligature-induced periodontitis with local administration of the LP17 or with PBS sham control. Five days after placement of the ligatures, mice treated with LP17 developed significantly less alveolar bone loss as compared to the sham-treated mice ($p < 0.05$) (Figure 2A,B), indicating that TREM-1 signaling contributes to induction of alveolar bone loss.

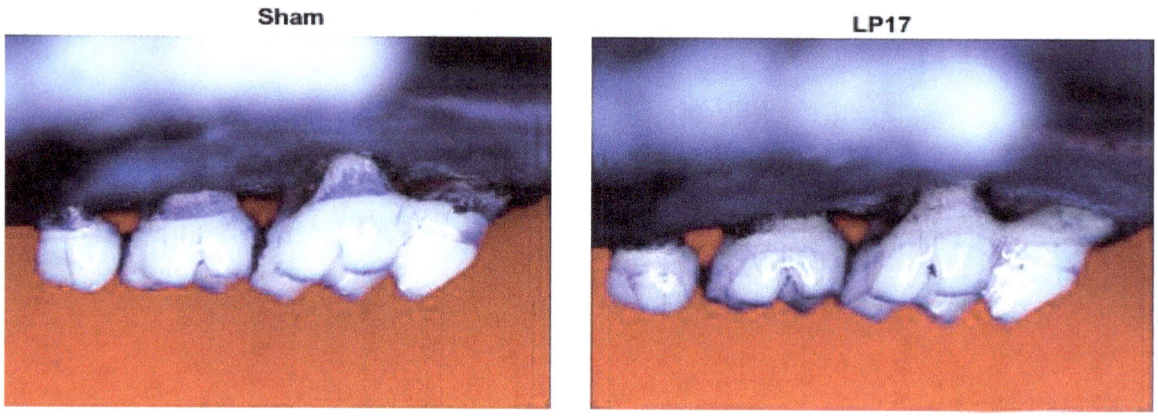

(A)

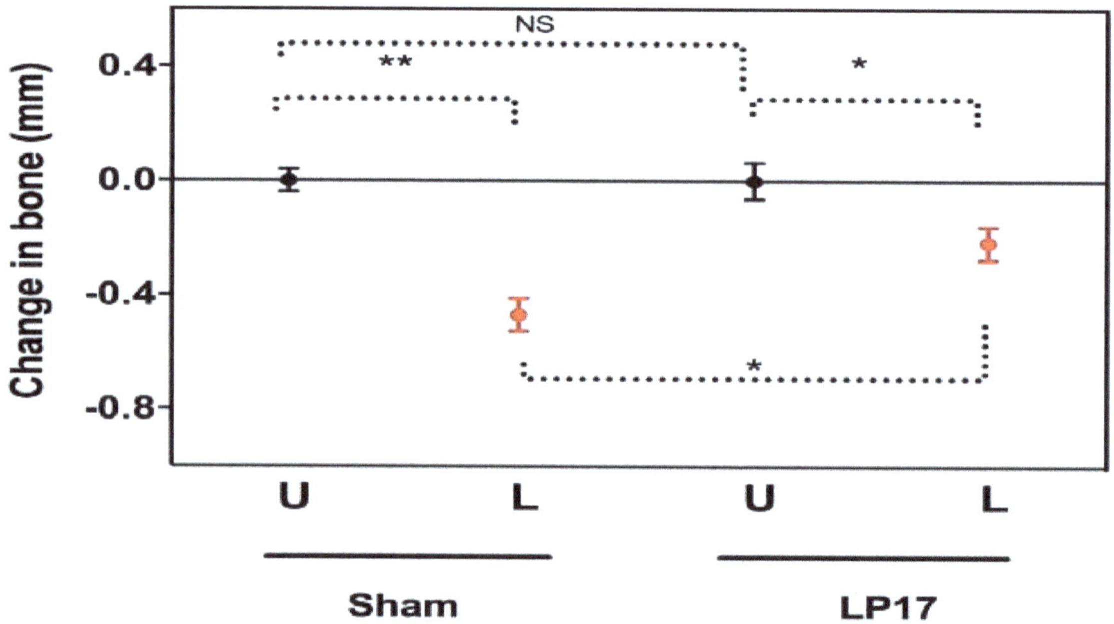

(B)

Figure 2. Inhibition of ligature-induced bone loss by LP17. Ligatures were placed on the left maxillary molars of C57BL/6 mice and then locally microinjected with 5 μg of TREM-1 blocking peptide (LP17) or with PBS sham 1 day before placing the ligature and every day thereafter until day 5. The distance between the cemento-enamel junction (CEJ) and alveolar bone crest (ABC) was measured at six predetermined points on the ligated side. Representative images of PBS sham- and LP17-treated maxillae exhibiting differential bone loss **(A).** To calculate bone loss, the six-site total CEJ–ABC distance for the ligated (L) side of each mouse was subtracted from the six-site total CEJ–ABC distance of the contralateral unligated (U) side. The results are presented in millimeters, and negative values indicate bone loss relative to the unligated control **(B).** Data are means ± SEM (n = 4–5 mice/group). * $p < 0.05$ and ** $p < 0.01$ between the indicated groups.

3.3. Investigation of Potential LP17 Antimicrobial Activity

To determine whether the protective effects of LP17 in ligature-induced periodontitis could, in part, be attributed to potential antimicrobial effects, we determined the microbial load of the treated mice from the above-described in vivo experiment (Figure 2). To this end, bacteria were extracted from the recovered ligatures (day 5) and cultivated anaerobically for 7 days on blood agar plates. To normalize the data, the counted CFUs were divided by the length of corresponding suture, and the results revealed that sutures from the LP17-treated mice yielded similar CFUs, as compared to the PBS sham-treated group ($p > 0.05$) (Figure 3A). Furthermore, the potential antimicrobial impact of LP17 was tested in vitro on a 6-species biofilm model for 5 days. A 1.3-fold reduction in total CFUs was observed, compared to the saline sham-treated group ($p > 0.05$). These results suggested that the LP17 peptide preferentially acted by regulating the host response rather than bacterial growth. Hence, we next investigated the host-modulating activity of LP17.

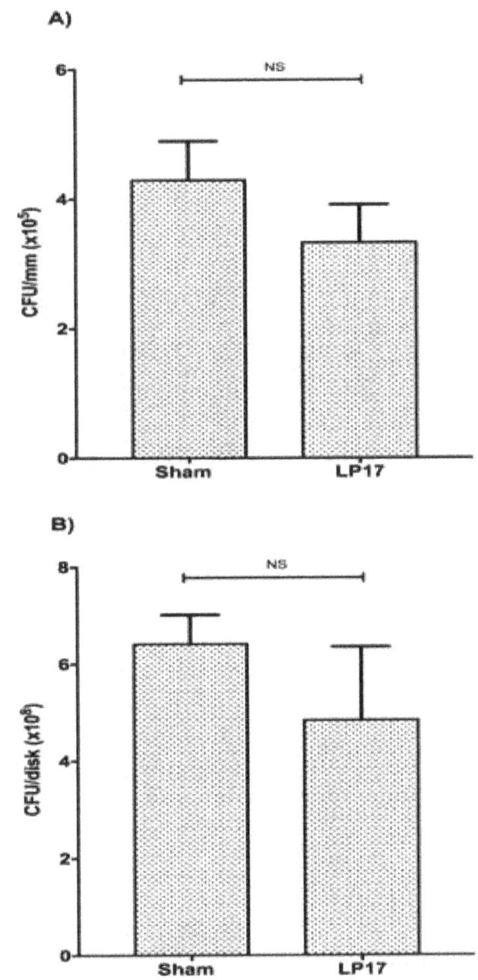

Figure 3. LP17 does not affect the microbial load in vivo. (**A**) Detached material from the recovered ligatures at day 5 from mice used in Figure 2 were cultivated anaerobically for 7 days on blood agar plates, followed by total colony forming unit (CFU) determination. To normalize the data, the counted CFUs were divided by the length of corresponding suture. Data are means ± SEM ($n = 5$ mice/group). NS: Not significant, $p > 0.05$. (**B**) LP17 does not affect the microbial load in vitro. The in vitro biofilms were grown in the presence of LP17 or 0.9% NaCl (sham). After 5 days of biofilm growth under anaerobic conditions, biofilm bacteria were harvested from the discs and cultivated anaerobically for 3 days on blood agar plates, followed by total CFU determination. The CFUs are given per hydroxyapatite (HA) disc. Data are means ± SEM ($n = 3$ disc /group). NS: Not significant, $p > 0.05$.

3.4. Modulation of Immunoregulatory Genes by TREM-1

To understand how TREM-1 signaling regulates the host periodontal response, the defleshed gingival tissues were analyzed for the expression of a number of immunoregulatory genes at day 5, by using a mouse immune response qPCR Array profiling for 92 individual genes (Table S1). Differential expression analysis was done by the following pair-wise comparisons: (a) unligated sites versus ligated sites and (b) PBS sham-treated ligated sites versus LP17-treated ligated sites. Although a basal expression level was detected for all studied genes at unligated control sites, a total of 38 genes were differentially transcribed by more than two-fold during the experimental infection period (Table S1). Among those, 27 genes were induced in the ligature-induced gingival sites, 7 of which reached statistical significance ($p < 0.05$). Another 11 genes were repressed more than two-fold, 7 of which also reached statistical significance ($p < 0.05$). The significantly upregulated genes were *IL-17A, IL-1β, CD80, CCR4, HMOX1, VEGFA,*and *CD68*, whereas the significantly downregulated ones were *SKI, SMAD 7, IL-7, NFATC 3, FAS, IL-15,* and *SMAD 3* (Figure 4A).

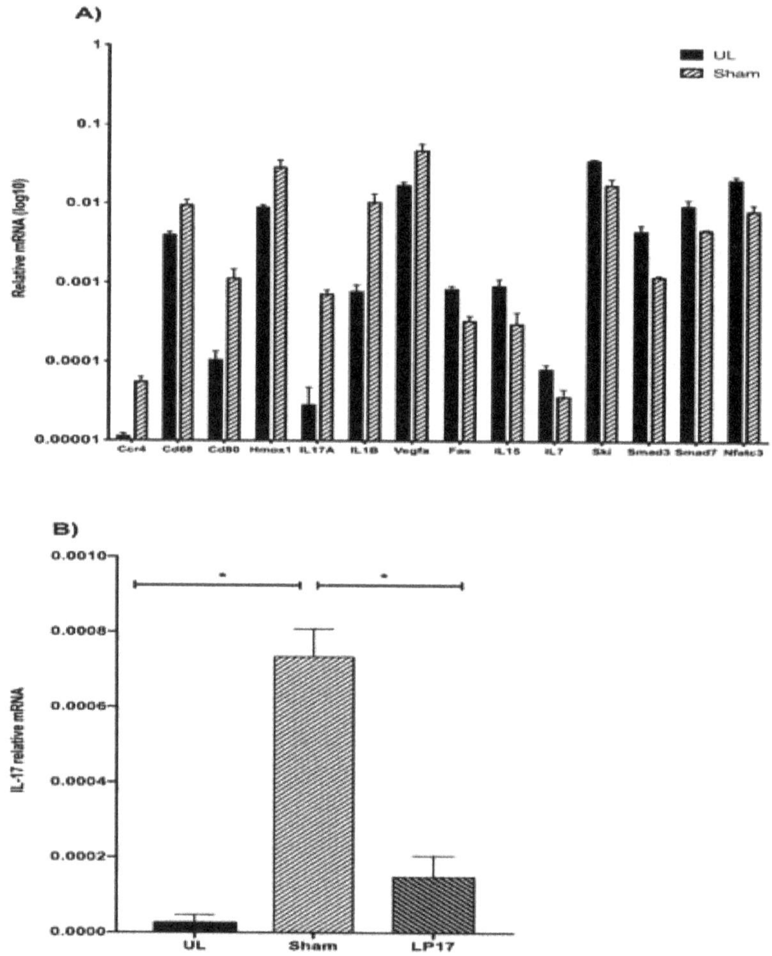

Figure 4. Modulation of immunoregulatory genes by TREM-1. Dissected gingiva from unligated control sites (UL) and ligated shame treated sites (Sham) for 5 days. The mRNA expression of 92 key genes mediating the immune response and four endogenous control genes including *GAPDH, HPRT, GUSB and 18S RNA mRNA* were assessed by qPCR. The gene expression levels were calibrated against the expression of housekeeping genes (detailed list provided in Table S2). The significantly regulated genes are presented (fold-change ≥ 2 and * $p < 0.05$). **(A).** Dissected gingiva from unligated control sites (UL), or ligated sites from PBS sham-treated sites (Sham) or sites treated with 5 μg synthetic TREM-1 inhibitor (LP17) for 5 days. The mRNA expression of IL-17 is presented (fold-change ≥ 2 and * $p < 0.05$). **(B).** Data are means ± SEM ($n = 3$ mice/group).

Treatment with the LP17 peptide altered the expression of 27 genes by more than two-fold (23 downregulated, 4 upregulated) (Supplement Table S2). Although the expression of proinflammatory cytokines associated with periodontal disease pathogenesis (such as, IL-1β, IL-6, IL-17A, and TNF) was inhibited, statistical significance was reached only for IL-17A, which was downregulated by 4.9-fold (Figure 4B). Taken together, these data indicate that ligature-induced periodontitis is associated with upregulation of a number of proinflammatory genes that seem to be inhibited by LP17, which predominantly targets IL-17A expression, a signature cytokine of Th17 cells that were shown to drive inflammatory bone loss in mice and humans [24].

3.5. Regulation of the RANKL/OPG Axis by TREM-1

The upregulation of IL-17A expression, a cytokine associated with chronic inflammatory tissue destruction and alveolar bone loss [25,26], prompted us to investigate further the involvement of TREM-1 in the molecular regulatory mechanisms of bone resorption, particularly the RANKL/OPG system. RANKL was significantly induced at the sham-treated ligated sites (39-fold), whereas administration of LP17 inhibited this upregulatory effect by 8.9-fold (Figure 5A). The expression of OPG also increased at the sham-treated ligated sites (2.7-fold) but was not significantly affected by administration of LP17 (Figure 5B). As a result, the relative RANKL/OPG ratio, a molecular determinant of bone resorption, was significantly reduced in response to LP17 treatment by five-fold as compared to PBS sham treatment (Figure 5C).

As IL-6 and COX-2 that are produced in high levels during inflammation are considered as key regulators of RANKL expression [4,27,28], we assessed their regulation by TREM-1. Interestingly, the expressions of COX-2 and IL-6 were not significantly affected by LP17 treatment, indicating that the regulation of RANKL in this model may not be dependent on COX-2 (Figure 6A) or IL-6 (Figure 6B).

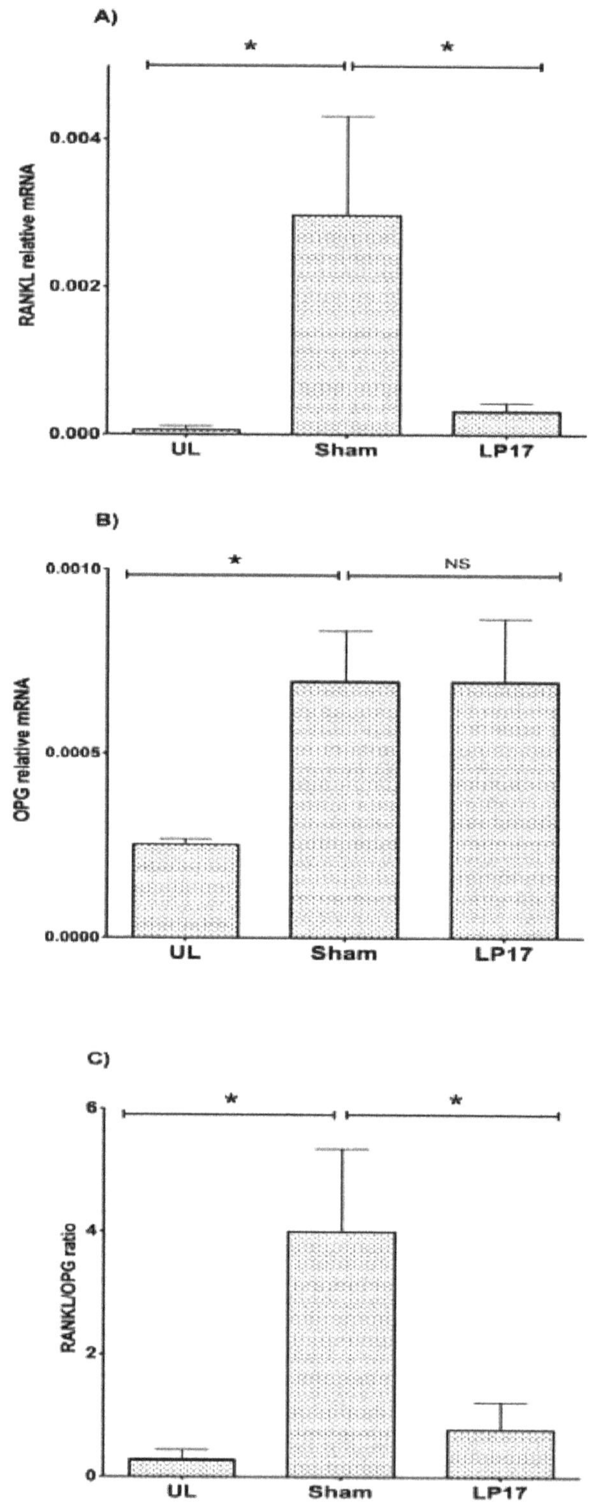

Figure 5. Inhibition of receptor activator of nuclear factor kappa-B-ligand (RANKL)/osteoprotegerin (OPG) ratio by LP17. Gingival tissue samples were dissected at day 5 from mice used in Figure 2 and were processed for gene expression of RANKL **(A)** and OPG **(B)** by qPCR. The relative RANKL/OPG ratio was also calculated **(C)**. The expression of the indicated molecules was determined in unligated (UL) control gingiva and in ligated gingival tissues treated with 5 μg synthetic TREM-1 inhibitor (LP17) or PBS sham. The gene expression levels were detected by TaqMan real-time qPCR and calibrated against the expression of the housekeeping gene *β-actin*. Results are means ± SEM (n = 4 mice/group). * $p < 0.05$ and ** $p < 0.01$ between the indicated groups. NS: Not significant, $p > 0.05$.

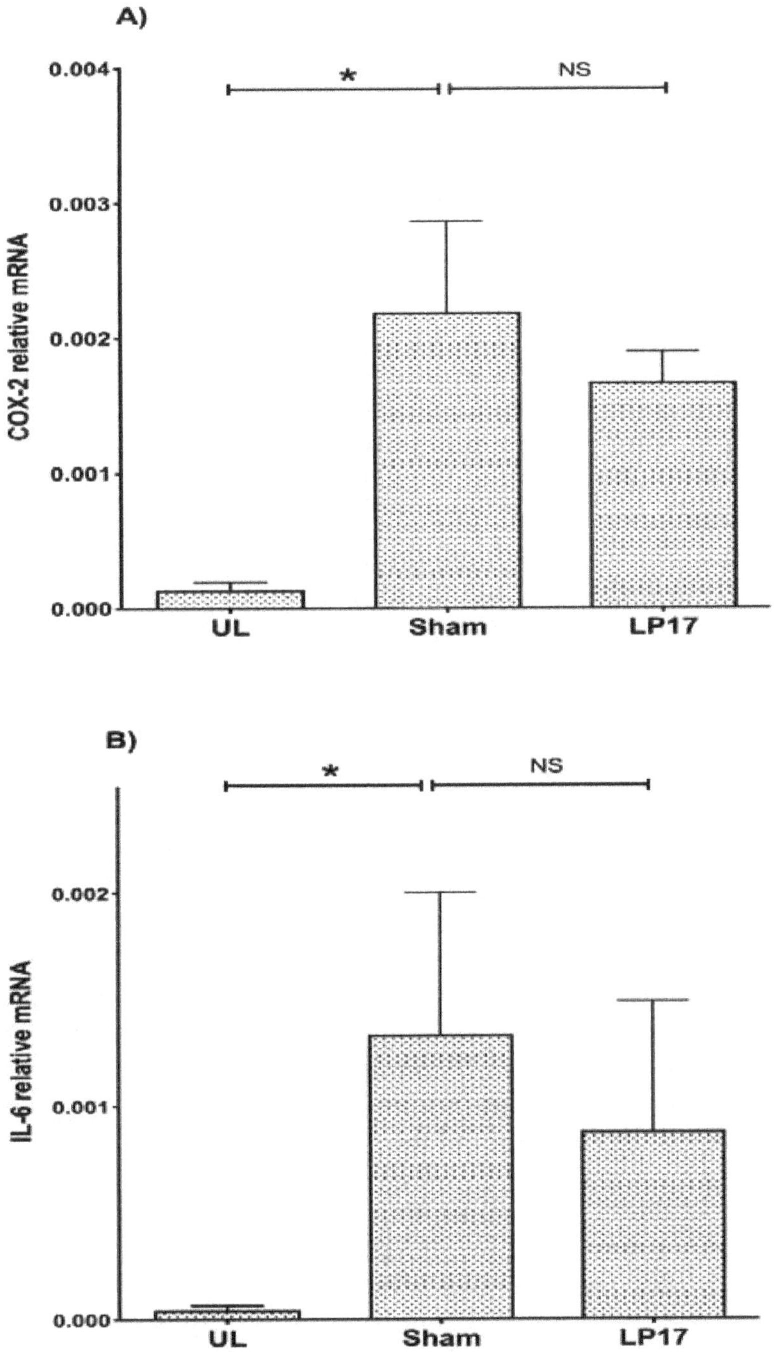

Figure 6. LP17 does not affect COX-2 and IL-6 levels. Gingival tissue samples were dissected at day 5 from mice used in Figure 2 and were processed for gene expression of COX-2 **(A)** and IL-6 **(B)** by qPCR. The expression of the indicated molecules was determined in unligated (UL) control gingiva and in ligated gingival tissues treated with 5 μg synthetic TREM-1 inhibitor (LP17) or PBS sham. The gene expression levels were detected by TaqMan real-time qPCR and calibrated against the expression of the housekeeping gene *β-actin*. Results are means ± SEM (n = 4 mice/group). NS: Not significant, $p > 0.05$.

4. Discussion

Our present study shows for the first time that TREM-1 regulates alveolar bone loss in experimental periodontitis and paves the way for a novel approach to treat human periodontitis. In line with earlier observations in humans demonstrating upregulated TREM-1 gingival expression in periodontitis patients, as compared to healthy controls [19], our study showed progressively increased induction of TREM-1 gingival expression during the course of experimental periodontitis in response to biofilm accumulation. TREM-1 propagates proinflammatory cytokine expression, representatively demonstrated by IL-1β in the present study. These findings are in accordance with our previous studies showing a positive correlation between subgingival biofilms and TREM-1 levels in gingival tissue or gingival crevicular fluid of individuals with periodontitis [16,19]. Although the cellular distribution of TREM-1 in gingival tissue was not investigated in the present experimental setting, monocytes/resident macrophages and polymorphonuclear neutrophilic leukocytes (PMNs) are known to be a major source of TREM-1 in inflammation [9,29–31]. In this respect, our earlier work presented that multispecies oral biofilms [19] or the keystone pathogen *Porphyromonas gingivalis* is able to induce TREM-1 gene expression in monocytes or in PMNs in the tissue culture systems [20,32].

The major novel finding of this in vivo study is that local (gingival) injection of a TREM-1 blocking peptide, namely LP17, substantially reduced the RANKL/OPG osteoclastogenic ratio and alveolar bone loss, thus providing preclinical support for a new therapeutic target for periodontitis. Clinical studies have demonstrated that the RANKL/OPG ratio as well as IL-17 gingival tissue expression are upregulated in human periodontitis [33–36]. Intriguingly, LP17 selectively downregulated IL-17 expression among all studied immune response markers. Given that IL-17 regulates the expression of RANKL [37], it is possible that the capacity of LP17 to downregulate the RANKL/OPG ratio may be mediated through its ability to inhibit IL-17. Similarly, inhibition of IL-17 by its antagonist Del-1 has been shown to efficiently block osteoclastogenesis and subsequent periodontitis [38,39]. Thus, our study lends further support to the concept that IL-17 is a key driver of periodontal bone loss, although this is the first time that TREM-1 signaling is linked to IL-17 in the context of periodontitis.

Our present data are also consistent with a recent in vitro study, demonstrating that the LR12 TREM-1 inhibitor LR12 could prevent monocytic activation by *P. gingivalis* LPS [40], as well as our earlier in vitro findings demonstrating that LP17 can reduce cytokine release by monocytes in response to *P. gingivalis* whole bacteria [20,21]. Moreover, an earlier study in a psoriasis model showed that TREM-1 blockade in vitro and ex vivo significantly reduced the number of Th17 cells and decreased the secretion of IL-17, suggesting that TREM-1 positively regulates Th17 responses [41]. The COX-2 pathway and IL-6 are also important regulators of the RANKL/OPG ratio [27]. However, it is unlikely that TREM-1 regulates the RANKL/OPG ratio via COX-2 or IL-6 since LP17 failed to affect the expression of either gene. Thus, it is concluded that the alveolar bone resorptive effects of TREM-1 are, at least in part, mediated through activation of the IL-17-RANKL axis.

Although the impact of TREM-1 signaling on microbial control has been controversial in several bacterial challenge models [13], in the experimental periodontitis model, LP17 did not show a significant effect on oral bacterial load. This finding suggests that TREM-1 inhibition protects against periodontitis predominantly through host-modulation effects and is in line with earlier work indicating that LP17 did not alter the in vitro levels of *P. gingivalis* [20,32,42].

Moreover, TREM-1-deficient mice used in colitis and other experimental models of infection-driven inflammatory diseases exhibited no alterations in microbial clearance efficiency [13]. On the other hand, studies on lung infection models (e.g., *Pseudomonas aeruginosa*-induced pneumonia) indicated that administration of LP17 peptide reduced the bacterial load at an early stage of infection while increasing it at later stages; these effects, however, were attributed to indirect antimicrobial effects of TREM-1 related to early enhancement of neutrophil influx and consequent increase in phagocytic activity [43]. These observations are in line with the main function of TREM-1 as an inflammation fine-tuner [44], rather than a direct eliminator of infection, as is the case, for instance, for TNF-alpha. Yet, the use of anti-TNF antibody may be complicated because of the increased risk for reactivation of latent infection [45].

5. Conclusions

The present study conclusively demonstrated the involvement of TREM-1 in alveolar bone resorption during the course of experimental periodontitis in mice. Mechanistically, TREM-1 reduced the RANKL/OPG osteoclastogenic ratio, presumably via the inhibition of IL-17. Importantly, our findings also reveal a previously unidentified TREM-1-driven axis for inflammatory bone loss that could be targeted via small-molecule antagonists for therapeutic intervention in human periodontitis.

Author Contributions: Conceptualization, N.B. and G.H.; Methodology, N.B., T.A,. G.N.B., and N.B.; Validation, N.B., G.N.B. and G.H.; Formal Analysis, T.A., N.B.; Resources, N.B., G.N.B., G.H.; Writing—Original Draft Preparation, N.B.; Writing—Review & Editing, G.H., G.N.B.; Visualization, T.A.; Supervision, G.H.; Funding Acquisition, N.B., G.N.B. and G.H.

References

1. Lamont, R.J.; Hajishengallis, G. Polymicrobial synergy and dysbiosis in inflammatory disease. *Trends Mol. Med.* **2015**, *21*, 172–183. [CrossRef] [PubMed]
2. Hajishengallis, G.; Korostoff, J.M. Revisiting the Page & Schroeder model: The good, the bad and the unknowns in the periodontal host response 40 years later. *Periodontol. 2000* **2017**, *75*, 116–151. [PubMed]
3. Garlet, G.P. Destructive and Protective Roles of Cytokines in Periodontitis: A Re-appraisal from Host Defense and Tissue Destruction Viewpoints. *J. Dent. Res.* **2010**, *89*, 1349–1363. [CrossRef] [PubMed]
4. Lerner, U. Inflammation-induced bone remodeling in periodontal disease and the influence of post-menopausal osteoporosis. *J. Dent. Res.* **2006**, *85*, 596–607. [CrossRef] [PubMed]
5. Belibasakis, G.N.; Bostanci, N. The RANKL-OPG system in clinical periodontology. *J. Clin. Periodontol.* **2012**, *39*, 239–248. [CrossRef] [PubMed]
6. Belibasakis, G.N.; Meier, A.; Guggenheim, B.; Bostanci, N. The RANKL-OPG system is differentially regulated by supragingival and subgingival biofilm supernatants. *Cytokine* **2011**, *55*, 98–103. [CrossRef]
7. Gibot, S.; Cravoisy, A. Soluble Form of the Triggering Receptor Expressed on Myeloid Cells-1 as a Marker of Microbial Infection. *Clin. Med. Res.* **2004**, *2*, 181–187. [CrossRef]
8. Colonna, M.; Facchetti, F. TREM-1 (Triggering Receptor Expressed on Myeloid Cells): A New Player in Acute Inflammatory Responses. *J. Infect. Dis.* **2003**, *187*, S397–S401. [CrossRef]
9. Schenk, M.; Bouchon, A.; Seibold, F.; Mueller, C. TREM-1–expressing intestinal macrophages crucially amplify chronic inflammation in experimental colitis and inflammatory bowel diseases. *J. Clin. Investig.* **2007**, *117*, 3097–3106. [CrossRef]
10. Gibot, S.; Kolopp-Sarda, M.-N.; Bene, M.-C.; Bollaert, P.-E.; Lozniewski, A.; Mory, F.; Lévy, B.; Faure, G.C. A Soluble Form of the Triggering Receptor Expressed on Myeloid Cells-1 Modulates the Inflammatory Response in Murine Sepsis. *J. Exp. Med.* **2004**, *200*, 1419–1426. [CrossRef]
11. Bouchon, A.; Facchetti, F.; Weigand, M.A.; Colonna, M. TREM-1 amplifies inflammation and is a crucial mediator of septic shock. *Nature* **2001**, *410*, 1103–1107. [CrossRef] [PubMed]
12. Boechat, N.; Bouchonnet, F.; Bonay, M.; Grodet, A.; Pelicic, V.; Gicquel, B.; Hance, A.J. Culture at High Density Improves the Ability of Human Macrophages to Control Mycobacterial Growth. *J. Immunol.* **2001**, *166*, 6203–6211. [CrossRef] [PubMed]
13. Weber, B.; Schuster, S.; Zysset, D.; Rihs, S.; Dickgreber, N.; Schurch, C.; Riether, C.; Siegrist, M.; Schneider, C.; Pawelski, H.; et al. TREM-1 Deficiency Can Attenuate Disease Severity without Affecting Pathogen Clearance. *PLoS Pathog.* **2014**, *10*, e1003900. [CrossRef] [PubMed]
14. Bostanci, N.; Öztürk, V.Ö.; Emingil, G.; Belibasakis, G.N. Elevated oral and systemic levels of soluble triggering receptor expressed on myeloid cells-1 (sTREM-1) in periodontitis. *J. Dent. Res.* **2013**, *92*, 161–165. [CrossRef] [PubMed]
15. Nylund, K.M.; Ruokonen, H.; Sorsa, T.; Heikkinen, A.M.; Meurman, J.H.; Ortiz, F.; Tervahartiala, T.; Furuholm, J.; Bostanci, N. Association of the Salivary Triggering Receptor Expressed on Myeloid Cells/its Ligand Peptidoglycan Recognition Protein 1 Axis with Oral Inflammation in Kidney Disease. *J. Periodontol.* **2018**, *89*, 117–129. [CrossRef]

16. Belibasakis, G.N.; Öztürk, V.; Emingil, G.; Bostanci, N. Soluble Triggering Receptor Expressed on Myeloid Cells 1 (sTREM-1) in Gingival Crevicular Fluid: Association with Clinical and Microbiologic Parameters. *J. Periodontol.* **2014**, *85*, 204–210. [CrossRef]
17. Bisson, C.; Massin, F.; Lefevre, P.A.; Thilly, N.; Miller, N.; Gibot, S. Increased gingival crevicular fluid levels of soluble triggering receptor expressed on myeloid cells (sTREM) -1 in severe periodontitis. *J. Clin. Periodontol.* **2012**, *39*, 1141–1148. [CrossRef]
18. Öztürk, V.Ö.; Belibasakis, G.N.; Emingil, G.; Bostanci, N. Impact of aging on TREM-1 responses in the periodontium: A cross-sectional study in an elderly population. *BMC Infect. Dis.* **2016**, *16*, 429.
19. Willi, M.; Belibasakis, G.N.; Bostanci, N. Expression and regulation of triggering receptor expressed on myeloid cells 1 in periodontal diseases. *Clin. Exp. Immunol.* **2014**, *178*, 190–200. [CrossRef]
20. Bostanci, N.; Thurnheer, T.; Belibasakis, G.N. Involvement of the TREM-1/DAP12 pathway in the innate immune responses to Porphyromonas gingivalis. *Mol. Immunol.* **2011**, *49*, 387–394. [CrossRef]
21. Bostanci, N.; Belibasakis, G.N. Doxycycline inhibits TREM-1 induction by Porphyromonas gingivalis. *FEMS Immunol. Med. Microbiol.* **2012**, *66*, 37–44. [CrossRef] [PubMed]
22. Abe, T.; Hajishengallis, G. Optimization of the ligature-induced periodontitis model in mice. *J. Immunol. Methods* **2013**, *394*, 49–54. [CrossRef] [PubMed]
23. Pelham, C.J.; Pandya, A.N.; Agrawal, D.K. Triggering receptor expressed on myeloid cells receptor family modulators: A patent review. *Expert Opin. Ther. Patents* **2014**, *24*, 1383–1395. [CrossRef] [PubMed]
24. Dutzan, N.; Kajikawa, T.; Abusleme, L.; Greenwell-Wild, T.; Zuazo, C.E.; Ikeuchi, T.; Brenchley, L.; Abe, T.; Hurabielle, C.; Martin, D.; et al. A dysbiotic microbiome triggers TH17 cells to mediate oral mucosal immunopathology in mice and humans. *Sci. Transl. Med.* **2018**, *10*, 0797. [CrossRef] [PubMed]
25. Gaffen, S.; Hajishengallis, G. A new inflammatory cytokine on the block: Re-thinking periodontal disease and the Th1/Th2 paradigm in the context of Th17 cells and IL-17. *J. Dent. Res.* **2008**, *87*, 817–828. [CrossRef] [PubMed]
26. Zenobia, C.; Hajishengallis, G. Basic biology and role of interleukin-17 in immunity and inflammation. *Periodontol. 2000* **2015**, *69*, 142–159. [CrossRef]
27. Belibasakis, G.N.; Guggenheim, B. Induction of prostaglandin E 2 and interleukin-6 in gingival fibroblasts by oral biofilms. *FEMS Immunol. Med. Microbiol.* **2011**, *63*, 381–386. [CrossRef] [PubMed]
28. Reddi, D.; Bostanci, N.; Hashim, A.; Aduse-Opoku, J.; Curtis, M.A.; Hughes, F.J.; Belibasakis, G.N. Porphyromonas gingivalis regulates the RANKL-OPG system in bone marrow stromal cells. *Microbes Infect.* **2008**, *10*, 1459–1468. [CrossRef]
29. Arts, R.J.; Joosten, L.A.; Dinarello, C.A.; Kullberg, B.J.; Van Der Meer, J.W.; Netea, M.G. TREM-1 interaction with the LPS/TLR4 receptor complex. *Eur. Cytokine Netw.* **2011**, *22*, 11–14. [CrossRef]
30. Alflen, A.; Stadler, N.; Lopez, P.A.; Teschner, D.; Theobald, M.; Heß, G.; Radsak, M.P. Idelalisib impairs TREM-1 mediated neutrophil inflammatory responses. *Sci. Rep.* **2018**, *8*, 5558. [CrossRef]
31. Fortin, C.F.; Lesur, O.; Fulop, T., Jr. Effects of TREM-1 activation in human neutrophils: Activation of signaling pathways, recruitment into lipid rafts and association with TLR4. *Int. Immunol.* **2007**, *19*, 41–50. [CrossRef] [PubMed]
32. Bostanci, N.; Thurnheer, T.; Aduse-Opoku, J.; Curtis, M.A.; Zinkernagel, A.S.; Belibasakis, G.N. Porphyromonas gingivalis Regulates TREM-1 in Human Polymorphonuclear Neutrophils via Its Gingipains. *PLoS ONE* **2013**, *8*, e75784. [CrossRef] [PubMed]
33. Takahashi, K.; Azuma, T.; Motohira, H.; Kinane, D.F.; Kitetsu, S. The potential role of interleukin-17 in the immunopathology of periodontal disease. *J. Clin. Periodontol.* **2005**, *32*, 369–374. [CrossRef] [PubMed]
34. Bostanci, N.; Ilgenli, T.; Emingil, G.; Afacan, B.; Han, B.; Töz, H.; Berdeli, A.; Atilla, G.; McKay, I.J.; Hughes, F.J.; et al. Differential expression of receptor activator of nuclear factor-kappaB ligand and osteoprotegerin mRNA in periodontal diseases. *J. Periodontal Res.* **2007**, *42*, 287–293. [CrossRef] [PubMed]
35. Dutzan, N.; Konkel, J.E.; Greenwell-Wild, T.; Moutsopoulos, N.M. Characterization of the human immune cell network at the gingival barrier. *Mucosal Immunol.* **2016**, *9*, 1163–1172. [CrossRef]
36. Moutsopoulos, N.M.; Konkel, J.; Sarmadi, M.; Eskan, M.A.; Wild, T.; Dutzan, N.; Abusleme, L.; Zenobia, C.; Hosur, K.B.; Abe, T.; et al. Defective neutrophil recruitment in leukocyte adhesion deficiency type I disease causes local IL-17-driven inflammatory bone loss. *Sci. Transl. Med.* **2014**, *6*, 229ra40. [CrossRef]

37. Koenders, M.I.; Lubberts, E.; Oppers-Walgreen, B.; Bersselaar, L.V.D.; Helsen, M.M.; Di Padova, F.E.; Boots, A.M.; Gram, H.; Joosten, L.A.; Berg, W.B. Blocking of Interleukin-17 during Reactivation of Experimental Arthritis Prevents Joint Inflammation and Bone Erosion by Decreasing RANKL and Interleukin-1. *Am. J. Pathol.* **2005**, *167*, 141–149. [CrossRef]
38. Shin, J.; Maekawa, T.; Abe, T.; Hajishengallis, E.; Hosur, K.; Pyaram, K.; Mitroulis, I.; Chavakis, T.; Hajishengallis, G. DEL-1 restrains osteoclastogenesis and inhibits inflammatory bone loss in nonhuman primates. *Sci. Transl. Med.* **2015**, *7*, 307ra155. [CrossRef]
39. Eskan, M.A.; Jotwani, R.; Abe, T.; Chmelar, J.; Lim, J.-H.; Liang, S.; Ciero, P.A.; Krauss, J.L.; Li, F.; Rauner, M.; et al. The leukocyte integrin antagonist Del-1 inhibits IL-17-mediated inflammatory bone loss. *Nat. Immunol.* **2012**, *13*, 465–473. [CrossRef]
40. Dubar, M.; Carrasco, K.; Gibot, S.; Bisson, C. Effects of Porphyromonas gingivalis LPS and LR12 peptide on TREM-1 expression by monocytes. *J. Clin. Periodontol.* **2018**, *45*, 799–805. [CrossRef]
41. Hyder, L.A.; Gonzalez, J.; Harden, J.L.; Johnson-Huang, L.M.; Zaba, L.C.; Pierson, K.C.; Eungdamrong, N.J.; Lentini, T.; Gulati, N.; Fuentes-Duculan, J.; et al. TREM-1 as a potential therapeutic target in psoriasis. *J. Investig. Dermatol.* **2013**, *133*, 1742–1751. [CrossRef]
42. Hajishengallis, G.; Liang, S.; Payne, M.A.; Hashim, A.; Jotwani, R.; Eskan, M.A.; McIntosh, M.L.; Alsam, A.; Kirkwood, K.L.; Lambris, J.D.; et al. Low-abundance biofilm species orchestrates inflammatory periodontal disease through the commensal microbiota and complement. *Cell Host Microbe* **2011**, *10*, 497–506. [CrossRef] [PubMed]
43. Klesney-Tait, J.; Keck, K.; Li, X.; Gilfillan, S.; Otero, K.; Baruah, S.; Meyerholz, D.K.; Varga, S.M.; Knudson, C.J.; Moninger, T.O.; et al. Transepithelial migration of neutrophils into the lung requires TREM-1. *J. Clin. Investig.* **2013**, *123*, 138–149. [CrossRef] [PubMed]
44. Silbereisen, A.; Hallak, A.; Nascimento, G.; Sorsa, T.; Belibasakis, G.; Lopez, R.; Bostanci, N. Regulation of PGLYRP1 and TREM-1 during Progression and Resolution of Gingival Inflammation. *JDR Clin. Transl. Res.* **2019**, *4*, 352–359. [CrossRef]
45. Keane, J.; Gershon, S.; Wise, R.P.; Mirabile-Levens, E.; Kasznica, J.; Schwieterman, W.D.; Siegel, J.N.; Braun, M.M. Tuberculosis associated with infliximab, a tumor necrosis factor alpha-neutralizing agent. *N. Engl. J. Med.* **2001**, *345*, 1098–1104. [CrossRef] [PubMed]

12

Exposure to *Porphyromonas gingivalis* Induces Production of Proinflammatory Cytokine via TLR2 from Human Respiratory Epithelial Cells

Norihisa Watanabe [1,2], Sho Yokoe [1,2], Yorimasa Ogata [3], Shuichi Sato [1] and Kenichi Imai [2,*]

[1] Department of Periodontology, Nihon University School of Dentistry, Chiyoda-ku, Tokyo 101-8310, Japan; watanabe.norihisa@nihon-u.ac.jp (N.W.); desh18040@g.nihon-u.ac.jp (S.Y.); satou.shuuichi@nihon-u.ac.jp (S.S.)

[2] Department of Microbiology, Nihon University School of Dentistry, 1-8-13 Kanda-Surugadai, Chiyoda-ku, Tokyo 101-8310, Japan

[3] Department of Periodontology, Nihon University School of Dentistry at Matsudo, Chiba 271-8587, Japan; ogata.yorimasa@nihon-u.ac.jp

* Correspondence: imai.kenichi@nihon-u.ac.jp

Abstract: Aspiration pneumonia is a major health problem owing to its high mortality rate in elderly people. The secretion of proinflammatory cytokines such as interleukin (IL)-8 and IL-6 by respiratory epithelial cells, which is induced by infection of respiratory bacteria such as *Streptococcus pneumoniae*, contributes to the onset of pneumonia. These cytokines thus play a key role in orchestrating inflammatory responses in the lower respiratory tract. In contrast, chronic periodontitis, a chronic inflammatory disease caused by the infection of periodontopathic bacteria, typically *Porphyromonas gingivalis*, is one of the most prevalent microbial diseases affecting humans globally. Although emerging evidence has revealed an association between aspiration pneumonia and chronic periodontitis, a causal relationship between periodontopathic bacteria and the onset of aspiration pneumonia has not been established. Most periodontopathic bacteria are anaerobic and are therefore unlikely to survive in the lower respiratory organs of humans. Therefore, in this study, we examined whether simple contact by heat-inactivated *P. gingivalis* induced proinflammatory cytokine production by several human respiratory epithelial cell lines. We found that *P. gingivalis* induced strong IL-8 and IL-6 secretion by BEAS-2B bronchial epithelial cells. *P. gingivalis* also induced strong IL-8 secretion by Detroit 562 pharyngeal epithelial cells but not by A549 alveolar epithelial cells. Additionally, Toll-like receptor (TLR) 2 but not TLR4 was involved in the *P. gingivalis*-induced proinflammatory cytokine production. Furthermore, *P. gingivalis* induced considerably higher IL-8 and IL-6 production than heat-inactivated *S. pneumoniae*. Our results suggest that *P. gingivalis* is a powerful inflammatory stimulant for human bronchial and pharyngeal epithelial cells and can stimulate TLR2-mediated cytokine production, thereby potentially contributing to the onset of aspiration pneumonia.

Keywords: aspiration pneumonia; chronic periodontitis; *Porphyromonas gingivalis*; proinflammatory cytokines; TLR2

---

1. Introduction

Aspiration pneumonia is a major health problem because of its high mortality rates in elderly people who are frequently immunocompromised [1]. This occurs because of inflammation in the lower respiratory tract that is stimulated by mis-swallowed saliva entering through the pharynx [1]. Pneumonia is characterized by increased number of infiltrated inflammatory cells such as neutrophils and elevated levels of proinflammatory cytokines, including chemokines, in the lower respiratory tract [2,3]. The so-called respiratory bacteria, such as *Streptococcus pneumoniae*, are exogenous; hence, they initially infect lower respiratory epithelia and subsequently induce proinflammatory cytokine production [3]. In turn, secreted cytokines such as interleukin (IL)-8 recruit neutrophils to infected tissues, and IL-6 exerts proinflammatory effects on respiratory epithelial cells [3–7]. These cytokines thus play a key role in orchestrating inflammatory responses in the lower respiratory tract in the development of pneumonia.

Chronic periodontitis is defined as an endogenous microflora-associated chronic inflammatory disease that develops as a result of poor oral hygiene [8]. The disease which causes the destruction of the periodontium, including alveolar bone, is one of the most prevalent infectious diseases worldwide [8]. Chronic periodontitis is caused by increased inflammatory responses, including proinflammatory cytokine production executed by host local immunity that is triggered by and amplified in relation to an increase in the number of periodontopathic bacteria [8]. Among them, the most pathogenic bacterium is *Porphyromonas gingivalis*, a Gram-negative black-pigmented anaerobe that predominantly colonizes periodontal pockets and is detected on the tongue dorsum and in the saliva of patients with advanced chronic periodontitis [9]. *P. gingivalis* exerts its virulence by interacting with several host pattern recognition receptors such as Toll-like receptor (TLR) 2 and TLR4 [10].

Accumulating evidence indicates that chronic periodontitis is a risk factor for several systemic diseases such as pre-term birth, heart diseases, diabetes, and atherosclerosis [8]. In this regard, we have reported that a major metabolite of *P. gingivalis* possibly induces the reactivation of latently infected viruses, namely human immunodeficiency virus and Epstein–Barr virus [11,12]. Over the last two decades, chronic periodontitis has also been identified as a risk factor for aspiration pneumonia in the elderly [13,14]. *P. gingivalis* is isolated from bronchoalveolar lavage fluid (BALF) or sputum from patients with pneumonia [15–18]. In fact, an increase in teeth with periodontal pockets in the elderly is associated with increased mortality from aspiration pneumonia [19]. Furthermore, periodontal interventions such as oral hygiene instruction reduce the occurrence of aspiration pneumonia, even among high-risk individuals [20]. Further, in the elderly, there is an increased risk of aspiration because these individuals have reduced laryngopharyngeal sensitivity [21]. Thus, these observations suggest that periodontopathic bacteria present in saliva are aspirated through the pharynx into the lower respiratory tract, thereby contributing to the onset of aspiration pneumonia. Despite its importance, a causal relationship between *P. gingivalis* and aspiration pneumonia remains unexamined.

Based on the aforementioned observations, we have hypothesized that increased number of *P. gingivalis* in the aspiration may induce proinflammatory cytokine production by human respiratory epithelia. However, *P. gingivalis is* anaerobic, and it is therefore unlikely to exhibit stable virulence in the respiratory tract. In addition, the duration of *P. gingivalis* survival in vitro and in vivo remains unclear. Therefore, in this study, we used heat-inactivated bacterial cells to examine whether *P. gingivalis* induced the production of proinflammatory cytokines such as IL-8 and IL-6 by human bronchial, alveolar, and pharyngeal epithelial cells via TLR2 or TLR4. To the best of our knowledge, we have delineated for the first time a putative mechanism by which *P. gingivalis* induces inflammation in human respiratory epithelia, thereby potentially contributing to the onset of aspiration pneumonia.

2. Materials and Methods

2.1. Cell Culture and Reagents

Human bronchial (BEAS-2B), pharyngeal (Detroit 562), and alveolar (A549) epithelial cells were purchased from ATCC (Manassas, VA, USA) and maintained at 37 °C in Dulbecco's modified Eagle's medium (Sigma, St. Louis, MO, USA) containing 10% heat-inactivated fetal bovine serum (Thermo Fisher Scientific, Rockford, IL, USA), penicillin (100 U/mL), and streptomycin (100 µg/mL), as described previously. HEK293 human embryonic kidney cells stably transfected with an expression plasmid for either human TLR2 (293-TLR2; InvivoGen, San Diego, CA, USA) or human TLR4 (293-TLR4; InvivoGen) were purchased and maintained at 37 °C in Dulbecco's modified Eagle's medium (Sigma) containing 10% heat-inactivated fetal bovine serum (Thermo Fisher Scientific) in the presence of the antibiotic blasticidin (10 μg/mL) to maintain selection for these transfectants. Neutralizing antibodies against human TLR2 and TLR4 were obtained from R&D Systems (Minneapolis, MN, USA). Lipoteichoic acid (LTA) derived from *Staphylococcus aureus* as a TLR2 ligand and lipopolysaccharide (LPS) derived from *Escherichia coli* as a TLR4 ligand were also purchased from Sigma.

2.2. *Bacterial Culture and Sample Adjustment*

P. gingivalis ATCC 33,277 was cultured in brain heart infusion broth (BHIB: Becton, Dickinson and Company, Sparks, MD, USA) supplemented with 5 μg/mL hemin and 0.5 μg/mL menadione. *S. pneumoniae* ATCC 6303 was cultured in BHIB. The cultures were incubated at 37 °C for 24–72 h and grown in an anaerobic chamber (Te-Her Anaerobox, Hirasawa Co. Ltd., Tokyo, Japan) under an anaerobic condition of 10% H_2, 10% CO_2, and 80% N_2. The bacterial cell density was adjusted to 1.0×10^{10} CFU/mL, and the bacterial suspension was heat-inactivated at 60 °C for 1 h and stored at −80 °C until use.

2.3. *mRNA Preparation and Real-Time Polymerase Chain Reaction (PCR)*

The experimental procedures for RNA purification and real-time PCR were performed as previously described [22]. Briefly, the cells were washed once with ice-cold phosphate-buffered saline and homogenized using QIAshredder (QIAGEN, Alameda, CA, USA), and total RNA was purified using an RNeasy Mini Kit (QIAGEN). For cDNA synthesis, total RNA (1 μg) was reverse-transcribed using an RNA PCR kit (PrimeScript; Takara Bio, Shiga, Japan). The resulting cDNA mixture was subjected to real-time PCR analysis using Premix Ex *Taq* solution (Takara Bio) containing 5 μM sense and antisense primers. The primer sequences used for the amplification of each gene were as follows: IL-8, forward (5′-CTT GTC ATT GCC AGC TGT GT-3′) and reverse (5′-TGA CTG TGG AGT TTT GGC TG-3′); IL-6, forward (5′-TTC GGT CCA GTT GCC TTC TC-3′) and reverse (5′-GAG GTG AGT GGC TGT CTG TG-3′); and glyceraldehyde-3-phosphate dehydrogenase (GAPDH), forward (5′-ACC AGC CCC AGC AAG AGC ACA AG-3′) and reverse (5′-TTC AAG GGG TCT ACA TGG CAA CTG-3′). PCR assays were performed using a TP-800 Thermal Cycler Dice Real-Time System (Takara Bio) and analyzed using the software provided by the device manufacturer. The thermal cycling conditions were 40 cycles of 95 °C for 5 s, 60 °C for 30 s, and 72 °C for 1 min. All real-time PCR experiments were performed in triplicate, and the specificity of each product was verified via melting curve analysis. Calculated gene expression levels were normalized to GAPDH mRNA levels.

2.4. *Cytokine Measurements*

IL-8 and IL-6 concentrations in the cell culture supernatants were measured using an enzyme-linked immunosorbent assay (ELISA) kit (R&D Systems) according to the manufacturer's recommendations. All experiments were performed in triplicate, and data are presented as the mean ± SD.

2.5. *Transfection and Luciferase Assay*

For NF-κB reporter assays, HEK293, 293-TLR2, or 293-TLR4 cells were plated in 12-well plates (4×10^5 cells/mL) and grown overnight. These cells were transfected with reporter plasmids using a Lipofectamine 2000 transfection reagent (Thermo Fisher Scientific) according to the manufacturer's instructions. Further, 200 ng of 5xκB-luc, a plasmid in which luciferase gene expression is under the control of NF-κB, and 10 ng of an internal control plasmid pRL-TK, which expresses *Renilla reniformis* luciferase under the control of the TK promoter, were used for each transfection. Twenty-four hours after transfection, the cells were incubated in the presence of heat-inactivated *P. gingivalis*, LTA, and LPS for 24 h. Cells were harvested using Passive Lysis Buffer (Promega, Madison, WI, USA), and the extracts were assessed for luciferase activity using a Dual-Luciferase Assay System (Promega) as described previously [12]. Luciferase activity was normalized to *R. reniformis* luciferase activity, which acted as an as an internal control for transfection efficiency.

3. Results

3.1. *P. gingivalis* Induced IL-8 and IL-6 mRNA Expression and Protein Production by Human Bronchial Epithelial Cells

P. gingivalis is considered to orchestrate dysbiosis of periodontal flora, which triggers inflammatory responses including cytokine production in the periodontium and in turn causes alveolar bone-destruction as a major symptom of chronic periodontitis [8]. We therefore first examined the mRNA induction of IL-8 and IL-6 by BEAS-2B bronchial epithelial cells and pertinent protein release using real-time PCR and ELISA, respectively.

As shown in Figure 1A, *P. gingivalis* markedly upregulated IL-8 and IL-6 mRNA expression in BEAS-2B cells. The levels of both mRNAs rose after a 1 h exposure to *P. gingivalis* and peaked at 3 h of incubation (151 ± 21- and 24 ± 3- fold, respectively). As shown in Figure 1B, *P. gingivalis* elicited the release of both cytokines between 1 and 12 h in a time-dependent manner. To clarify the cause-and-effect relationship between the density of bacteria and the extent of cytokine mRNA expression and protein production levels, we used *P. gingivalis* at densities equivalent to 1×10^7–1×10^8 CFU/mL. As shown in Figure 1C,D, *P. gingivalis* induced cytokine production as well as mRNA expression in a density-dependent manner.

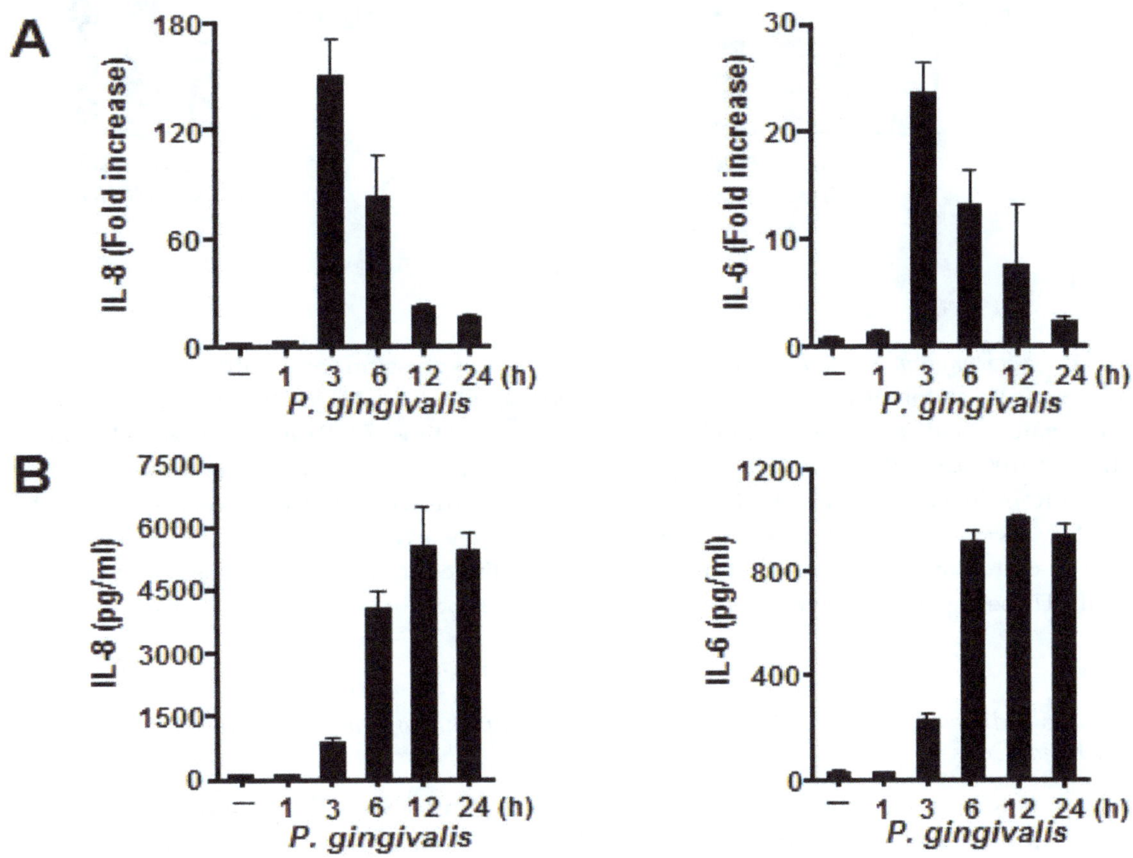

(a)

Figure 1. *Cont.*

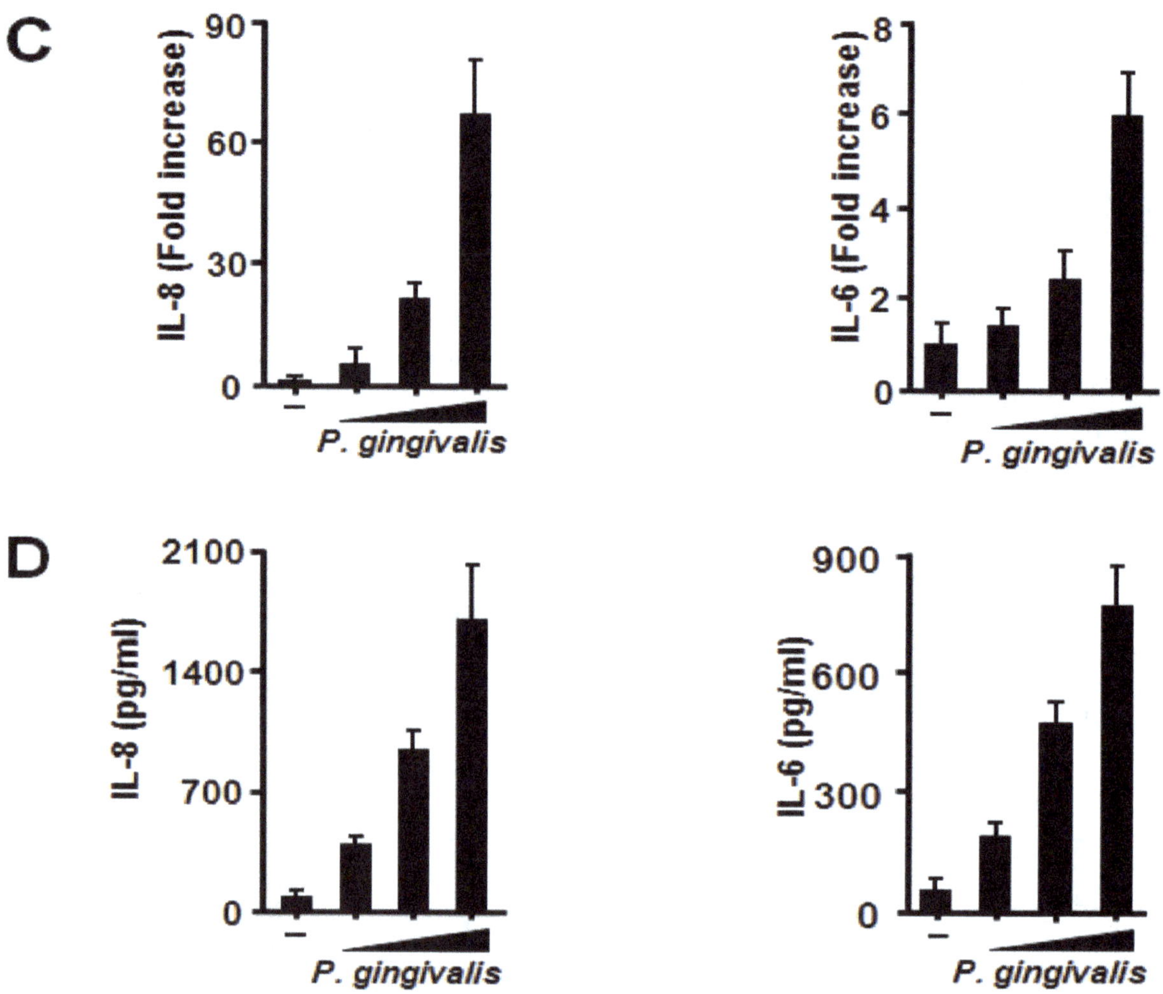

(**b**)

Figure 1. *Porphyromonas gingivalis*-induced mRNA expression and protein production of proinflammatory cytokines by human bronchial epithelial cells. BEAS-2B cells were exposed to heat-inactivated *P. gingivalis* (1×10^8 CFU/mL) for the indicated times (**A**,**B**) and at different bacterial cell densities (1×10^7, 0.5×10^8, or 1×10^8 CFU/mL) for 3 h (**C**) or 12 h (**D**). The cells were harvested, and IL-8 and IL-6 mRNA levels were measured using real-time polymerase chain reaction with specific primers. The mRNA levels were normalized to the GAPDH mRNA level and expressed as fold increases. IL-8 and IL-6 protein levels were determined by enzyme-linked immunosorbent assay and expressed as pg/mL. These experiments were performed in triplicate, and data are presented as the mean ± SD.

3.2. P. gingivalis Induced IL-8 and IL-6 Production by Human Pharyngeal Epithelial Cells but not by Human Alveolar Epithelial Cells

Because *P. gingivalis*-induced IL-8 and IL-6 production by BEAS-2B bronchial epithelial cells was observed, we examined whether pharyngeal epithelial cell line was also reactive to the stimulation with *P. gingivalis* because every material to be swallowed is retained in the pharynx for a while. As expected, stronger IL-8 production and much weaker IL-6 production than those by BEAS-2B cells were observed in Detroit 562 pharyngeal epithelial cells, which was in a density-dependent manner (Figure 2A). In contrast, proinflammatory cytokine production by *P. gingivalis* was not observed in A549 alveolar epithelial cells (Figure 2B).

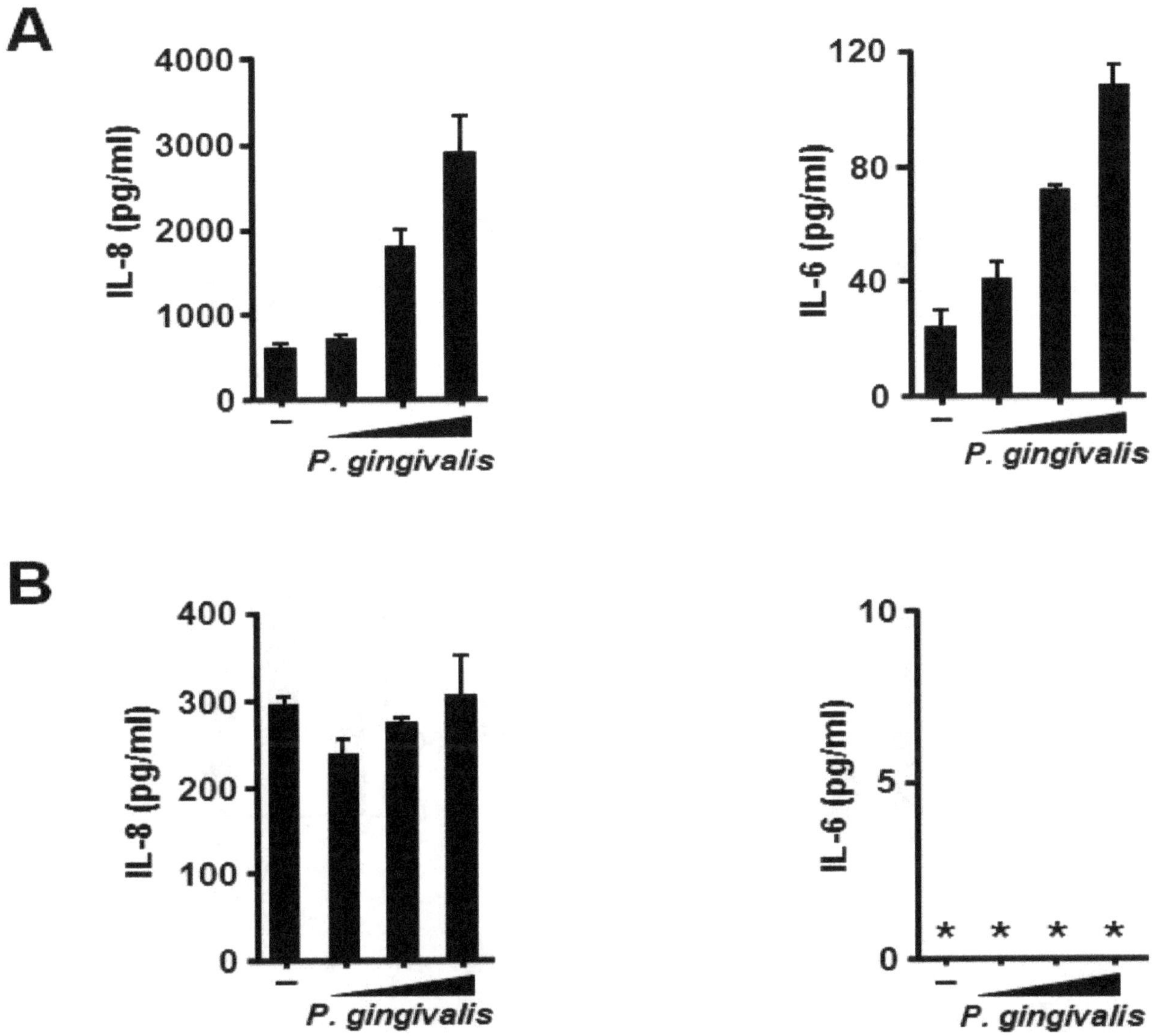

Figure 2. Effects of *Porphyromonas gingivalis* on interleukin (IL)-8 and IL-6 production by two human respiratory epithelial cells. Human pharyngeal (Detroit 562) (**A**) or alveolar (A549) (**B**) epithelial cells were incubated with heat-inactivated *P. gingivalis* (1×10^8 CFU/mL) for 12 h. IL-8 and IL-6 protein levels in the cell culture supernatants were determin ed by enzyme-linked immunosorbent assay. These experiments were performed in triplicate, and data are presented as the mean ± SD. *; below the detection limit.

3.3. P. gingivalis More Strongly Induced IL-8 and IL-6 Production than S. pneumoniae by Human Bronchial Epithelial Cells

S. pneumoniae contributes to the onset of aspiration pneumonia by inducing proinflammatory cytokines release. We therefore compared the inducibility of heat-inactivated bacterial cells between *P. gingivalis* and *S. pneumoniae* by human bronchial and pharyngeal epithelial cells. As shown in Figure 3A, *S. pneumoniae* induced IL-8 and IL-6 release by BEAS-2B cells but at much lower levels than *P. gingivalis*. Much stronger IL-8 production and much weaker IL-6 production were observed with Detroit 562 cells (Figure 3B), whereas no significant cytokine release was observed with A549 cells (Figure 3C).

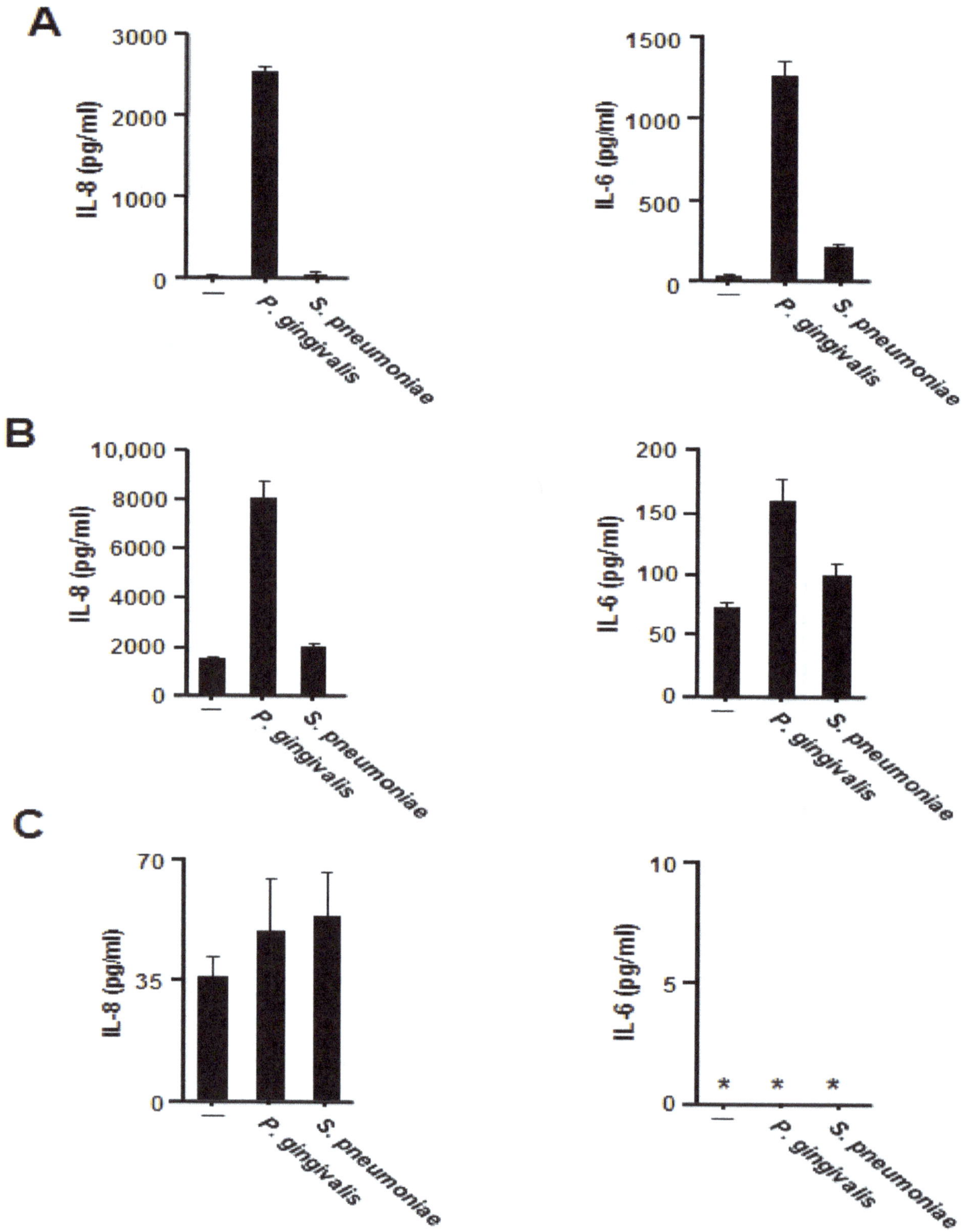

Figure 3. Comparison between the induction of proinflammatory cytokines by *Porphyromonas gingivalis* and by *Streptococcus pneumoniae*. BEAS-2B (**A**), Detroit 562 (**B**) or A549 (**C**) cells were incubated in the presence of heat-inactivated cells (1×10^8 CFU/mL) of *P. gingivalis* or *S. pneumoniae* for 12 h. IL-8 and IL-6 levels in the culture supernatants were then determined using enzyme-linked immunosorbent assay. These experiments were performed in triplicate, and data are presented as the mean ± SD. *; below the detection limit.

3.4. *Involvement of TLR2 in P. gingivalis-Induced Proinflammatory Cytokine Production*

Several studies have demonstrated TLR2 and TLR4 are important host receptors for recognizing *P. gingivalis* [10]. Eventually, these TLRs are reported to express on BASE-2B cells as well as on human bronchial epithelium and on Detroit 562 cells [23–25]. However, no study has yet examined whether human respiratory epithelial cells recognize *P. gingivalis* with their TLR2 or TLR4. In parallel, for producing IL-8 and IL-6, NF-κB is known to be an important transcription factor [26]. We therefore first examined whether these TLRs were involved in the NF-κB activation in *P. gingivalis*-stimulated epithelial cells using a luciferase assay. For this purpose, TLR-null HEK293 cells and HEK293 cells stably expressing either TLR2 or TLR4 cells were transfected with NF-κB reporter plasmids. As expected, NF-κB in 293-TLR2 cells were activated only by the stimulation with its specific ligand LTA from *S. aureus*, and likewise, 293-TLR4 cells were activated only by LPS from *E. coli*, whereas HEK293 cells were not activated by the both ligands (Figure 4A). When these cells were stimulated with *P. gingivalis*, 293-TLR2 cells alone were activated in a density-dependent manner (Figure 4A). These findings suggest that the observed cytokine production by BEAS-2B and Detroit 562 cells is induced via TLR2 but not via TLR4. To confirm this, BEAS-2B and Detroit 562 cells were treated with anti-TLR2 or anti-TLR4 antibodies prior to the stimulation with *P. gingivalis*. As shown in Figure 4B,C, anti-TLR4 antibodies had no effect on IL-8 and IL-6 production by either cell line following exposure to *P. gingivalis*, whereas the anti-TLR2 antibody significantly abrogated the production of both cytokines.

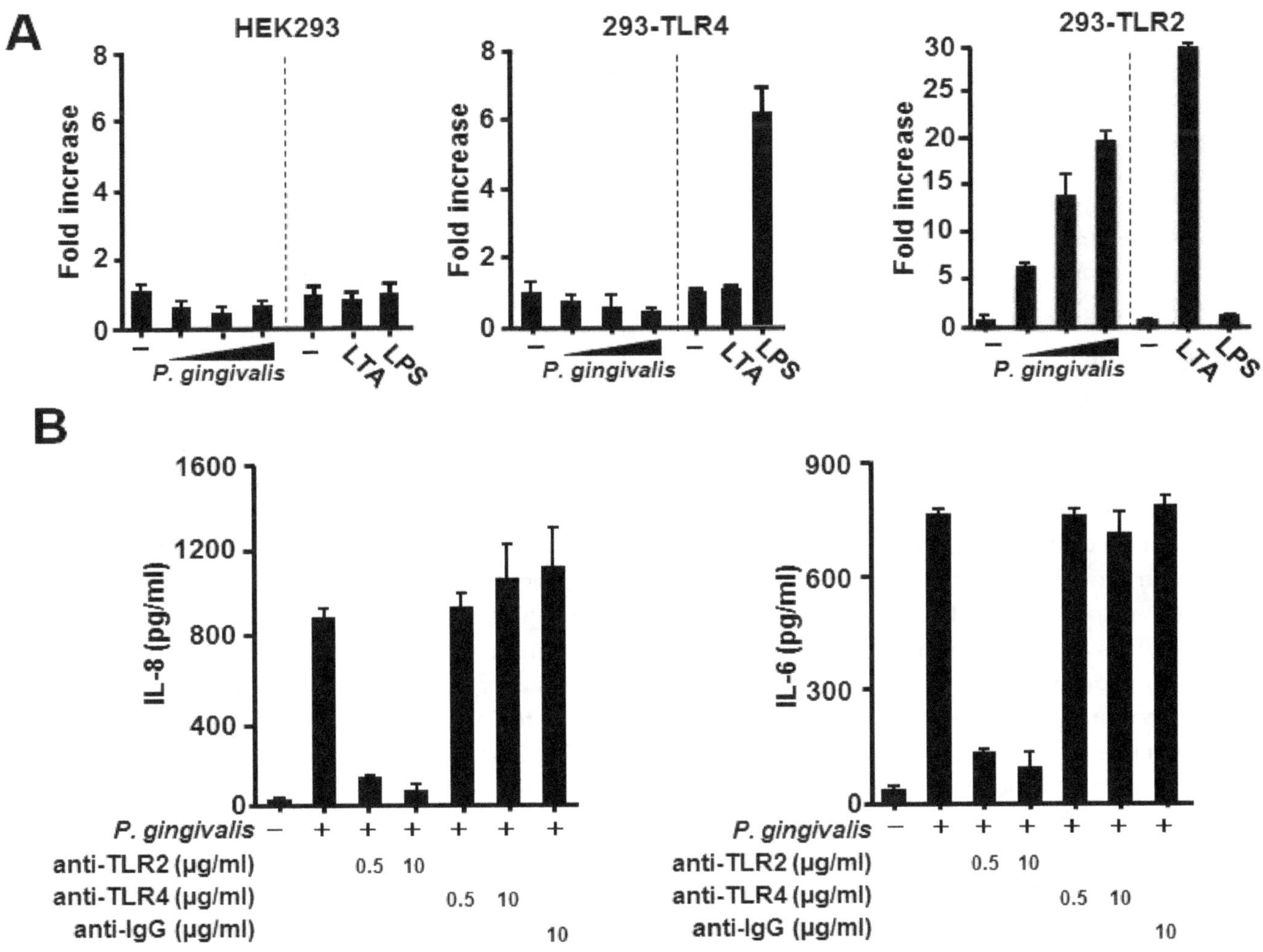

(a)

Figure 4. *Cont.*

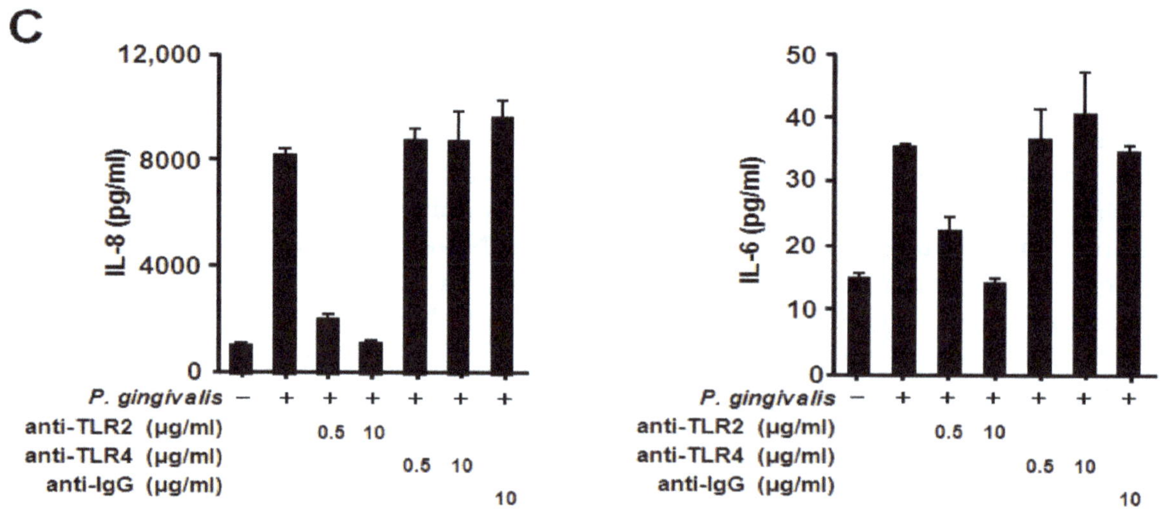

(b)

Figure 4. Involvement of Toll-like receptor (TLR)2 but not TLR4 in *Porphyromonas gingivalis*-induced proinflammatory cytokine production. (**A**) HEK293 cells, 293-TLR4 cells, or 293-TLR2 cells were transfected with a 5xκB-luc reporter plasmid together with an internal pRL-TK control plasmid. Twenty-four hours after transfection, these cells were stimulated with heat-inactivated *P. gingivalis* (1×10^7, 0.5×10^8, or 1×10^8 CFU/mL), *S. aureus* LTA (5 μg/mL), or *E. coli* LPS (200 ng/mL) for 24 h. Luciferase activity in the whole cell lysate was then determined. The data are presented as the fold increase in luciferase activity relative to that in control transfected cells (no stimulation). Data are presented as the mean ± SD of three independent transfections.BEAS-2B (**B**) and Detroit 562 (**C**) cells were pretreated with the indicated concentrations of anti-TLR2, anti-TLR4, or control antibodies for 1 h and then stimulated with or without *P. gingivalis* (1×10^8 CFU/mL). After 12 h incubation, culture supernatants were collected, and IL-8 and IL-6 levels were measured using enzyme-linked immunosorbent assay. These experiments were performed in triplicate, and data are presented as the mean ± SD.

4. Discussion

Because bacteria in saliva are aspirated into the lower respiratory tract, many studies have revealed an association between chronic periodontitis and aspiration pneumonia. In fact, *P. gingivalis* has been isolated from BALF or sputum in patients with aspiration pneumonia [15–18]. However, the mechanism by which the bacterium triggers the development of aspiration pneumonia has not been delineated. By contrast, *S. pneumoniae* is a major exogenous respiratory pathogen that infects the bronchial epithelium. This subsequently induces the release of proinflammatory cytokines, thereby contributing to the development of pneumonia [2,3]. In the present study, we found that *P. gingivalis* is a significant inflammatory stimulant for bronchial and pharyngeal epithelial cells.

IL-8, a potent neutrophil chemoattractant and activator, is associated with the pathogenesis of pneumonia. It accumulates and subsequently degranulates neutrophils, resulting in the destruction of normal tissues [2,3]. In fact, IL-8 levels are markedly elevated in BALF or sputum from patients with pneumonia in relation to an increase of neutrophil counts [4–6]. Interestingly, the extent of IL-8 release by respiratory epithelia is positively correlated with the bacterial load in the lower respiratory tract, which consequently contributes to lung injury [27,28]. In this regard, secreted IL-6 is involved in the stimulation of acute-phase protein synthesis, leukocyte recruitment, B-cell differentiation, and T-cell activation in many chronic inflammatory diseases [2,3]. IL-6 levels are also increased in the plasma and BALF of patients with pneumonia [7]. We observed that the release of IL-8 and IL-6 by bronchial and pharyngeal epithelial cells, both of which were induced by the exposure by *P. gingivalis*, was stronger than that by *S. pneumoniae*. Because IL-8 and IL-6 exert their proinflammatory effects in paracrine and autocrine manners, they must elicit inflammatory responses in neighboring host cells.

Our results thus suggest that inflammation in the lower respiratory epithelial cells is caused by an exposure to *P. gingivalis* itself and additionally by the absorption of paracrine proinflammatory cytokines released from the pharyngeal epithelium, which is induced by a precedent exposure to *P. gingivalis*. Therefore, these results may provide the novel insight that *P. gingivalis* contributes to the onset of aspiration pneumonia by inducing proinflammatory cytokine-production by bronchial and pharyngeal epithelial cells without infection.

From the aforementioned viewpoint, it should be also noted that elderly people have an increased risk of salivary aspiration because of their reduced laryngopharyngeal sensitivity and swallowing reflex impairment, both of which are ascribable to mild cognitive impairment [21]. In addition, an average person generates and ingests up to 1.5 L of saliva per day, which contains 1×10^8/mL bacteria released from oral biofilms, indicating more than 1×10^{11} bacteria are swallowed daily [29,30]. Moreover, a high incidence of silent aspiration during sleep is eventually recorded in the elderly [31,32]. These observations along with our findings support our hypothesis that increased number of *P. gingivalis* in saliva because of poor oral hygiene raises the risk of the onset of aspiration pneumonia.

Respiratory epithelia represent the first line of defense against exogenous respiratory pathogens. Respiratory epithelia are surely exposed to aspirated *P. gingivalis*, after which the bacterium presumably attaches to epithelial surfaces via several interactions between epithelial receptors and bacterial ligands such as fimbriae and LPS [10]. However, recognition of bacterial attachment by the epithelium alone might induce cytokine production. The present findings of proinflammatory secretion by bronchial and pharyngeal epithelial cells exposed to heat-inactivated *P. gingivalis* indicate that infection is not necessarily required for the observed induction of cytokine production. In this connection, several studies have indicated that heat-inactivated *P. gingivalis* appears capable of modulating the expression of inflammatory cytokines in several types of human cells other than respiratory epithelial cells, such as monocytes, whole blood cells, and gingival epithelial cells [33–36]. These observations are reminiscent of the manner how *S. pneumoniae* induces pneumonia.

Significant involvement of TLR2 but not TLR4 of several types of human cells, such as periodontal ligament cells, gingival fibroblasts, and monocytes, gingival epithelial cells, in proinflammatory cytokine production induced by *P. gingivalis* is also reported [35–37]. Although both BEAS-2B and Detroit 562 cells express TLR2 and TLR4, to the best of our knowledge, we found for the first time that only anti-TLR2 antibody significantly and concentration-dependently reduced *P. gingivalis*-induced IL-8 and IL-6 production by these cells. In parallel with these findings, *P. gingivalis* can elicit high levels of proinflammatory cytokine production in wild-type or TLR4-deficient mice, but not TLR2-deficient mice [38,39]. This suggests that without heat inactivation, TLR2 is necessary for *P. gingivalis* to induce proinflammatory cytokine production by host cells. These observations along with our findings suggest that bronchial and pharyngeal epithelia secrete some proinflammatory cytokines via TLR2 stimulation and become inflamed quickly when they are exposed to *P. gingivalis* irrespective of bacterial vitality.

Although *P. gingivalis* LPS and Fim A, a major fimbriae of *P. gingivalis*, have been widely accepted as TLR2 ligands [40–42], the stimulation of neither BEAS-2B nor Detroit 562 cells by these bacterial surface structures alone elicited IL-8 and IL-6 protein secretion. Therefore, the necessity of other surface structures or the whole *P. gingivalis* cell for the observed cytokine production is currently under study. In addition, in the human phagocytes, TLR2 is an essential molecule for sensing *P. gingivalis* and appears to be paired often by TLR1 and sometimes by TLR6 for arranging subsequent intracellular signaling due to imminent immunological necessity [40,43]. Because this has not been investigated in human respiratory epithelia, it would be interesting to see how blocking of TLR1 or TLR6 influences the *P. gingivalis*-induced IL-8 and IL-6 production. Further studies are therefore needed. However, it would be important that our findings have revealed a putatively causal relationship between *P. gingivalis* as a proinflammatory stimulant to several human respiratory epithelia and the onset of aspiration pneumonia.

Author Contributions: N.W., S.Y., and K.I. performed the experiments, analyzed the data, contributed reagents/materials/analytical tools, prepared the figures, and reviewed drafts of the article. Y.O. and S.S. contributed to the discussion, analyzed the data, and reviewed the drafts of the article. K.I. conceived, designed the experiments, authored or reviewed drafts of the article. All authors have read and agreed to the published version of the manuscript.

References

1. Okazaki, T.; Ebihara, S.; Mori, T.; Izumi, S.; Ebihara, T. Association between sarcopenia and pneumonia in older people. *Geriatr. Gerontol. Int.* **2019**, *20*, 7–13. [CrossRef]
2. Strieter, R.M.; Belperio, J.; Keane, M.P. Host innate defenses in the lung: The role of cytokines. *Curr. Opin. Infect. Dis.* **2003**, *16*, 193–198. [CrossRef]
3. Gomez, M.I.; Prince, A. Airway epithelial cell signaling in response to bacterial pathogens. *Pediatr. Pulmonol.* **2007**, *43*, 11–19. [CrossRef] [PubMed]
4. Boutten, A.; Dehoux, M.S.; Seta, N.; Ostinelli, J.; Venembre, P.; Crestani, B.; Dombret, M.C.; Durand, G.; Aubier, M. Compartmentalized IL-8 and elastase release within the human lung in unilateral pneumonia. *Am. J. Respir. Crit. Care Med.* **1996**, *153*, 336–342. [CrossRef] [PubMed]
5. Schütte, H.; Lohmeyer, J.; Rosseau, S.; Ziegler, S.; Siebert, C.; Kielisch, H.; Pralle, H.; Grimminger, F.; Morr, H.; Seeger, W. Bronchoalveolar and systemic cytokine profiles in patients with ARDS, severe pneumonia and cardiogenic pulmonary oedema. *Eur. Respir. J.* **1996**, *9*, 1858–1867. [CrossRef] [PubMed]
6. Chollet-Martin, S.; Montravers, P.; Gibert, C.; Elbim, C.; Desmonts, J.M.; Fagon, J.Y.; A Gougerot-Pocidalo, M. High levels of interleukin-8 in the blood and alveolar spaces of patients with pneumonia and adult respiratory distress syndrome. *Infect. Immun.* **1993**, *61*, 4553–4559. [CrossRef] [PubMed]
7. Montón, C.; Ewig, S.; Torres, A.; El-Ebiary, M.; Filella, X.; Rañó, A.; Xaubet, A. Role of glucocorticoids on inflammatory response in nonimmunosuppressed patients with pneumonia: A pilot study. *Eur. Respir. J.* **1999**, *14*, 218–220. [CrossRef]
8. Pihlstrom, B.L.; Michalowicz, B.S.; Johnson, N.W. Periodontal diseases. *Lancet* **2005**, *366*, 1809–1820. [CrossRef]
9. Bostanci, N.; Belibasakis, G.N. Porphyromonas gingivalis: An invasive and evasive opportunistic oral pathogen. *FEMS Microbiol. Lett.* **2012**, *333*, 1–9. [CrossRef] [PubMed]
10. Iii, F.C.G.; Genco, C.A. Porphyromonas gingivalis Mediated Periodontal Disease and Atherosclerosis: Disparate Diseases with Commonalities in Pathogenesis Through TLRs. *Curr. Pharm. Des.* **2007**, *13*, 3665–3675. [CrossRef]
11. Imai, K.; Ochiai, K.; Okamoto, T. Reactivation of Latent HIV-1 Infection by the Periodontopathic BacteriumPorphyromonas gingivalisInvolves Histone Modification. *J. Immunol.* **2009**, *182*, 3688–3695. [CrossRef] [PubMed]
12. Imai, K.; Inoue, H.; Tamura, M.; Cueno, M.E.; Inoue, H.; Takeichi, O.; Kusama, K.; Saito, I.; Ochiai, K. The periodontal pathogen Porphyromonas gingivalis induces the Epstein–Barr virus lytic switch transactivator ZEBRA by histone modification. *Biochimie* **2012**, *94*, 839–846. [CrossRef] [PubMed]
13. Van Der Maarel-Wierink, C.D.; Vanobbergen, J.N.O.; Bronkhorst, E.M.; Schols, J.M.G.A.; De Baat, C. Oral health care and aspiration pneumonia in frail older people: A systematic literature review. *Gerodontology* **2012**, *30*, 3–9. [CrossRef] [PubMed]
14. Terpenning, M.S.; Taylor, G.W.; Lopatin, D.E.; Kerr, C.K.; Dominguez, B.L.; Loesche, W.J. Aspiration Pneumonia: Dental and Oral Risk Factors in an Older Veteran Population. *J. Am. Geriatr. Soc.* **2001**, *49*, 557–563. [CrossRef]
15. Nagaoka, K.; Yanagihara, K.; Harada, Y.; Yamada, K.; Migiyama, Y.; Morinaga, Y.; Izumikawa, K.; Kohno, S. Quantitative detection of periodontopathic bacteria in lower respiratory tract specimens by real-time PCR. *J. Infect. Chemother.* **2017**, *23*, 69–73. [CrossRef] [PubMed]
16. Yatera, K.; Noguchi, S.; Mukae, H. The microbiome in the lower respiratory tract. *Respir. Investig.* **2018**, *56*, 432–439. [CrossRef]
17. Bartlett, J.G.; Finegold, S.M. Anaerobic infections of the lung and pleural space. *Am. Rev. Respir. Dis.* **1974**, *110*, 56–77. [CrossRef]
18. Bartlett, J.G. Anaerobic bacterial infection of the lung. *Anaerobe* **2012**, *18*, 235–239. [CrossRef]

19. Awano, S.; Ansai, T.; Takata, Y.; Soh, I.; Akifusa, S.; Hamasaki, T.; Yoshida, A.; Sonoki, K.; Fujisawa, K.; Takehara, T. Oral Health and Mortality Risk from Pneumonia in the Elderly. *J. Dent. Res.* **2008**, *87*, 334–339. [CrossRef]
20. Scannapieco, F.A.; Bush, R.B.; Paju, S. Associations Between Periodontal Disease and Risk for Nosocomial Bacterial Pneumonia and Chronic Obstructive Pulmonary Disease. A Systematic Review. *Ann. Periodontol.* **2003**, *8*, 54–69. [CrossRef]
21. Faverio, P.; Aliberti, S.; Bellelli, G.; Suigo, G.; Lonni, S.; Pesci, A.; Restrepo, M.I. The management of community-acquired pneumonia in the elderly. *Eur. J. Intern. Med.* **2014**, *25*, 312–319. [CrossRef]
22. Imai, K.; Kamio, N.; Cueno, M.E.; Saito, Y.; Inoue, H.; Saito, I.; Ochiai, K. Role of the histone H3 lysine 9 methyltransferase Suv39 h1 in maintaining Epsteinn-Barr virus latency in B95-8 cells. *FEBS J.* **2014**, *281*, 2148–2158. [CrossRef]
23. Liu, X.; Wetzler, L.M.; Nascimento, L.E.O.; Massari, P. Human Airway Epithelial Cell Responses to Neisseria lactamica and Purified Porin via Toll-Like Receptor 2-Dependent Signaling. *Infect. Immun.* **2010**, *78*, 5314–5323. [CrossRef]
24. Rydberg, C.; Månsson, A.; Uddman, R.; Riesbeck, K.; Cardell, L.-O. Toll-like receptor agonists induce inflammation and cell death in a model of head and neck squamous cell carcinomas. *Immunology* **2009**, *128*, e600–e611. [CrossRef]
25. Dogan, S.; Zhang, Q.; Pridmore, A.C.; Mitchell, T.J.; Finn, A.; Murdoch, C. Pneumolysin-induced CXCL8 production by nasopharyngeal epithelial cells is dependent on calcium flux and MAPK activation via Toll-like receptor 4. *Microbes Infect.* **2011**, *13*, 65–75. [CrossRef]
26. Hayden, M.S.; Ghosh, S. Signaling to NF-KappaB. *Genes Dev.* **2004**, *18*, 2195–2224. [CrossRef]
27. Hill, A.T.; Campbell, E.J.; Hill, S.L.; Bayley, D.L.; Stockley, R.A. Association between airway bacterial load and markers of airway inflammation in patients with stable chronic bronchitis. *Am. J. Med.* **2000**, *109*, 288–295. [CrossRef]
28. Nocker, R.E.; Schoonbrood, D.F.; Graaf, E.A.v.d.G.; Hack, C.E.; Lutter, R.; Jansen, H.M.; Out, T.A. Interleukin-8 in airway inflammation in patients with asthma and chronic obstructive pulmonary disease. *Int. Arch. Allergy Immunol.* **1996**, *109*, 183–191. [CrossRef]
29. Boutaga, K.; Savelkoul, P.H.M.; Winkel, E.G.; Van Winkelhoff, A.J. Comparison of Subgingival Bacterial Sampling with Oral Lavage for Detection and Quantification of Periodontal Pathogens by Real-Time Polymerase Chain Reaction. *J. Periodontol.* **2007**, *78*, 79–86. [CrossRef]
30. Von Troil-Linden, B.; Torkko, H.; Alaluusua, S.; Jousimies-Somer, H.; Asikainen, S. Salivary Levels of Suspected Periodontal Pathogens in Relation to Periodontal Status and Treatment. *J. Dent. Res.* **1995**, *74*, 1789–1795. [CrossRef]
31. Marik, P.E.; Kaplan, D. Aspiration Pneumonia and Dysphagia in the Elderly. *Chest* **2003**, *124*, 328–336. [CrossRef] [PubMed]
32. Ebihara, S.; Ebihara, T.; Kohzuki, M. Effect of Aging on Cough and Swallowing Reflexes: Implications for Preventing Aspiration Pneumonia. *Lung* **2011**, *190*, 29–33. [CrossRef] [PubMed]
33. Hamedi, M.; Belibasakis, G.N.; Cruchley, A.T.; Rangarajan, M.; Curtis, M.A.; Bostanci, N. Porphyromonas gingivalis culture supernatants differentially regulate interleukin-1beta and interleukin-18 in human monocytic cells. *Cytokine* **2009**, *45*, 99–104. [CrossRef] [PubMed]
34. Takahashi, N.; Honda, T.; Domon, H.; Nakajima, T.; Tabeta, K.; Yamazaki, K. Interleukin-1 receptor-associated kinase-M in gingival epithelial cells attenuates the inflammatory response elicited byPorphyromonas gingivalis. *J. Periodontal Res.* **2010**, *45*, 512–519. [CrossRef] [PubMed]
35. Sun, Y.; Shu, R.; Li, C.-L.; Zhang, M.-Z. Gram-Negative Periodontal Bacteria Induce the Activation of Toll-Like Receptors 2 and 4, and Cytokine Production in Human Periodontal Ligament Cells. *J. Periodontol.* **2010**, *81*, 1488–1496. [CrossRef]
36. Tietze, K.; Dalpke, A.; Morath, S.; Mutters, R.; Heeg, K.; Nonnenmacher, C. Differences in innate immune responses upon stimulation with gram-positive and gram-negative bacteria. *J. Periodontal Res.* **2006**, *41*, 447–454. [CrossRef]
37. Andrukhov, O.; Ertlschweiger, S.; Moritz, A.; Bantleon, H.P.; Rausch-Fan, X. Different effects of P. gingivalis LPS and E. coli LPS on the expression of interleukin-6 in human gingival fibroblasts. *Acta Odontol. Scand.* **2014**, *72*, 337–345. [CrossRef]

38. Burns, E.; Bachrach, G.; Shapira, L.; Nussbaum, G. Cutting Edge: TLR2 Is Required for the Innate Response toPorphyromonas gingivalis: Activation Leads to Bacterial Persistence and TLR2 Deficiency Attenuates Induced Alveolar Bone Resorption. *J. Immunol.* **2006**, *177*, 8296–8300. [CrossRef]
39. Hayashi, C.; Madrigal, A.G.; Liu, X.; Ukai, T.; Goswami, S.; Gudino, C.V.; Gibson, F.C.; Genco, C.A.; Gibson, I.F.C. Pathogen-mediated inflammatory atherosclerosis is mediated in part via Toll-like receptor 2-induced inflammatory responses. *J. Innate Immun.* **2010**, *2*, 334–343. [CrossRef]
40. Hajishengallis, G.; Tapping, R.I.; Harokopakis, E.; Nishiyama, S.-I.; Ratti, P.; Schifferle, R.E.; Lyle, E.A.; Triantafilou, M.; Triantafilou, K.; Yoshimura, F. Differential interactions of fimbriae and lipopolysaccharide from Porphyromonas gingivalis with the Toll-like receptor 2-centred pattern recognition apparatus. *Cell Microbiol.* **2006**, *8*, 1557–1570. [CrossRef]
41. Jain, S.; Coats, S.R.; Chang, A.M.; Darveau, R.P. A Novel Class of Lipoprotein Lipase-Sensitive Molecules Mediates Toll-Like Receptor 2 Activation by Porphyromonas gingivalis. *Infect. Immun.* **2013**, *81*, 1277–1286. [CrossRef]
42. Nichols, F.C.; Bajrami, B.; Clark, R.B.; Housley, W.; Yao, X. Free Lipid A Isolated from Porphyromonas gingivalis Lipopolysaccharide Is Contaminated with Phosphorylated Dihydroceramide Lipids: Recovery in Diseased Dental Samples. *Infect. Immun.* **2011**, *80*, 860–874. [CrossRef]
43. Kawai, T.; Akira, S. The role of pattern-recognition receptors in innate immunity: Update on Toll-like receptors. *Nat. Immunol.* **2010**, *11*, 373–384. [CrossRef] [PubMed]

13

Periodontitis: A Multifaceted Disease of Tooth-Supporting Tissues

Eija Könönen [1,2,*], Mervi Gursoy [1] and Ulvi Kahraman Gursoy [1]

1 Department of Periodontology, Institute of Dentistry, University of Turku, 20520 Turku, Finland
2 Oral Health Care, Welfare Division, City of Turku, 20101 Turku, Finland
* Correspondence: eija.kononen@utu.fi

Abstract: Periodontitis is an infection-driven inflammatory disease in which the composition of biofilms plays a significant role. Dental plaque accumulation at the gingival margin initiates an inflammatory response that, in turn, causes microbial alterations and may lead to drastic consequences in the periodontium of susceptible individuals. Chronic inflammation affects the gingiva and can proceed to periodontitis, which characteristically results in irreversible loss of attachment and alveolar bone. Periodontitis appears typically in adult-aged populations, but young individuals can also experience it and its harmful outcome. Advanced disease is the major cause of tooth loss in adults. In addition, periodontitis is associated with many chronic diseases and conditions affecting general health.

Keywords: periodontal disease; alveolar bone loss; gingiva; bacteria; biofilm; immunity; inflammation; smoking

---

1. Introduction

Periodontitis is an infection-driven inflammatory disease in tooth-supporting tissues (i.e., the periodontium). Moreover, genetics and environmental and behavioral factors are involved in the development of the disease, the exposure of susceptible individuals to its initiation, and the speed of progression. The structure of the periodontium is diverse; it is composed of the gingiva, the underlying connective tissue, cement on the root surface, alveolar bone, and the periodontal ligament between the cementum and alveolar bone (Figure 1A,B). The junctional epithelium of the gingiva is a unique structure, located at the bottom of the gingival sulcus, which controls the constant presence of bacteria at this site. The most characteristic feature of periodontitis is the activation of osteoclastogenesis and the destruction of alveolar bone as its consequence, which is irreversible and leads to loss of tooth support.

Periodontal disease, especially its mild and moderate forms, is highly prevalent in adult-aged populations all over the world, with prevalence rates around 50% [1], while its severe form increases especially between the third and fourth decades of life, with the global prevalence being around 10% [2]. Certain demographic characteristics, such as age, gender, ethnicity, and socioeconomic status, influence the prevalence of periodontitis. Other strongly contributing factors include smoking, diabetes mellitus, metabolic syndrome, and obesity [3,4]. It is noteworthy that smoking and diabetes can expose individuals to the advanced form of periodontal disease already in adolescence and early adulthood [5–7]. There is also a strong relation of smoking to tooth loss in young individuals [8]. Severe periodontitis, the major cause of tooth loss in adults (https://www.nidcr.nih.gov/research/data-statistics/periodontal-disease), is typically complicated by the drifting and hypermobility of teeth, eventually resulting in the collapsed bite function of an affected individual [9,10]. Moreover, periodontal disease as well as tooth loss are considered to have an association with a variety of chronic diseases and conditions affecting general health.

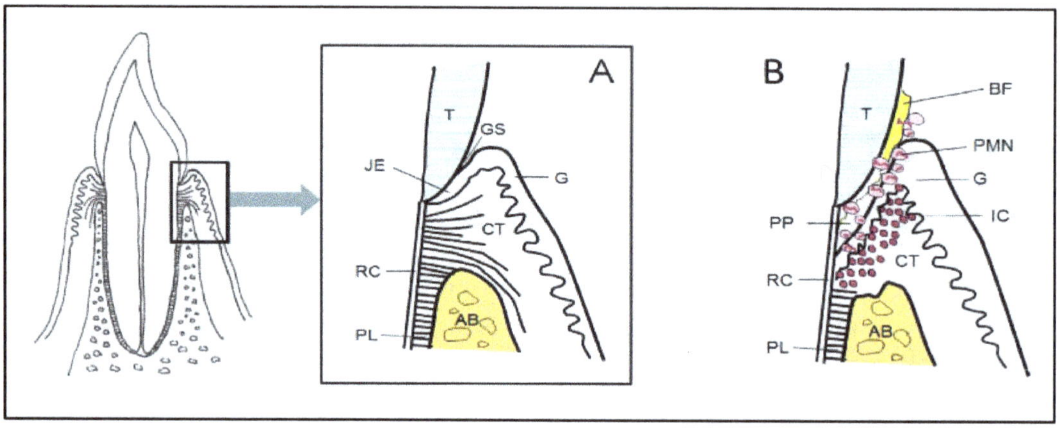

Figure 1. The anatomical structure of the periodontium in health (**A**) and in periodontitis (**B**). Abbreviations: Alveolar bone (AB), bacterial biofilm (BF), connective tissue (CT), gingiva (G), gingival sulcus (GS), inflammatory cells (IC), junctional epithelium (JE), polymorphonuclear neutrophils (PMN), periodontal ligament (PL), periodontal pocket (PP), root cementum (RC), and tooth (T).

Even in periodontal health, immune cells are constantly present in the gingiva, thus supporting the balance between oral biofilms and the host [11]. This constant communication keeps the immune response active, being a reciprocal, synergistic, and dynamic interaction. In the periodontium, the immune response carries characteristics of that of any other part of the body; the first action against microbes is due to non-specific innate response, while extended pathogenic challenge activates specific adaptive responses.

Excessive dental plaque accumulation at the gingival margin leads to inflammation and increasing proportions of proteolytic and often obligately anaerobic species [12]. The presence of periodontal species with pathogenic potential in the gingival sulcus initiates an inflammatory response in gingival tissue. When allowed to become chronic, this can have drastic consequences in the periodontium of susceptible individuals. Interactions between the components and metabolic activities of the oral microbiota and the host either support the balance (homeostasis) or result in disturbance (dysbiosis) within the microbiota [12]. Periodontal health-associated commensals are important in protecting the balance, for example, by inhibiting the growth of periodontitis-associated pathogens. However, qualitative and quantitative alterations within subgingival biofilms can result in disrupted homeostasis, which consequently can lead to the onset of disease with various degrees of periodontal tissue destruction.

2. Pathogenic Biofilms

Multispecies biofilm formation and maturation occur on tooth surfaces via intergeneric interactions, where coaggregations occur between different bacterial taxa, and highly diverse bacterial communities are formed at supragingival (above the gumline) and subgingival (below the gumline) sites [13,14]. *Fusobacterium nucleatum*, which belongs to the core anaerobic microbiota of the oral cavity from early years of life onwards [15,16], is seen as an important bridging organism of maturing dental biofilms, allowing late-colonizing species with virulent properties to be colonized [13]. This gradual maturation and shifts in the microbial composition influence the pathogenicity of subgingival biofilms where metabolically highly specialized microorganisms function in physical proximity as interactive microbial communities [12]. Focusing on only its adherence capabilities may lead to the underestimation of other important virulence characteristics of *F. nucleatum*, a relevant bacterium in the initiation and progression of periodontal disease. In a biofilm, this obligate anaerobe can survive and increase its numbers in aerobic environments [17]. Indeed, recent evidence indicates that *F. nucleatum* induces an environmental change through hypoxia [18], which can support the colonization of anaerobic pathogens in dental biofilms. The effects of *F. nucleatum*-induced hypoxia are not limited to the shifts in the biofilm composition—this hypoxia also directs endothelial cells to an inflammatory state and activates angiogenesis [18].

In subgingival biofilms, anaerobic gram-negative species with their biologically active lipopolysaccharide (LPS)-containing cell wall structure may be essential in awakening the inflammatory reaction in the gingiva and culprits of periodontal destruction to occur in periodontitis-susceptible individuals [11]. Subgingival plaque samples collected from periodontitis patients and periodontitis-free individuals differ from each other. *Porphyromonas gingivalis*, *Tannerella forsythia*, and *Treponema denticola*, the so-called red complex, have shown the strongest association with periodontal disease [19]. In another study by using 454 pyrosequencing of 16S rRNA genes, *P. gingivalis* and *T. denticola* but also *Filifactor alocis*, a gram-positive anaerobe, formed the top three species [20]. Of these, *P. gingivalis* is suggested to be the principal pathogen in the process, causing a disturbed interplay between the subgingival biofilm and the host response [21]. Even as a minor constituent of the subgingival microbiota, it is able to severely affect the ecosystem by influencing the numbers and community organization of commensal bacteria at the site and dysregulate innate immunity pathways. *P. gingivalis*, a highly proteolytic gram-negative anaerobe, is a common recovery from deepened periodontal pockets of adult periodontitis patients. While *P. gingivalis* is rather rare in children and adolescents, its salivary carriage rates increase significantly with aging, and it is detected in the majority of the Finnish population after the age of 55 years [22]. Different from *P. gingivalis*, the carriage of *Aggregatibacter actinomycetemcomitans* was less frequent, without any connection to age. This gram-negative capnophilic coccobacillus and an established periodontal pathogen has been linked to aggressive forms of periodontal disease [23]. Besides these traditional pathogens, open-ended molecular methods have significantly enlarged the list of pathogenic species within periodontitis-associated subgingival biofilms [24].

Many periodontitis-associated species, among those *A. actinomycetemcomitans*, *P. gingivalis*, and *F. nucleatum*, or even polymicrobial aggregates, are capable of invading periodontal tissues [25–27], thus evading many defense mechanisms of the host. This, in turn, has an impact on the persistence of inflammation and progression of periodontal tissue destruction.

For periodontal disease to occur, it is not the presence of a single periodontal pathogen, but the interplay between the composition of the subgingival biofilm and the host response where host factors and specific niches play an important role. In dysbiotic biofilms, there is abundance of immunostimulatory pathobionts and their virulence factors, but also a reduced inhibitory effect of commensal bacteria, thus resulting in an increased inflammatory response [28,29]. In gingival epithelia, cellular responses are especially elicited against polymicrobial biofilms due to their interbacterial metabolic and virulence synergisms [30], leading the way to initial pocket formation and attachment loss. Deepening periodontal pockets with an anaerobic environment, inflammatory conditions, and a large amount of substrates originating from tissue destruction all favor the growth of inflammophilic periodontal pathogens and pathobionts [21]. Notably, daily smoking contributes to further disturbances in the subgingival microbiota, facilitating an abundance of periodontal pathogens and the reduction of beneficial commensals, thus exposing smokers to periodontal disease [31].

There have been intensive research activities targeting periodontitis-associated bacteria and/or the antibodies working against them, with the aim of revealing their involvement in various systemic diseases and conditions. Major periodontal pathogens raise local and systemic antibody responses; it has been shown in multivariate analyses that the main determinant of the systemic antibody response to *P. gingivalis* and *A. actinomycetemcomitans* is the carriage of the pathogen, whereas the presence or degree of periodontal disease has only a modest modifying effect [32]. High serum IgG antibodies to major periodontal pathogens act as risk factors for future cardiovascular events [33–35]. Also, the circulation of LPS of virulent gram-negative pathogens (endotoxemia) accompanied by exaggerated proinflammatory responses is connected to risk for these events [33]. Subgingival bacteria, including *P. gingivalis* and *A. actinomycetemcomitans*, have also been associated with the prevalence of prediabetes in young diabetes-free adults [36]. Interestingly, associations between bacterial measures and prediabetes are consistently stronger than those between periodontitis and prediabetes. Furthermore, there is accumulating evidence on the role of *P. gingivalis* in rheumatoid arthritis [37,38]. A prospective study on the association between pancreatic cancer and the oral microbiome revealed that the carriage of *P. gingivalis* and *A. actinomycetemcomitans* is a subsequent risk for this highly lethal cancer type [39]. Besides the impact of *F. nucleatum* as the key organism in dental biofilms and its involvement in oral and extra-oral polymicrobial infections [40], recent research has shown its significant carcinogenic potential. Its ability to tolerate oxygen, create hypoxia, and induce an inflammatory environment may explain the role of *F. nucleatum* in the development and progression of colorectal adenocarcinoma [41].

3. Immunologic Players of the Periodontium

Due to the constant interaction with bacteria, immune cells (neutrophils, macrophages, and lymphocytes) are present in the periodontium to take part in maintaining a healthy equilibrium. Neutrophils continuously transmigrate through the junctional epithelium to gingival sulcus and release antimicrobial peptides (α-defensins) against invading bacteria, while they also stimulate adhesion and the spread of keratinocytes on the tooth surface [42]. Resident cells of the periodontium (keratinocytes, fibroblasts, dendritic cells, and osteoblasts) are not passive barriers against bacterial invasion, but they initiate innate immune response and regulate adaptive immune response [43,44]. An essential component is the complement pathway, which activates, amplifies, and synchronizes innate immune response by opsonizing and killing bacteria as well as activating mast cells, neutrophils, and macrophages of the periodontium [45].

Keratinocytes, which form the majority of the gingival epithelium, are capable of producing and secreting various immune response mediators, among them human β-defensins (hBDs), cathelicidins, proinflammatory cytokines, chemokines, and angiogenetic proteins [46,47]. In the healthy gingiva, innate response is mainly regulated by keratinocytes and neutrophils; keratinocytes secrete hBDs to protect the oral and sulcular epithelium (Figure 2A), whereas neutrophils secrete α-defensins to protect the junctional epithelium (Figure 2B). Gingival keratinocytes recognize pathogen-associated molecular patterns (PAMPs) by their pattern recognition receptors, such as toll-like receptors (TLRs). mRNA expressions of TLR 1–9 are detected in connective tissue and epithelial layers of the gingiva [48]. In addition, bacterial signaling molecules (cyclic dinucleotides and quorum signaling molecules) activate cytokine response in gingival keratinocytes [49,50]. There is also a reciprocal interaction between innate-immune proteins and keratinocytes. For example, proinflammatory interleukins (IL-1α, IL-1β, IL-6) activate the protein expression and secretion of hBDs from keratinocytes [46,51], while keratinocytes can suppress the inflammatory response by secreting monocyte chemotactic protein-induced protein-1 [52].

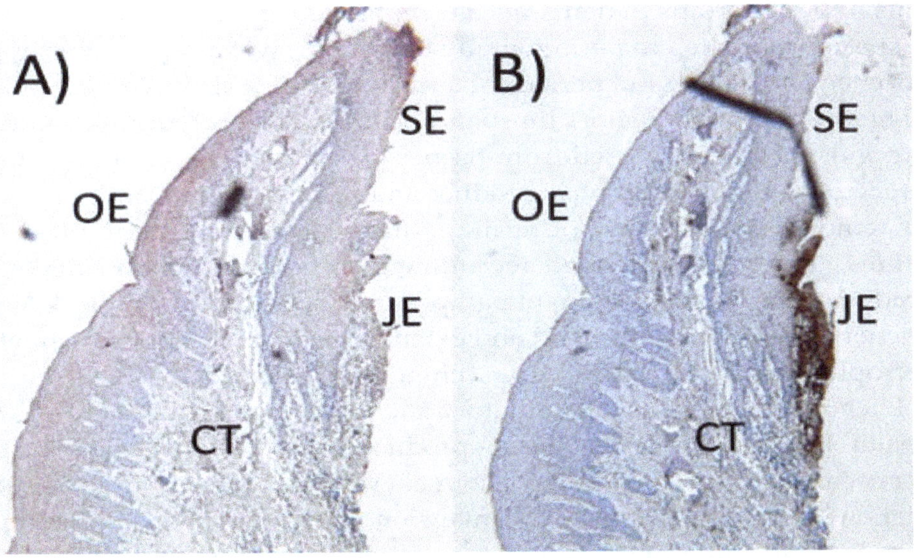

Figure 2. In a healthy gingiva, epithelial defensins (human β-defensins (hBD-2) in red color) are located in the oral (OE) and sulcular (SE) epithelia (**A**), while neutrophilic antimicrobial peptides (α-defensins in brown color) are located in the junctional epithelium (JE) and partly in connective tissue (CT) (**B**). (An original figure by U.K.G.)

Gingival connective tissue, periodontal ligament, and the organic component of the bone are formed of collagen. Fibroblasts are responsible for the synthesis of new collagen bundles and they remove the old collagen by secreting matrix metalloproteinases (MMPs). Overexpression of MMPs by gingival fibroblasts may either induce the release of cytokines and chemokines from the extracellular matrix or cleave cytokines and interrupt immune response signaling cascades [53]. The interplay between neutrophils and gingival fibroblasts is a good example of the bidirectional interactions between resident and immune cells.

Dendritic cells differ from keratinocytes and fibroblasts by acting as phagocytes and antigen-presenting cells. In a healthy environment, dendritic cells are in their immature forms and have high phagocytic capacity against invading microorganisms, but during infection they initiate a maturation process that involves their migration to lymph nodes to activate $CD4^+$ T cells [54] and promote the polarization of T-helper (Th)1, Th2, Th17, and B cells [55]. Uncontrolled upregulation of Th1 and Th17 cell pathways enhances alveolar bone loss via the induction of osteoclastogenesis [56]. There is also evidence that dendritic cells can differentiate to osteoclasts [57]; however, it is unknown how much of the bone resorption seen in periodontitis is actually induced by dendritic cell-derived osteoclasts.

Neutrophils form the primary defense system in periodontal tissues. Notably, their migration through the junctional epithelium into the gingival sulcus is a continuous process, which may differ from other organs, where transmigration is a hallmark of infection [58]. In the healthy oral cavity, neutrophil populations tend to be parainflammatory, while proinflammatory neutrophil phenotypes are present in periodontal disease [59]. Severe forms of periodontitis can be connected to diseases with neutrophil function defects, such as leukocyte adhesion deficiency 1 (LAD-1). Lack of neutrophil surveillance against bacterial infection is considered the cause of excessive periodontal degradation in neutrophil function deficiencies. However, recent evidence indicates that the absence of neutrophils in LAD-1 leads to the overproduction of IL-17, which eventually enhances the proliferation and differentiation of B cells [60]. Chronic granulomatous disease (CGD) is another genetic disease, which is characterized by defective neutrophilic respiratory burst and bacterial elimination. Although CGD patients are prone to developing bacterial and fungal infections, their periodontitis prevalence does not differ from that of the general population. In the highlights of these two examples, the presence of neutrophils in the periodontal immune response cascade seems to be more important than their ability to kill bacteria, as other phagocytes can take care of bacterial killing [60]. Interestingly, peripheral blood neutrophils of periodontitis patients release higher levels of proinflammatory cytokines and reactive oxygen species compared to periodontally healthy individuals, and this hyperinflammatory response persists even after successful periodontal treatment [61,62].

Neutrophils have a relatively short lifespan and they are programmed to die via apoptosis. Apoptotic neutrophils are phagocytosed from tissues by macrophages and are eliminated through lymphatics (efferocytosis). Since neutrophils produce and secrete a significant number of inflammatory molecules, their removal is a hallmark of healing. In inflamed periodontal tissues, partly due to pathogenic biofilms, there is an extended recruitment of neutrophils and delayed apoptotic cell death [63]. Instead of enhanced elimination of pathogens, however, neutrophils demonstrate impaired antibacterial function with this uncontrolled and extended immune response activation [64].

Tissue macrophages derive either from circulating monocytes or from embryo-derived precursors [65]. Phenotyping them as inflammatory and resolving macrophages will define their roles in disease and health. Inflammatory macrophages produce and secrete a large group of cytokines (IL-1β, IL-23, IL-6, tumor necrosis factor (TNF)-α) and enzymes (MMPs) that take part in osteoclastogenesis and collagen degradation in periodontitis [66]. A conversion from a destructive inflammatory phenotype to a resolving and bone-forming phenotype requires both signaling molecules and the presence of apoptotic neutrophils [67]. *P. gingivalis* can reverse the conversion of inflammatory macrophages to resolving macrophages by inducing inflammatory cytokines [68]. Impaired elimination of neutrophils by macrophages and defects in the activation of resolving macrophages may in turn lead to the initiation and progression of periodontitis.

Innate immune cells present intra- and extracellular pathogens to lymphocytes. In the gingiva, the most common subset of lymphocytes is $CD4^+$ T cells, followed by $CD8^+$ T cells, which are further subgrouped as Th1, Th2, Th17, Th9, regulatory (Treg), and unconventional $\gamma\delta$ T cells [69]. Recent evidence indicates the role of Th17 cells as one main regulator of T cell response and bone resorption in the periodontium [70]. In addition, Treg cells can limit the progression of periodontal disease without suppressing the immune response. When chronic gingivitis progresses to periodontitis, there is a shift from T cell dominance to B and plasma cells. Different types of B cells include naive B cells, memory B cells, and antibody-secreting B cells. Antibodies produced against periodontitis-associated pathogens can be found in saliva and in serum as well [32].

Finally, periodontitis is a complex disease with a nonlinear character, and its effects on immune response are rather disproportional [71]. Although knowledge about immune cell functions has considerably increased, it is still difficult to fully understand cellular interactions in periodontal disease pathogenesis due to its multicausal etiology.

4. Inflammatory Process and Periodontal Tissue Destruction

The junctional epithelium forms a unique seal between the root surface and gingiva, and its main function is to provide protection to the underlying tissues against the constant exposure of oral microbes and their by-products [72]. Various molecular factors involved in adhesion, cell–cell interactions, chemotaxis, proinflammatory cytokines, epithelial growth, MMP activation, and antimicrobial peptide production contribute to the function of the junctional epithelium. If this elegant and well-adapted defense system is overwhelmed by bacterial virulence factors (e.g., *P. gingivalis* gingipains) and prolonged inflammation (clinically seen as gingival bleeding and changes in soft tissue contour and color), the junctional epithelium migrates apically on the root surface and activates collagen destruction, which eventually leads to periodontal pocket formation [72]. It is noteworthy that although gingival inflammation is the precursor of periodontitis and a clinically relevant risk factor for disease progression, not all gingivitis lesions lead to periodontitis [73]. During periodontal pocket formation, new tissue formation by resident cells (keratinocytes, fibroblasts, osteoblasts) is suppressed, whereas tissue degradation by neutrophils, macrophages, and osteoclasts is stimulated; thus, the balance between tissue removal and regeneration is disrupted [74].

Proinflammatory cytokines (IL-1β, IL-6, IL-23, TNF-α), chemokines (IL-8), and antimicrobial peptides produced by keratinocytes, fibroblasts, and dendritic cells are chemoattractant gradients for neutrophils, which migrate into inflamed tissues and stimulate the chemotaxis of nonresident cells (macrophages, lymphocytes, plasma cells, and mast cells) to the site of infection [43,44]. Phagocytic cells mainly aim to eliminate invading pathogens by producing and secreting antimicrobial agents, reactive oxygen species, and enzymes. However, abundant tissue concentrations of collagenolytic MMPs and elastase activate the degradation of type I collagen in the connective tissue and periodontal ligament [75]. During disease, MMP-8 is the major collagenase in periodontal tissues. Irreversible periodontal destruction occurs when the inflammatory cell infiltrate, predominantly containing plasma cells, extends deeper into the connective tissue, leading to tissue damage in periodontal ligament and alveolar bone [76].

Alveolar bone resorption is the principal pathological characteristic of periodontitis. The activation of osteoclasts, multi-nucleated bone-resorbing cells, is regulated by a cascade of inflammatory proteins (cytokines) and enzymes (MMPs). IL-1β, IL-6, and TNF-α are the major proinflammatory cytokines in osteoclastogenesis activation, which is achieved by upregulating the receptor of nuclear factor-kappa ligand (RANKL) expression and inhibiting the differentiation of osteoblasts as well as decreasing osteocalcin production and new bone formation [77]. Due to the upregulated RANKL (stimulator of mature osteoclast formation) and downregulated osteoprotegerin (blocker of RANKL action), degradation of the bone is enabled to progress. MMP-1, -8, and -13 are especially involved in alveolar bone destruction by degrading type I collagen (the main type of collagen in the periodontium), while two gelatinases (MMP-2 and -9) accomplish the degradation of denatured collagen [78]. Furthermore, MMP-9 assists in osteoclast migration and MMP-13 triggers osteoclast activation, which all facilitate type I collagen degradation.

The disease development with fast or slow progress and with stable periods varies among periodontal sites and among individuals. Diagnosis of periodontitis is based on clinical and radiographic information on periodontal attachment and alveolar bone loss. In the current classification system, staging estimates the severity of the disease, while grading aims to estimate the rate of its progression, taking the known risk factors into account [10]. At the early phase of periodontal disease, the clinical signs and symptoms can be lacking or very mild. When periodontal tissue destruction proceeds, deepened pocket depths with alveolar bone loss result in tooth mobility, drifting, flaring, and finally loss of the affected tooth. In advanced cases, where several teeth are affected, these abnormalities lead to the collapse of the bite function.

5. Periodontal Therapy—Impact on Oral and General Health

The primary goal of periodontal therapy is to reduce the infectious and inflammatory challenge and to halt the progressing tissue destruction. Removal of pathogenic biofilms and suppression of inflammation can discontinue the periodontal tissue degradation; however, only limited regain of lost tissues occurs, depending on the form of tissue defects, systemic health status, and age [79]. In advanced cases, the active anti-infective treatment phase is often combined with surgery to eliminate residual pockets—with the aim of improving the ecology at periodontal sites—or sometimes with adjunctive systemic antimicrobials to reduce pathogen burden. In smokers, however, the treatment outcome is compromised, which makes smoking cessation an essential part of their periodontal therapy [80,81]. The beneficial influence of quitting may partly be due to decreased pathogen numbers and increased abundance of health-associated commensals in subgingival biofilms [82]. Although anti-infective treatment reduces total bacterial counts, proportions of periodontal pathogens, as well as the number of sites colonized with pathogens, many of the species return with time [83]. Therefore, daily oral hygiene of the patient and continuing professional supportive periodontal therapy are necessary to maintain the outcome and strengthen the long-term success of the treatment [84,85]. Moreover, patients with advanced disease and masticatory dysfunction and bite collapse due to severe tooth loss have an obvious need for complex rehabilitation of the bite function as well as esthetic treatment. After treatment, however, periodontitis patients with prosthodontic reconstructions have still an increased risk for tooth loss, and many patient-related factors such as age, socioeconomic status, non-compliance, and diabetes are associated with abutment tooth loss [86].

Since untreated periodontitis increases systemic low-grade inflammation, another treatment goal is to improve this condition [87]. Although intensive mechanical periodontal treatment of patients with severely damaged periodontal tissues can cause an acute systemic inflammatory response and impair endothelial function, this occurs only transiently and, after six months, a significantly improved endothelial function is reached [88]. Furthermore, periodontal treatment has been shown to reduce atherosclerotic biomarkers (e.g., IL-6, TNF-α) of individuals with cardiovascular disease and/or diabetes [89] as well as to improve the glycemic status (Hba1c levels) of diabetic patients [90,91].

6. Future Considerations

Periodontal disease is multifactorial and the imbalance between tissue loss and gain can occur due to various reasons, including aggressive infection, uncontrolled chronic inflammation, weakened healing, or all of the above simultaneously. Thus, successful disease management requires an understanding of different elements of the disease at the individual level and the design of personalized treatment modalities, including immunotherapies and modulators of inflammation [92,93]. With the aid of newly developed omics technologies, these novel strategies may become available for clinicians.

Author Contributions: Conceptualization: E.K., U.K.G.; Writing: E.K., M.G., U.K.G.; Visualization: M.G., U.K.G.

References

1. Eke, P.I.; Dye, B.A.; Wei, L.; Thornton-Evans, G.O.; Genco, R.J. Prevalence of periodontitis in adults in the United States: 2009 and 2010. *J. Dent. Res.* **2012**, *91*, 914–920. [CrossRef] [PubMed]
2. Kassebaum, N.J.; Bernabé, E.; Dahiya, M.; Bhandari, B.; Murray, C.J.; Marcenes, W. Global burden of severe periodontitis in 1990–2010: A systematic review and meta-regression. *J. Dent. Res.* **2014**, *93*, 1045–1053. [CrossRef] [PubMed]
3. Genco, R.J.; Borgnakke, W.S. Risk factors for periodontal disease. *Periodontol. 2000* **2013**, *62*, 59–94. [CrossRef] [PubMed]
4. Lalla, E.; Papapanou, P.N. Diabetes mellitus and periodontitis: A tale of two common interrelated diseases. *Nat. Rev. Endocrinol.* **2011**, *7*, 738–748. [CrossRef] [PubMed]
5. Lalla, E.; Cheng, B.; Lal, S.; Kaplan, S.; Softness, B.; Greenberg, E.; Goland, R.S.; Lamster, I.B. Diabetes mellitus promotes periodontal destruction in children. *J. Clin. Periodontol.* **2007**, *34*, 294–298. [CrossRef] [PubMed]
6. Heikkinen, A.M.; Pajukanta, R.; Pitkäniemi, J.; Broms, U.; Sorsa, T.; Koskenvuo, M.; Meurman, J.H. The effect of smoking on periodontal health of 15- to 16-year-old adolescents. *J. Periodontol.* **2008**, *79*, 2042–2047. [CrossRef] [PubMed]
7. Thomson, W.M.; Shearer, D.M.; Broadbent, J.M.; Foster Page, L.A.; Poulton, R. The natural history of periodontal attachment loss during the third and fourth decades of life. *J. Clin. Periodontol.* **2013**, *40*, 672–680. [CrossRef] [PubMed]
8. Ylöstalo, P.; Sakki, T.; Laitinen, J.; Järvelin, M.R.; Knuuttila, M. The relation of tobacco smoking to tooth loss among young adults. *Eur. J. Oral Sci.* **2004**, *112*, 121–126. [CrossRef] [PubMed]
9. Kosaka, T.; Ono, T.; Yoshimuta, Y.; Kida, M.; Kikui, M.; Nokubi, T.; Maeda, Y.; Kokubo, Y.; Watanabe, M.; Miyamoto, Y. The effect of periodontal status and occlusal support on masticatory performance: The Suita study. *J. Clin. Periodontol.* **2014**, *41*, 497–503. [CrossRef]
10. Tonetti, M.S.; Greenwell, H.; Kornman, K.S. Staging and grading of periodontitis: Framework and proposal of a new classification and case definition. *J. Clin. Periodontol.* **2018**, *45* (Suppl. 20), S149–S161. [CrossRef]
11. Darveau, R.P. Periodontitis: A polymicrobial disruption of host homeostasis. *Nat. Rev. Microbiol.* **2010**, *8*, 481–490. [CrossRef] [PubMed]
12. Sanz, M.; Beighton, D.; Curtis, M.A.; Cury, J.A.; Dige, I.; Dommisch, H.; Ellwood, R.; Giacaman, R.A.; Herrera, D.; Herzberg, M.C.; et al. Role of microbial biofilms in the maintenance of oral health and in the

development of dental caries and periodontal diseases. Consensus report of group 1 of the joint EFP/ORCA workshop on the boundaries between caries and periodontal disease. *J. Clin. Periodontol.* **2017**, *44* (Suppl. 18), 5–11. [CrossRef] [PubMed]
13. Kolenbrander, P.E.; Palmer, R.J., Jr.; Periasamy, S.; Jakubovics, N.S. Oral multispecies biofilm development and the key role of cell-cell distance. *Nat. Rev. Microbiol.* **2010**, *8*, 471–480. [CrossRef] [PubMed]
14. Paster, B.J.; Boches, S.K.; Galvin, J.L.; Ericson, R.E.; Lau, C.N.; Levanos, V.A.; Sahasrabudhe, A.; Dewhirst, F.E. Bacterial diversity in human subgingival plaque. *J. Bacteriol.* **2001**, *183*, 3770–3783. [CrossRef]
15. Könönen, E. Development of oral bacterial flora in young children. *Ann. Med.* **2000**, *32*, 107–112. [CrossRef]
16. Haraldsson, G.; Holbrook, W.P.; Könönen, E. Clonal persistence of oral *Fusobacterium nucleatum* in infancy. *J. Dent. Res.* **2004**, *83*, 500–504. [CrossRef]
17. Gursoy, U.K.; Pöllänen, M.; Könönen, E.; Uitto, V.J. Biofilm formation enhances the oxygen tolerance and invasiveness of *Fusobacterium nucleatum* in an oral mucosa culture model. *J. Periodontol.* **2010**, *81*, 1084–1091. [CrossRef]
18. Mendes, R.T.; Nguyen, D.; Stephens, D.; Pamuk, F.; Fernandes, D.; Hasturk, H.; Van Dyke, T.E.; Kantarci, A. Hypoxia-induced endothelial cell responses - possible roles during periodontal disease. *Clin. Exp. Dent. Res.* **2018**, *4*, 241–248. [CrossRef]
19. Socransky, S.S.; Haffajee, A.D.; Cugini, M.A.; Smith, C.; Kent, R.L., Jr. Microbial complexes in subgingival plaque. *J. Clin. Periodontol.* **1998**, *25*, 134–144. [CrossRef]
20. Griffen, A.L.; Beall, C.J.; Campbell, J.H.; Firestone, N.D.; Kumar, P.S.; Yang, Z.K.; Podar, M.; Leys, E.J. Distinct and complex bacterial profiles in human periodontitis and health revealed by 16S pyrosequencing. *ISME J.* **2012**, *6*, 1176–1185. [CrossRef]
21. Hajishengallis, G. The inflammophilic character of the periodontitis-associated microbiota. *Mol. Oral Microbiol.* **2014**, *29*, 248–257. [CrossRef] [PubMed]
22. Könönen, E.; Paju, S.; Pussinen, P.J.; Hyvönen, M.; Di Tella, P.; Suominen-Taipale, L.; Knuuttila, M. Population-based study of salivary carriage of periodontal pathogens in adults. *J. Clin. Microbiol.* **2007**, *45*, 2446–2451. [CrossRef]
23. Könönen, E.; Müller, H.P. Microbiology of aggressive periodontitis. *Periodontol. 2000* **2014**, *65*, 46–78. [CrossRef] [PubMed]
24. Curtis, M.A. Periodontal microbiology - the lid's off the box again. *J. Dent. Res.* **2014**, *93*, 840–842. [CrossRef] [PubMed]
25. Saglie, F.R.; Marfany, A.; Camargo, P. Intragingival occurrence of *Actinobacillus actinomycetemcomitans* and *Bacteroides gingivalis* in active destructive periodontal lesions. *J. Periodontol.* **1988**, *59*, 259–265. [CrossRef] [PubMed]
26. Gursoy, U.K.; Könönen, E.; Uitto, V.J. Intracellular replication of fusobacteria requires new actin filament formation of epithelial cells. *APMIS* **2008**, *116*, 1063–1070. [CrossRef] [PubMed]
27. Baek, K.; Ji, S.; Choi, Y. Complex intratissue microbiota forms biofilms in periodontal lesions. *J. Dent. Res.* **2018**, *97*, 192–200. [CrossRef] [PubMed]
28. Jiao, Y.; Hasegawa, M.; Inohara, N. The role of oral pathobionts in dysbiosis during periodontitis development. *J. Dent. Res.* **2014**, *93*, 539–546. [CrossRef] [PubMed]
29. Herrero, E.R.; Fernandes, S.; Verspecht, T.; Ugarte-Berzal, E.; Boon, N.; Proost, P.; Bernaerts, K.; Quirynen, M.; Teughels, W. Dysbiotic biofilms deregulate the periodontal inflammatory response. *J. Dent. Res.* **2018**, *97*, 547–555. [CrossRef]
30. Peyyala, R.; Kirakodu, S.S.; Novak, K.F.; Ebersole, J.L. Oral microbial biofilm stimulation of epithelial cell responses. *Cytokine* **2012**, *58*, 65–72. [CrossRef]
31. Mason, M.R.; Preshaw, P.M.; Nagaraja, H.N.; Dabdoub, S.M.; Rahman, A.; Kumar, P.S. The subgingival microbiome of clinically healthy current and never smokers. *ISME J.* **2015**, *9*, 268–272. [CrossRef] [PubMed]
32. Pussinen, P.J.; Könönen, E.; Paju, S.; Hyvärinen, K.; Gursoy, U.K.; Huumonen, S.; Knuuttila, M.; Suominen, A.L. Periodontal pathogen carriage, rather than periodontitis, determines the serum antibody levels. *J. Clin. Periodontol.* **2011**, *38*, 405–411. [CrossRef] [PubMed]
33. Pussinen, P.J.; Tuomisto, K.; Jousilahti, P.; Havulinna, A.S.; Sundvall, J.; Salomaa, V. Endotoxemia, immune response to periodontal pathogens, and systemic inflammation associate with incident cardiovascular disease events. *Arterioscler. Thromb. Vasc. Biol.* **2007**, *27*, 1433–1439. [CrossRef] [PubMed]

34. Damgaard, C.; Reinholdt, J.; Enevold, C.; Fiehn, N.E.; Nielsen, C.H.; Holmstrup, P. Immunoglobulin G antibodies against *Porphyromonas gingivalis* or *Aggregatibacter actinomycetemcomitans* in cardiovascular disease and periodontitis. *J. Oral Microbiol.* **2017**, *9*, 1374154. [CrossRef] [PubMed]
35. Palm, F.; Lahdentausta, L.; Sorsa, T.; Tervahartiala, T.; Gokel, P.; Buggle, F.; Safer, A.; Becher, H.; Grau, A.J.; Pussinen, P. Biomarkers of periodontitis and inflammation in ischemic stroke: A case-control study. *Innate Immun.* **2014**, *20*, 511–518. [CrossRef]
36. Demmer, R.T.; Jacobs, D.R., Jr.; Singh, R.; Zuk, A.; Rosenbaum, M.; Papapanou, P.N.; Desvarieux, M. Periodontal bacteria and prediabetes prevalence in ORIGINS: The oral infections, glucose intolerance, and insulin resistance study. *J. Dent. Res.* **2015**, *94*, 201–211. [CrossRef]
37. Scher, J.U.; Ubeda, C.; Equinda, M.; Khanin, R.; Buischi, Y.; Viale, A.; Lipuma, L.; Attur, M.; Pillinger, M.H.; Weissmann, G.; et al. Periodontal disease and the oral microbiota in new-onset rheumatoid arthritis. *Arthritis Rheum.* **2012**, *64*, 3083–3094. [CrossRef]
38. Eriksson, K.; Fei, G.; Lundmark, A.; Benchimol, D.; Lee, L.; Hu, Y.O.O.; Kats, A.; Saevarsdottir, S.; Catrina, A.I.; Klinge, B.; et al. Periodontal health and oral microbiota in patients with rheumatoid arthritis. *J. Clin. Med.* **2019**, *8*, 630. [CrossRef]
39. Fan, X.; Alekseyenko, A.V.; Wu, J.; Peters, B.A.; Jacobs, E.J.; Gapstur, S.M.; Purdue, M.P.; Abnet, C.C.; Stolzenberg-Solomon, R.; Miller, G.; et al. Human oral microbiome and prospective risk for pancreatic cancer: A population-based nested case-control study. *Gut* **2018**, *67*, 120–127. [CrossRef]
40. Han, Y.W. *Fusobacterium nucleatum*: A commensal-turned pathogen. *Curr. Opin. Microbiol.* **2015**, *23*, 141–147. [CrossRef]
41. Abed, J.; Maalouf, N.; Parhi, L.; Chaushu, S.; Mandelboim, O.; Bachrach, G. Tumor targeting by *Fusobacterium nucleatum*: A pilot study and future perspectives. *Front. Cell. Infect. Microbiol.* **2017**, *7*, 295. [CrossRef] [PubMed]
42. Gursoy, U.K.; Könönen, E.; Luukkonen, N.; Uitto, V.J. Human neutrophil defensins and their effect on epithelial cells. *J. Periodontol.* **2013**, *84*, 126–133. [CrossRef] [PubMed]
43. Benakanakere, M.; Kinane, D.F. Innate cellular responses to the periodontal biofilm. *Front. Oral Biol.* **2012**, *15*, 41–55. [PubMed]
44. Cekici, A.; Kantarci, A.; Hasturk, H.; Van Dyke, T.E. Inflammatory and immune pathways in the pathogenesis of periodontal disease. *Periodontol. 2000* **2014**, *64*, 57–80. [CrossRef] [PubMed]
45. Damgaard, C.; Holmstrup, P.; Van Dyke, T.E.; Nielsen, C.H. The complement system and its role in the pathogenesis of periodontitis: Current concepts. *J. Periodontal Res.* **2015**, *50*, 283–293. [CrossRef]
46. Liu, J.; Du, X.; Chen, J.; Hu, L.; Chen, L. The induction expression of human β-defensins in gingival epithelial cells and fibroblasts. *Arch. Oral Biol.* **2013**, *58*, 1415–1421. [CrossRef]
47. Kasnak, G.; Könönen, E.; Syrjänen, S.; Gürsoy, M.; Zeidán-Chuliá, F.; Firatli, E.; Gürsoy, U.K. NFE2L2/NRF2, OGG1, and cytokine responses of human gingival keratinocytes against oxidative insults of various origin. *Mol. Cell. Biochem.* **2019**, *452*, 63–70. [CrossRef]
48. Song, B.; Zhang, Y.L.; Chen, L.J.; Zhou, T.; Huang, W.K.; Zhou, X.; Shao, L.Q. The role of Toll-like receptors in periodontitis. *Oral Dis.* **2017**, *23*, 168–180. [CrossRef]
49. Elmanfi, S.; Zhou, J.; Sintim, H.O.; Könönen, E.; Gürsoy, M.; Gürsoy, U.K. Regulation of gingival epithelial cytokine response by bacterial cyclic dinucleotides. *J. Oral Microbiol.* **2018**, *11*, 1538927. [CrossRef]
50. Fteita, D.; Könönen, E.; Gürsoy, M.; Ma, X.; Sintim, H.O.; Gürsoy, U.K. Quorum sensing molecules regulate epithelial cytokine response and biofilm-related virulence of three *Prevotella* species. *Anaerobe* **2018**, *54*, 128–135. [CrossRef]
51. Hiroshima, Y.; Bando, M.; Kataoka, M.; Inagaki, Y.; Herzberg, M.C.; Ross, K.F.; Hosoi, K.; Nagata, T.; Kido, J. Regulation of antimicrobial peptide expression in human gingival keratinocytes by interleukin-1α. *Arch. Oral Biol.* **2011**, *56*, 761–767. [CrossRef] [PubMed]
52. Jura, J.; Skalniak, L.; Koj, A. Monocyte chemotactic protein-1-induced protein-1 (MCPIP1) is a novel multifunctional modulator of inflammatory reactions. *Biochim. Biophys. Acta* **2012**, *1823*, 1905–1913. [CrossRef] [PubMed]
53. Cavalla, F.; Hernández-Rios, P.; Sorsa, T.; Biguetti, C.; Hernández, M. Matrix metalloproteinases as regulators of periodontal inflammation. *Int. J. Mol. Sci.* **2017**, *18*, 440.
54. Wilensky, A.; Segev, H.; Mizraji, G.; Shaul, Y.; Capucha, T.; Shacham, M.; Hovav, A.H. Dendritic cells and their role in periodontal disease. *Oral Dis.* **2014**, *20*, 119–126. [CrossRef] [PubMed]

55. Song, L.; Dong, G.; Guo, L.; Graves, D.T. The function of dendritic cells in modulating the host response. *Mol. Oral Microbiol.* **2018**, *33*, 13–21. [CrossRef] [PubMed]
56. Cheng, W.C.; Hughes, F.J.; Taams, L.S. The presence, function and regulation of IL-17 and Th17 cells in periodontitis. *J. Clin. Periodontol.* **2014**, *41*, 541–549. [CrossRef] [PubMed]
57. Alnaeeli, M.; Penninger, J.M.; Teng, Y.T. Immune interactions with CD4+ T cells promote the development of functional osteoclasts from murine CD11c+ dendritic cells. *J. Immunol.* **2006**, *177*, 3314–3326. [CrossRef] [PubMed]
58. Parkos, C.A. Neutrophil-epithelial interactions: A double-edged sword. *Am. J. Pathol.* **2016**, *186*, 1404–1416. [CrossRef] [PubMed]
59. Fine, N.; Hassanpour, S.; Borenstein, A.; Sima, C.; Oveisi, M.; Scholey, J.; Cherney, D.; Glogauer, M. Distinct oral neutrophil subsets define health and periodontal disease states. *J. Dent. Res.* **2016**, *95*, 931–938. [CrossRef] [PubMed]
60. Hajishengallis, G.; Moutsopoulos, N.M.; Hajishengallis, E.; Chavakis, T. Immune and regulatory functions of neutrophils in inflammatory bone loss. *Semin. Immunol.* **2016**, *28*, 146–158. [CrossRef] [PubMed]
61. Matthews, J.B.; Wright, H.J.; Roberts, A.; Ling-Mountford, N.; Cooper, P.R.; Chapple, I.L. Neutrophil hyper-responsiveness in periodontitis. *J. Dent. Res.* **2007**, *86*, 718–722. [CrossRef] [PubMed]
62. Ling, M.R.; Chapple, I.L.; Matthews, J.B. Peripheral blood neutrophil cytokine hyper-reactivity in chronic periodontitis. *Innate Immun.* **2015**, *21*, 714–725. [CrossRef] [PubMed]
63. Olsen, I.; Hajishengallis, G. Major neutrophil functions subverted by *Porphyromonas gingivalis*. *J. Oral Microbiol.* **2016**, *8*, 30936. [CrossRef] [PubMed]
64. Sochalska, M.; Potempa, J. Manipulation of neutrophils by *Porphyromonas gingivalis* in the development of periodontitis. *Front. Cell. Infect. Microbiol.* **2017**, *7*, 197. [CrossRef] [PubMed]
65. Davies, L.C.; Rosas, M.; Jenkins, S.J.; Liao, C.T.; Scurr, M.J.; Brombacher, F.; Fraser, D.J.; Allen, J.E.; Jones, S.A.; Taylor, P.R. Distinct bone marrow-derived and tissue-resident macrophage lineages proliferate at key stages during inflammation. *Nat. Commun.* **2013**, *4*, 1886. [CrossRef] [PubMed]
66. Hajishengallis, G.; Sahingur, S.E. Novel inflammatory pathways in periodontitis. *Adv. Dent. Res.* **2014**, *26*, 23–29. [CrossRef] [PubMed]
67. Garlet, G.P.; Giannobile, W.V. Macrophages: The bridge between inflammation resolution and tissue repair? *J. Dent. Res.* **2018**, *97*, 1079–1081. [CrossRef] [PubMed]
68. Papadopoulos, G.; Shaik-Dasthagirisaheb, Y.B.; Huang, N.; Viglianti, G.A.; Henderson, A.J.; Kantarci, A.; Gibson, F.C. Immunologic environment influences macrophage response to *Porphyromonas gingivalis*. *Mol. Oral Microbiol.* **2017**, *32*, 250–261. [CrossRef] [PubMed]
69. Dutzan, N.; Konkel, J.E.; Greenwell-Wild, T.; Moutsopoulos, N.M. Characterization of the human immune cell network at the gingival barrier. *Mucosal Immunol.* **2016**, *9*, 1163–1172. [CrossRef] [PubMed]
70. Campbell, L.; Millhouse, E.; Malcolm, J.; Culshaw, S. T cells, teeth and tissue destruction - what do T cells do in periodontal disease? *Mol. Oral Microbiol.* **2016**, *31*, 445–456. [CrossRef] [PubMed]
71. Loos, B.G.; Papantonopoulos, G.; Jepsen, S.; Laine, M.L. What is the contribution of genetics to periodontal risk? *Dent. Clin. North Am.* **2015**, *59*, 761–780. [CrossRef]
72. Bosshardt, D.D.; Lang, N.P. The junctional epithelium: From health to disease. *J Dent. Res.* **2005**, *84*, 9–20. [CrossRef]
73. Lang, N.P.; Schätzle, M.A.; Löe, H. Gingivitis as a risk factor in periodontal disease. *J. Clin. Periodontol.* **2009**, *36* (Suppl. 10), 3–8. [CrossRef]
74. Henderson, B.; Kaiser, F. Bacterial modulators of bone remodeling in the periodontal pocket. *Periodontol. 2000* **2018**, *76*, 97–108. [CrossRef]
75. Sorsa, T.; Tjäderhane, L.; Konttinen, Y.T.; Lauhio, A.; Salo, T.; Lee, H.M.; Golub, L.M.; Brown, D.L.; Mäntylä, P. Matrix metalloproteinases: Contribution to pathogenesis, diagnosis and treatment of periodontal inflammation. *Ann. Med.* **2006**, *38*, 306–321. [CrossRef]
76. Kurgan, S.; Kantarci, A. Molecular basis for immunohistochemical and inflammatory changes during progression of gingivitis to periodontitis. *Periodontol. 2000* **2018**, *76*, 51–67. [CrossRef]
77. Belibasakis, G.N.; Bostanci, N. The RANKL-OPG system in clinical periodontology. *J. Clin. Periodontol.* **2012**, *39*, 239–248. [CrossRef]

78. Gursoy, U.K.; Könönen, E.; Huumonen, S.; Tervahartiala, T.; Pussinen, P.J.; Suominen, A.L.; Sorsa, T. Salivary type I collagen degradation end-products and related matrix metalloproteinases in periodontitis. *J. Clin. Periodontol.* **2013**, *40*, 18–25. [CrossRef]
79. Reynolds, M.A.; Kao, R.T.; Camargo, P.M.; Caton, J.G.; Clem, D.S.; Fiorellini, J.P.; Geisinger, M.L.; Mills, M.P.; Nares, S.; Nevins, M.L. Periodontal regeneration - intrabony defects: A consensus report from the AAP regeneration workshop. *J. Periodontol.* **2015**, *86* (Suppl. 2), 105–107. [CrossRef]
80. Bunaes, D.F.; Lie, S.A.; Enersen, M.; Aastrøm, A.N.; Mustafa, K.; Leknes, K.N. Site-specific treatment outcome in smokers following non-surgical and surgical periodontal therapy. *J. Clin. Periodontol.* **2015**, *42*, 933–942. [CrossRef]
81. Ryder, M.I.; Couch, E.T.; Chaffee, B.W. Personalized periodontal treatment for the tobacco- and alcohol-using patient. *Periodontol. 2000* **2018**, *78*, 30–46. [CrossRef]
82. Delima, S.L.; McBride, R.K.; Preshaw, P.M.; Heasman, P.A.; Kumar, P.S. Response of subgingival bacteria to smoking cessation. *J. Clin. Microbiol.* **2010**, *48*, 2344–2449. [CrossRef]
83. Haffajee, A.D.; Teles, R.P.; Socransky, S.S. The effect of periodontal therapy on the composition of the subgingival microbiota. *Periodontol* **2006**, *42*, 219–258. [CrossRef]
84. Axelsson, P.; Nyström, B.; Lindhe, J. The long-term effect of a plaque control program on tooth mortality, caries and periodontal disease in adults. Results after 30 years of maintenance. *J. Clin. Periodontol.* **2004**, *31*, 749–757. [CrossRef]
85. Rosling, B.; Serino, G.; Hellström, M.K.; Socransky, S.S.; Lindhe, J. Longitudinal periodontal tissue alterations during supportive therapy. Findings from subjects with normal and high susceptibility to periodontal disease. *J. Clin. Periodontol.* **2001**, *28*, 241–249. [CrossRef]
86. Müller, S.; Eickholz, P.; Reitmeir, P.; Eger, T. Long-term tooth loss in periodontally compromised but treated patients according to the type of prosthodontic treatment. A retrospective study. *J. Oral Rehabil.* **2013**, *40*, 358–367. [CrossRef]
87. Paraskevas, S.; Huizinga, J.D.; Loos, B.G. A systematic review and meta-analyses on C-reactive protein in relation to periodontitis. *J. Clin. Periodontol.* **2008**, *35*, 277–290. [CrossRef]
88. Tonetti, M.S.; D'Aiuto, F.; Nibali, L.; Donald, A.; Storry, C.; Parkar, M.; Suvan, J.; Hingorani, A.D.; Vallance, P.; Deanfield, J. Treatment of periodontitis and endothelial function. *N. Engl. J. Med.* **2007**, *356*, 911–920. [CrossRef]
89. Teeuw, W.J.; Slot, D.E.; Susanto, H.; Gerdes, V.E.; Abbas, F.; D'Aiuto, F.; Kastelein, J.J.; Loos, B.G.J. Treatment of periodontitis improves the atherosclerotic profile: A systematic review and meta-analysis. *J. Clin. Periodontol.* **2014**, *41*, 70–79. [CrossRef]
90. Wang, X.; Han, X.; Guo, X.; Luo, X.; Wang, D. The effect of periodontal treatment on hemoglobin A1c levels of diabetic patients: A systematic review and meta-analysis. *PLoS ONE* **2014**, *9*, e108412. [CrossRef]
91. D'Aiuto, F.; Gkranias, N.; Bhowruth, D.; Khan, T.; Orlandi, M.; Suvan, J.; Masi, S.; Tsakos, G.; Hurel, S.; Hingorani, A.D.; et al. Systemic effects of periodontitis treatment in patients with type 2 diabetes: A 12 month, single-centre, investigator-masked, randomised trial. *Lancet Diabetes Endocrinol.* **2018**, *6*, 954–965.
92. Morand, D.N.; Davideau, J.L.; Clauss, F.; Jessel, N.; Tenenbaum, H.; Huck, O. Cytokines during periodontal wound healing: Potential application for new therapeutic approach. *Oral Dis.* **2017**, *23*, 300–311. [CrossRef]
93. Alvarez, C.; Rojas, C.; Rojas, L.; Cafferata, E.A.; Monasterio, G.; Vernal, R. Regulatory T lymphocytes in periodontitis: A translational view. *Mediators Inflamm.* **2018**, *2018*, 7806912. [CrossRef]

14

Rheumatoid Arthritis-Associated Mechanisms of *Porphyromonas gingivalis* and *Aggregatibacter actinomycetemcomitans*

Eduardo Gómez-Bañuelos, Amarshi Mukherjee, Erika Darrah and Felipe Andrade *

Division of Rheumatology, The Johns Hopkins University School of Medicine, Baltimore, MD 21224, USA
* Correspondence: andrade@jhmi.edu

Abstract: Rheumatoid arthritis (RA) is an autoimmune disease of unknown etiology characterized by immune-mediated damage of synovial joints and antibodies to citrullinated antigens. Periodontal disease, a bacterial-induced inflammatory disease of the periodontium, is commonly observed in RA and has implicated periodontal pathogens as potential triggers of the disease. In particular, *Porphyromonas gingivalis* and *Aggregatibacter actinomycetemcomitans* have gained interest as microbial candidates involved in RA pathogenesis by inducing the production of citrullinated antigens. Here, we will discuss the clinical and mechanistic evidence surrounding the role of these periodontal bacteria in RA pathogenesis, which highlights a key area for the treatment and preventive interventions in RA.

Keywords: Rheumatoid arthritis; *Porphyromonas gingivalis*; *Aggregatibacter actinomycetemcomitans*; periodontitis; periodontal disease; citrullination; peptidylarginine deiminase; ACPA; anti-CCP

---

1. Introduction

Rheumatoid arthritis (RA) is an autoimmune disease of unknown etiology characterized by synovial inflammation, joint destruction, and high titer autoantibodies [1]. The disease affects 0.5–1% of the adult population worldwide and is associated with increased mortality rates compared with the general population [2]. A microbial origin in RA has been hypothesized for more than a century [3–6], yet, different to chronic diseases that have an infectious origin, a causal agent for RA has not been identified. Instead, numerous studies support the idea that the etiology of RA is multifactorial with a complex interplay between genetic and environmental factors [7]. Multiple risk factors have been associated with RA, including specific HLA (human leukocyte antigen) alleles, female sex, smoking, obesity, infections, and menopause, among others [8]. Nevertheless, these factors are also common in the general population, which makes it difficult to understand why only few individuals develop RA and not others with similar risk. Even in monozygotic twins, the disease concordance is rather low, varying between 8.8 and 21% [9–12]. Although stochastic events may explain the discordance in disease development among individuals at risk, the current model of RA relies on the contribution of an environmental factor, most likely a microbial agent, which may be responsible for triggering the disease in susceptible individuals.

Assuming that a microorganism is involved in RA pathogenesis, at least two hypotheses may explain why this causal agent has not yet been found. First, RA may be triggered by a rare pathogen that is exclusive to patients with RA, which has not yet been discovered because of the lack of proper technologies. Second, different to other chronic infectious diseases that are linked to a single pathogen, RA may result from the individual or interacting effects of different microbial agents likely unified by triggering common arthritogenic pathways. Moreover, like other risk factors in RA, microbial species with arthritogenic potential may also be common in the general population, but only drive RA in the perfect setting of other predisposing elements.

While it cannot be excluded that a single unknown pathogen may cause RA, current studies suggest that dysbiotic microbiomes may play a role in the pathogenesis of the disease [13–15]. In this regard, several bacterial candidates have been mechanistically linked to RA either by creating a pro-inflammatory environment or by inducing the production of autoantibodies [13–15]. Here, we will discuss the evidence surrounding the potential role of two of these microbial agents, *Porphyromonas gingivalis* (*P. gingivalis*) and *Aggregatibacter actinomycetemcomitans* (*Aa*), in the mechanistic model of RA. Importantly, these pathogens are not exclusive to RA. Indeed, they are causal agents of periodontitis, a common disease in the adult population initially associated with RA in the late 1800s [16].

2. The Focal Infection Theory, Oral Sepsis, and RA

In order to discuss the potential role of periodontal pathogens in the etiology of RA, it is important to first review the historical background leading to the link between the mouth and RA. In contrast to other arthritides known for several centuries, the first description of RA (initially termed "primary asthenic gout") was not made until 1800 by Augustin Jacob Landré-Beauvais [17]. Later, Alfred Garrod in 1859 proposed the name "rheumatoid arthritis" for diseases previously known as chronic rheumatic arthritis and rheumatic gout, and provided a detailed clinical description to distinguish RA from gout [18]. Once RA was established as an independent entity, numerous investigators tried to identify the etiology of this disease. Due to the inflammatory nature of RA, it was thought that the etiology was infectious, leading to the search for microbial organisms in the joints of patients with RA.

Between 1887 and the early 1900s, several investigators claimed to identify different bacteria in RA synovial fluid and tissue [3–6]. Although the results were inconsistent and not reproducible [19–22], these initial studies reinforced the idea that RA had an infectious origin, either due to bacteria within the joint itself or to a toxin produced by microorganisms in some other part of the body [23]. During the late 1800s, it was widely accepted that an infection in one part of the body may have effects on a different anatomical site (e.g., the syphilitic chancre is followed by systemic infection [24]). Thus, this notion fueled speculation that similar to other chronic diseases [25], RA was the result of microbial dissemination from distant sites of chronic focus of infection, including nasal sinuses, gut, lungs, genitourinary tract and the mouth [26–30]. This idea, known as the focal infection theory, defined the cause and treatment of a broad range of diseases, including RA, for several decades in the early 1900s [25,31,32].

In 1891, Willoughy D. Miller first conjectured that oral pathogens play a significant role in the production of local and systemic diseases [33,34]. This notion was further promoted by William Hunter in 1900, who was responsible for highlighting that the mouth was a major focus of infection driving diseases in other organs of the body. In particular, he reached the incorrect conclusion that pernicious anemia was the result of infective gastritis caused by oral sepsis [35–38]. Following these observations, oral sepsis (including caries, gingivitis, stomatitis, periodontitis, and tonsillitis) was considered a major focus of infection causing systemic diseases in which the etiology was unknown, such as RA [25,30,39,40]. This notion was further supported by anecdotal reports of patients with "rheumatism" cured after the removal of carious teeth [41], leading to the use of tonsillectomies and tooth extractions as the standard of treatment [29,31]. In the 1930s, this theory was refuted by the demonstration that neither tooth extraction nor tonsillectomy provided clinical benefit to patients with RA [42–44].

3. Periodontitis and RA

Among the different causes of oral sepsis that were linked to RA, an association with "pyorrhea alveolaris" was noticed in 1895 [16]. Pyorrhea alveolaris, also known as Riggs' disease and currently termed periodontal disease (PD) or periodontitis, was described by John W. Riggs in 1875 [45]. Periodontitis is a bacterial-induced chronic inflammatory disease affecting the tissues that support the teeth, including the alveolar bone. The disease results from dysbiosis of the oral microbiota and is associated with destruction of periodontal tissue, potentially leading to tooth loss [46]. Since the implantation site of the teeth is also an articulation, it was initially thought that the destruction of the periodontal membrane and alveolar bone in patients with RA and pyorrhea alveolaris was part of same RA-induced damage affecting the dentoalveolar joint [16]. Nevertheless, the establishment of the focal infection theory tilted the paradigm to underscore periodontitis as a cause (not as a consequence) of RA in the early 1900s [26–28].

However, after the downfall of the focal infection theory as the cause of RA in the 1930s, the study of periodontitis in the pathogenesis of RA was left behind. Later, at least two major advances renewed interest in periodontitis as a component of the mechanistic model of RA. The first occurred between the 1960s–1990s, when significant advances were made in the immunopathogenesis of periodontitis, which suggested important mechanistic similarities with autoimmune diseases [47], in particular RA [48]. These include common mechanisms of immune-mediated tissue damage, patterns of pro-inflammatory cytokines (e.g., interleukin (IL)-1, IL-6 and tumor necrosis factor α), immune complex deposition and complement activation [48–50]. Rapidly progressive periodontitis is also associated with *HLA-DRB1* alleles linked to RA [51,52]. Moreover, B cells and plasma cells predominate in the affected sites in chronic periodontitis [53–55], autoantibodies such as rheumatoid factor (RF) and anti-collagen antibodies are found in the periodontal lesion [56–59], and RF can be detected in dental periapical lesions from patients with RA [60]. The second advance was in 1999, when it was discovered that an important periodontal pathogen (*P. gingivalis*) secretes a peptidylarginine deiminase (PAD)-like enzyme [61], which was incorrectly thought to be equivalent to human PADs at the time [62]. As PAD enzymes are responsible for generating citrullinated proteins, major targets of autoantibodies in RA [63], it was hypothesized that periodontitis drives RA via the production of citrullinated antigens by *P. gingivalis* [62]. Together, these findings have provided the basis for the renewed theory that periodontitis and RA may be mechanistically related and potentially linked by a common etiologic factor.

In the last 10 years, numerous epidemiological studies, extensively reviewed elsewhere [64–66], have reported a positive association of RA with PD when compared to healthy (non-RA) controls. Overall, a recent meta-analysis found that patients with RA had a 13% greater risk of periodontitis compared to healthy controls, ranging from 4 to 23% (RR: 1.13; 95% CI: 1.04, 1.23; $p = 0.006$) [65]. In addition, a case-control study from the Medical Biobank of Northern Sweden found that periodontitis, characterized as marginal jawbone loss, precedes the clinical onset of RA [67], supporting a potential role for PD in RA pathogenesis. Not every study, however, has confirmed this association either by comparing RA with healthy controls [68,69] or with patients with osteoarthritis (OA) [65]. Although these studies have methodological differences that may explain their discrepancies, a causal relation between RA and periodontitis may be difficult to sustain based purely on association studies.

A major caveat in the epidemiological association between RA and periodontitis is that PD is likely the most frequent chronic infectious disease in humans worldwide. The overall rate of PD in the adult US population is 47%, with 38% over age 30 and 64% over age 65 having either severe or moderate periodontitis [70]. Moreover, severe forms of periodontitis affect 11.2% of the global adult population [71]. Considering that almost half of the adult population has some form of PD, it may be hard to demonstrate a causal relationship with RA, since its prevalence is only 0.5–1% of the adult population [2]. Indeed, the relative risk of periodontitis in patients with RA is only 1.13 when compared to healthy controls, and of 1.10 compared to OA [65]. Despite these potential shortcomings, additional studies have been centered on addressing whether periodontitis, and in particular periodontal pathogens, may have a mechanistic role in RA through the production of citrullinated antigens.

4. Citrullination and RA

The discovery that the majority of patients with RA have antibodies to citrullinated proteins (known as ACPAs) [63,72,73] marked an important advance in understanding potential pathogenic mechanisms in RA [1]. Citrullination is an enzymatic process mediated by the peptidylarginine deiminases (PADs) in which arginine residues are deiminated to generate citrulline residues [74]. Five PADs have been identified in humans (PAD1–4 and 6) [1], but only PAD1–4 have citrullinating activity [75]. PAD2 and PAD4 have gained prominence as potential candidates that drive citrullination of self-antigens in RA due to their increased expression in rheumatoid synovial tissue and fluid [76–78]. PADs are calcium dependent enzymes. Four, five, and six calcium-binding sites were identified in the structure of PAD1, PAD4, and PAD2, respectively, with calcium binding inducing conformational changes required to generate the active site cleft [79–81]. PADs are highly specific for peptidylarginine residues, requiring at least one additional amino acid residue N-terminal to the site of modification [74,82]. Thus, these enzymes can only citrullinate arginine residues within polypeptide chains but not at their termini (i.e., they are endodeiminases). Different from arginine deiminases (ADI), which catalyze the deimination of free L-arginine, PADs cannot generate citrulline from free L-arginine [74]. PADs 2, 3, and 4 form homodimers, whereas PAD1 is monomeric in solution [79–81]. Each PAD monomer contains a C-terminal catalytic domain and an N-terminal domain involved in substrate binding and protein–protein interactions [79–81]. The PADs are highly conserved and share 50%–55% sequence identity [79], but exhibit distinct substrate preferences and tissue expression [83,84].

Citrullination is a normal process across multiple tissues in humans [85]. More than 200 proteins are citrullinated in different healthy human tissues, with the highest levels found in the brain and lungs [85]. Together, this set of proteins is referred to as the citrullinome. Large amounts of citrullinated proteins are found in RA synovial fluid, including more than 100 proteins that are normally citrullinated among different normal tissues [85–91]. This unique pattern of citrullination that includes proteins spanning the range of molecular weights is termed hypercitrullination [87]. Similar to the RA joint, it is noteworthy that periodontitis is also characterized by the accumulation of large amounts of citrullinated proteins with similar patterns of hypercitrullination found in RA [92,93], supporting the notion that PD is a potential source of citrullinated autoantigens. Understanding which components in periodontitis are responsible for driving hypercitrullination may, therefore, provide important mechanistic insights into RA pathogenesis.

5. *P. gingivalis* in RA Pathogenesis

P. gingivalis was linked to periodontal disease in the early 1960s, initially named *Bacteroides melaninogenicus* (*B. melaninogenicus*) [94], which was later found to include two species, *B. melaninogenicus* (later *Prevotela melaninogenica*) and *B. asaccharolyticus* [95]. The name *B. gingivalis* was later proposed to distinguish oral from non-oral *B. asaccharolyticus* [96,97], and in the late 1980s, *B. gingivalis* was further reclassified in a new genus, the *Porphyromonas* [98]. *P. gingivalis* has been implicated in the pathogenesis of periodontitis by subverting host immune defenses, leading to overgrowth of oral commensal bacteria, which causes inflammatory tissue destruction [99,100].

Different approaches have been used to address a potential association between *P. gingivalis* and RA, many of which have shown inconsistent or inconclusive results. These include: (1) bacterial detection in gingival tissue, subgingival plaque and/or gingival crevicular fluid (GCF) either by staining using anti-*P. gingivalis* antibodies, bacterial culture, and/or DNA amplification (PCR) [101–107]; (2) metagenomic sequencing in saliva and subgingival plaque, which surveys complex microbial communities [103,106,108–112]; and (3) measuring antibodies to *P. gingivalis* in serum [101,113–125], which in contrast to the other assays that detect the existing bacteria in the mouth, it is an indirect test that determines past or present exposure to *P. gingivalis*.

Due to its convenience, the detection of antibodies to *P. gingivalis* (mainly IgG) has been the most widely used assay to study the relationship between this pathogen and RA. However, it is important to highlight that there is not a standard assay to measure such antibodies. All studies used in house ELISAs with different types of *P. gingivalis* antigens. These include bacterial cells either as intact bacteria (not fixed or fixed with formalin) or bacterial extracts generated by sonication [101,113–119], purified recombinant proteins (e.g., bacterial PAD, arginine gingipain (RgpB), or hemin binding protein 35 (HBP35)] [120–124,126], HtpG peptides (HSP90 homologue) [111], *P. gingivalis*-specific lipopolysaccharide or outer membrane antigens [125,127]. In regard to the bacterial strains, studies have included either laboratory strains or clinical isolates, which may have some antigenic differences [128]. Considering conflicting conclusions from these studies [101,113–125] and others not cited in this review, an association between anti-*P. gingivalis* antibodies and RA is difficult to sustain. However, based on a selected number of publications, two meta-analysis have reported a significant association between higher antibody titers to *P. gingivalis* and RA when compared to healthy controls with unknown PD status [129], and to healthy controls with and without PD [130]. Anti-*P. gingivalis* antibody levels also positively correlated with ACPAs in one study [129]. Nevertheless, a significant association was not found between antibodies to *P. gingivalis* and RA when compared to non-RA controls (e.g., population-based case-controls) [129]. This finding may be explained by the presence of individuals with chronic diseases and high prevalence of severe PD in the non-RA population, supporting the idea that the relative abundance of *P. gingivalis* is associated with PD severity regardless of RA [111]. Moreover, one meta-analysis showed that only antibodies to whole *P. gingivalis*, but not anti-RgpB antibodies, were positively associated with RA [129], highlighting that the anti-*P. gingivalis* antibody assays are not comparable. Interestingly, one study reported that anti-RgpB antibody concentrations increase before the onset of RA symptoms [123], suggesting a temporal relationship between *P. gingivalis* infection and the clinical onset of RA.

Unlike the detection of antibodies to *P. gingivalis*, which has shown some positive association with RA, a number of studies detecting *P. gingivalis* by PCR and metagenomic sequencing in saliva, subgingival plaque and/or GCF failed to confirm such an association [103–111]. In one of these studies, however, *P. gingivalis* was detected more frequently in a small subgroup of patients with recently diagnosed, never-treated RA, in comparison with patients with established RA or healthy controls; although this finding could be explained by a higher prevalence of severe periodontitis in those patients [111]. More recently, an increase in the relative abundance of *P. gingivalis* was found at healthy periodontal sites in at risk anti-CCP antibody positive individuals compared with anti-CCP negative healthy controls, though the significance of this finding is unclear [112].

From these studies, it is difficult to reach a definitive conclusion as to the relationship between RA and *P. ginigvalis*. A complicating factor is that every assay has different implications with regard to the status of *P. gingivalis* in the patient (e.g., carrier, active infection, or past and present exposure), and their significance is likely influenced by the source of antigen (in the case of antibodies), periodontal sample collection, and the control group used for comparison (e.g., OA, non-RA, healthy controls with or without PD). Overall, it is likely that positive associations with *P. gingivalis* may reflect PD severity rather than RA status, which importantly, neither supports nor excludes a pathogenic role for *P. gingivalis* in RA.

5.1. *P. gingivalis in Experimental Models of Arthritis*

In addition to epidemiological data, experimental studies using different animal models of immune-mediated arthritis (e.g., collagen-induced arthritis (CIA), methylated bovine serum albumin-induced arthritis, and the SKG mouse model) and different routes of bacterial inoculation (including oral, intraperitoneal and subcutaneous chambers) reached the conclusion that *P. gingivalis* can increase the incidence and/or exacerbate the disease [131–141].

However, many of these studies have important caveats. Several studies have reported that DBA/1 mice (a susceptible strain to induce CIA) are resistant to oral colonization by *P. gingivalis* and therefore, have recommended the use of non-oral routes of inoculation or different strains of mice to study the effect of *P. gingivalis* in experimental arthritis [131,136,142]. These findings contrast with others that have successfully induced PD with *P. gingivalis* in DBA/1 mice [132,134,135]. Among DBA/1 mice that developed periodontitis, however, there are also differences observed, with some studies showing that PD exacerbates CIA [132,134], but not others [135]. Using the SKG model of spontaneous arthritis, there are also discrepancies in the induction of PD by *P. gingivalis*, and whether this process aggravates arthritis [141,142]. Although these conflicting data may be explained by differences in mouse strains or environmental conditions that may affect the immune system in mice, the data certainly highlights the lack of reproducible mouse models to study the effect of periodontitis and *P. gingivalis* in autoimmune arthritis.

Using models of arthritis in rats, periodontitis induced by *P. gingivalis* had no effect in the development or severity of pristane-induced arthritis in Dark Agouti rats [143]. More recently, however, one study showed that *P. gingivalis*-associated periodontitis was sufficient to induce erosive arthritis in Lewis rats, providing the first direct evidence that *P. gingivalis* may have the capacity to induce arthritis [144].

Several mechanisms have been proposed by which *P. gingivalis* may promote autoimmune arthritis in humans and in experimental animals. These include the induction of a systemic Th17 cell response [132–134], induction of autoantibodies [131,138,143,144], cross-reactivity between bacterial and host antigens [145], by promoting C5a generation [141], through direct dissemination of *P. gingivalis* into the joints [136], and by swallowing the bacteria, which may alter the gut microbiota and gut immune system [137]. Nevertheless, the production of citrullinated autoantigens by a PAD enzyme released from *P. gingivalis* is considered the most important mechanistic evidence to support a role of *P. gingivalis* in RA pathogenesis [14,146].

5.2. *P. gingivalis PAD (PPAD)*

The existence of an arginine deiminase-like enzyme in *P. gingivalis* was suggested in the early 1990's [147], and the enzyme was purified and characterized in 1999 [61]. PPAD is not evolutionarily related to mammalian PADs. Structurally, it is a close relative of agmatine deiminases, which are found across bacteria [148]. Different to mammalian PADs, PPAD does not require calcium for catalysis, it is only composed of a ~40 kDa catalytic domain, and it can convert free L-arginine to free L-citrulline [61,148,149]. In addition, PPAD only modifies C-terminal arginine residues (i.e., an exodeiminase), as those generated after peptide cleavage by arginine gingipain (Rgp) [149], which is also secreted by *P. gingivalis*. Several PPAD variants have been identified through the analysis of *P. gingivalis* genomes and clinical isolates [150]. One of these variants (termed PPAD-T2) has two-fold higher catalytic activity compared with PPAD from the reference strain (PPAD-T1) [150]. Whether PPAD variants are relevant for *P. gingivalis* pathogenesis is unknown.

PPAD is detected in the outer membrane (OM) fractions of *P. gingivalis* and as a secreted enzyme, which is found in a soluble form and in association with outer membrane vesicles (OMVs) [120,151,152]. In most clinical isolates (termed type I isolates), extracellular PPAD is mainly found in secreted OMVs and to a minor extent in a soluble form. In contrast, a small subset of clinical isolates (termed type II isolates) showed minimal levels of PPAD in OMVs and most of the enzyme in the soluble form [152]. Type II isolates are associated with a lysine residue at position 373 in PPAD [152]. The clinical significance of *P. gingivalis* type I and type II subsets in the pathogenesis of PD and RA is unknown. Secreted PPAD is believed to be a major virulence factor of *P. gingivalis* due to its capacity to generate ammonia during deimination of arginine to citrulline. Ammonia may protect *P. gingivalis* during acidic cleansing in the mouth [153], and promote periodontal infection by inhibiting neutrophil function [154,155].

5.3. *PPAD-Mediated Citrullination of Bacterial and Host Proteins*

A potential association between PPAD and citrullination in RA was initially suggested as a hypothesis in 2004 [62]. The first experimental evidence, published in 2010, provided two major findings [156]. The first was that clinical isolates of *P. gingivalis* were highly enriched in citrullinated proteins, suggesting that Rgp and PPAD are actively cleaving and citrullinating a large number of substrates in *P. gingivalis*. The second was that after cleavage by Rgp, PPAD citrullinates C-terminal arginine residues in fibrinogen and α-enolase, two important targets of ACPAs in RA. Together, these data provided initial evidence to suggest that bacterial and host proteins citrullinated by PPAD might initiate the loss of tolerance to citrullinated autoantigens in RA [156].

Subsequent studies, however, did not confirm the abundant citrullination initially found in *P. gingivalis* [120,128]. Indeed, although PPAD may citrullinate some proteins in *P. gingivalis*, this feature appears to be exclusive to a few bacterial strains (it was only detectable in reference strain W83 and the clinical isolate MDS45), and potential citrullination seems to be limited to only six bacterial proteins [128]. Whether C-terminal citrullinated peptides derived from these bacterial proteins are specific targets of ACPAs is unknown. Interestingly, PPAD is stable at low pH, resistant to limited proteolysis, and retains significant activity after boiling [61]. Therefore, depending on the processing of *P. gingivalis* for protein analysis, it is possible that citrullination of bacterial proteins may occur in vitro following cell lysis [120]. As an artifact, this may explain the reports of abundant citrullination (including endocitrullination) in lysates from *P. gingivalis* [121,157], as well as the finding that some monoclonal ACPAs cross-react with citrullinated outer membrane antigens (OMAs) from *P. gingivalis* lysates [157].

Regarding autoantigen citrullination by *P. gingivalis* [156], it is important to highlight that neither Rgp nor PPAD have substrate specificity. The finding that fibrinogen and α-enolase are cleaved and citrullinated by these enzymes is, therefore, not surprising, as any other protein would be predicted to undergo the same processing when exposed to these enzymes. Since cleavage and citrullination by Rgp and PPAD is not specific for RA autoantigens, additional evidence is required to support a role of PPAD in the lack of tolerance to citrullinated autoantigens. For example, this could be achieved by demonstrating that C-terminal citrullination mediated by Rgp and PPAD enhances immunoreactivity to autoantigens in RA.

5.4. *Self-Endocitrullination of Pro-PPAD*

PPAD is expressed as a pro-enzyme (thereafter pro-PPAD) that contains four domains: an N-terminal pro-peptide, a catalytic domain, an immunoglobulin-superfamily (IgSF) domain and a C-terminal domain (CTD) [148,149]. The mature enzyme only contains the catalytic and IgSF domains [148]. N-terminal processing appears to maintain enzyme activity and stability [120,158], while C-terminal cleavage is required for cell surface translocation of PPAD [159,160]. During the production and immunogenic analysis of recombinant pro-PPAD, it was noticed that the pro-enzyme undergoes self-endocitrullination when expressed in *E. coli,* and that this modified protein was preferentially recognized by RA sera when compared with the native pro-enzyme [121]. Using 13 cyclic PPAD peptides (termed CPP1-CPP13, which should not be confused with cyclic citrullinated peptides or CCPs) encompassing 18 potential citrullination sites in pro-PPAD, the study further identified immunodominant endocitrullinated peptides recognized by RA antibodies [121]. Although these results were surprising, because PPAD has no endocitrullination activity, it was assumed that these findings were analogous to PPAD from *P. gingivalis*. Thus, the data were interpreted to suggest that loss of tolerance to citrullinated proteins in RA may originate from an antimicrobial immune response directed against citrullinated PPAD [121].

Nevertheless, further studies demonstrated that self-endocitrullination of pro-PPAD was an artifact that resulted from the lack of N-terminal processing of the enzyme expressed in *E. coli* [120]. The absence of endocitrullination in PPAD has been additionally confirmed in structural studies using processed PPAD expressed in *E. coli* or generated in *P. gingivalis* [148,149]. In accordance with these findings, it was also demonstrated that although patients with RA have antibodies to PPAD, these antibodies have no preferential reactivity to the citrullinated pro-enzyme made in *E. coli* [120]. Together, these data demonstrated that self-endocitrullination of pro-PPAD in *E. coli* and the serum reactivity to this modified protein are unlikely to reflect the function and immunogenicity of PPAD from *P. gingivalis* [14,120,161].

Although some RA sera appear to react with cyclic citrullinated peptides derived from pro-PPAD (i.e., CPPs) [121,162], it is unclear whether these peptides are recognized by antibodies to native PPAD or if similar to commercial CCPs, CPPs may function as non-specific targets to detect ACPAs [161]. In this regard, although it was justified that CPPs were generated without knowledge that endocitrullination of pro-PPAD in *E. coli* was an artifact, there is no scientific support to continue their use in the study of RA. Nevertheless, antibodies to CPPs are still being used as biomarkers to link PPAD self-endocitrullination and RA pathogenesis. In particular, serum reactivity against the peptide termed CPP3 has been used to define clinical associations between *P. gingivalis* and RA [122,123,163,164], and to demonstrate that *P. gingivalis* can induce antibodies to citrullinated PPAD in rats [143]. Since the significance of CPPs is unclear, the findings generated with these peptides should be taken with caution. More importantly, serum reactivity to CPPs should not be considered as a maker of citrullination induced by PPAD.

5.5. *PPAD in Experimental Models of Arthritis*

To establish a direct role of PPAD in the production of ACPAs in RA, several experimental models of arthritis have been used to demonstrate that *P. gingivalis* induces or exacerbates arthritis *via* PPAD-mediated autoantigen citrullination and ACPA production. However, while several studies appear to confirm this hypothesis [131,138,144], these studies also highlight important misunderstandings in the study of protein citrullination and ACPAs in RA. For example, in a model of *P. gingivalis* and CIA, citrullinated proteins were mistakenly quantified by a colorimetric method, which measures both free citrulline and peptidylcitrulline [131]. In addition, unconventional methods have been used to detect or define ACPAs. This include the quantification of IgG levels against ACPA (i.e., anti-ACPA antibodies) rather than antibodies to the citrullinated substrates themselves [138]. More recently, one study showed that *P. gingivalis* drives ACPAs (detected by the anti-CCP2 assay) and erosive arthritis in Lewis rats, providing the first evidence that this microbial agent may be arthritogenic [144]. However, it also demonstrated that the antibody response was not specific to the citrullinated forms of antigens [144].

The failure to demonstrate a role of PPAD in autoantigen citrullination and ACPA production in mice and rats is not surprising. Although these animal models express synovial citrullinated proteins and recapitulate several features of the human disease [140,165], they do not produce antibodies specific for citrullinated proteins as observed in RA [165–169]. Moreover, they have a high amount of false-positive reactivity toward citrullinated peptides [166], which is frequently misinterpreted as ACPA positivity when non-citrullinated peptide controls are not included to confirm specificity [131,139,140]. Considering these important shortcomings, even if PPAD plays a critical role in the induction of ACPAs in RA, this hypothesis will be hard to demonstrate using current models of immune-mediated arthritis. Indeed, the data from some animal models of arthritis strongly suggest that *P. gingivalis* may exacerbate or induce disease by mechanisms independent of ACPA production, which may involve the activity of PPAD as a virulence factor targeting either free L-citrulline or protein substrates [131]. Thus, although epidemiological and experimental data may suggest a potential role of *P. gingivalis* in RA pathogenesis, there is no experimental evidence to support that this process is mediated by the induction of ACPAs against host or bacterial proteins citrullinated by PPAD.

6. *Aa* in RA Pathogenesis

6.1. *Infection Due to Aa*

Aa, initially named *Bacterium actinomycetem comitans*, is a Gram-negative oral pathobiont first described in 1912 as a co-isolate from actinomycosis lesions [170]. It was reclassified as *Actinobacillus actinomycetemcomitans* and *Haemophilus actinomycetemcomitans* [171], and finally transferred in 2006 to a new genus, the *Aggregatibacter* [172]. For many years, it was thought that *Aa* was unable to cause infection, except in conjunction with *Actinomyces* [173,174]. This idea was initially supported by the finding that injection of a pure culture of *Aa* in the skin of a normal individual produced no infection [174]. In the 1960's, however, several cases of *Aa* infection not associated with actinomycosis were reported, which were mainly associated with endocarditis [175–177]. *Aa* is now considered part of the HACEK (*Haemophilus*, *Aggregatibacter* (previously *Actinobacillus*), *Cardiobacterium*, *Eikenella*, *Kingella*) group of bacteria that are an unusual cause of infective endocarditis [178]. In addition, it is recognized as a cause of serious infections that can affect almost any organ, although these are very uncommon [179,180].

Although *Aa* is a rare cause of infection, this bacterium has attracted special attention since the 1980s because of its strong association with severe forms of periodontitis [181–185], both localized aggressive periodontitis (LAP) and chronic periodontitis [181,182,186–195]. *Aa* expresses several virulence factors [196]. Among these, the production of leukotoxin A (LtxA) is considered the major pathogenic component in the progression of aggressive periodontitis [195]. LtxA is a member of the repeats-in-toxin (RTX) family of pore-forming proteins [197]. Lymphocyte function-associated antigen (LFA)-1 (CD11a/CD18), Mac-1 (CD11b/CD18) and $\alpha_X\beta_2$ (CD11c/CD18) act as receptors for LtxA (CD18 harbors the major binding site for LtxA), which accounts for the selective killing of human leukocytes [198]. By secreting LtxA, *Aa* induces cytolysis of target cells, thereby disabling host immune defenses and permitting escape from immune surveillance. *Aa* isolates exhibit variable virulence potential [195]. Strains of the serotype b JP2 genotype, characterized by a 530-bp deletion in the promoter region of the leukotoxin operon, has been shown to be highly virulent [199,200]. This genotype, which expresses 10- to 20-fold-higher levels of LtxA due to deletion of a transcriptional terminator [201], is associated with LAP primarily in subjects of African descent [202]. A more detailed analysis of the pathogenic mechanisms associated with the induction of periodontitis by *Aa* have been reviewed recently. [203]

6.2. Aa-Induced Hypercitrullination and the Production Citrullinated RA Autoantigens

A role of *Aa* in the pathogenesis of RA was suggested in 2016, during the search for periodontal pathogens that may explain the presence of hypercitrullination in periodontitis [92]. The study of gingival tissue from patients with PD using anti-citrulline antibodies provided initial evidence that protein citrullination is increased in PD [204,205], supporting the idea that periodontitis is a potential source of citrullinated autoantigens. In addition, the data suggested the possibility that this process was linked to the activity of PPAD [205]. However, although further analysis by mass spectrometry (MS) of GCF confirmed that protein citrullination is increased in PD, this approach also provided two novel findings [92]. First, GCF from patients with PD is highly enriched in citrullinated proteins, mimicking patterns of cellular hypercitrullination found in the rheumatoid joint [92]. Second, peptide spectra of citrullinated proteins in periodontitis were consistent with endocitrullination [92], suggesting that an abnormal activation of host PADs, rather than PPAD, may be responsible for this process. Importantly, the presence of endocitrullination in periodontitis has been further confirmed by MS in GCF and periodontal tissue from patients with PD, both with and without RA [93].

Among different microbial species associated with severe periodontitis, in vitro studies identified *Aa* as the only pathogen that could reproduce the citrullinome found in periodontitis and RA, including the production of well-known targets of ACPAs [92]. In contrast to *P. gingivalis*, however, *Aa* does not encode a PAD-like enzyme. Instead, *Aa* drives citrullination by hyperactivating host PADs through the activity of LtxA. This toxin targets neutrophils, which are enriched in PAD enzymes and constitute the major immune cells in PD and the RA joint [206–208]. Since PADs are calcium dependent, the prominent calcium influx generated by the lytic effect of LtxA hyperactivates these enzymes, driving global hypercitrullination of a wide range of cellular proteins [92]. During this process, cell membrane integrity is eventually lost and membrane rupture occurs with release of citrullinated contents into the extracellular space [92]. Interestingly, this process is similar to the induction of hypercitrullination by host immune-effector pathways (i.e., perforin and complement) in the RA joint [87], suggesting that membranolytic damage by pore-forming proteins may be a unifying mechanism in the production of citrullinated autoantigens [209]. The form of cell death induced by these pore-forming mechanisms has recently been named leukotoxic hypercitrullination (LTH) [209], to distinguish it from other forms of neutrophil death that do not induce hypercitrullination.

6.3. *Aa* Exposure and RA Pathogenesis

Similar to *P. gingivalis*, epidemiological studies to identify an association between *Aa* and RA have been done by detecting antibodies in serum. In particular, IgG antibodies to LtxA (used as markers of *Aa* infection) have been measured in two large cohorts of patients with RA [92,210]. In one study that included patients with established RA, anti-LtxA antibodies were significantly associated with RA when compared to healthy individuals without PD [92]. Similarly, anti-LtxA antibodies were associated with chronic periodontitis in patients without RA, and the strongest association was observed in individuals with severe periodontitis [92]. Antibodies to LtxA may, therefore, identify a subgroup of RA patients with moderate to severe PD. Interestingly, this study also found that the association between *HLA-DRB1* susceptibility alleles (known as shared epitope alleles) and RA autoantibodies was restricted to patients who had evidence of *Aa* exposure. This suggested that in susceptible individuals, LtxA-induced hypercitrullination may play a role in ACPA production [92]. In support of this hypothesis, ACPA production and RA-like symptoms were recently reported in a patient with *Aa* endocarditis who had strong a genetic susceptibility to RA conferred by three HLA alleles linked to ACPA-positive RA [211].

In a different study using a large cohort of patients with early RA, anti-LtxA antibodies were also significantly enriched in RA compared to healthy controls and patients with other inflammatory arthritides (in both groups PD status was unknown) [210], supporting the high prevalence of *Aa* exposure in RA, both in early and established disease. However, this study found that the interaction between *HLA-DRB1*-SE and anti-CCP positivity was not exclusive to anti-LtxA-positive patients with RA [210]. Major differences among these cohorts may explain this discrepancy [212].

Analogous to *P. gingivalis*, metagenomic sequencing and PCR analysis in subgingival plaque have not found a significant association between the presence of *Aa* and RA [104,105,108,110]. In one study, however, analysis of GCF using commercial DNA probes (micro-Ident) identified *Aa* as the only periodontal pathogen showing significant differences between RA and non-RA controls (both with and without PD) [107]. Thus, similar to *P. gingivalis*, positive associations with *Aa* likely indicate PD severity irrespective of RA status.

Few studies have explored the potential role of *Aa* in experimental arthritis [142,213]. However, defining the causal effect of *Aa* in animal models of arthritis has the same limitations as those described for the study of *P. gingivalis*. Moreover, LtxA is known to have activity against leukocytes in primates, with no toxicity on rodent cells [214]. Therefore, different to the human model, any effect that *Aa* may have in the induction of experimental arthritis in rodents is unlikely to be driven by LtxA-induced hypercitrullination and the production of ACPAs.

7. *P. gingivalis* and *Aa* in the Mechanistic Model of RA: Causal Agents, Risk Factors, Disease Modulators, or Research Distractors

Assuming that periodontitis has a mechanistic role in RA, *P. gingivalis* and *Aa* may influence disease pathogenesis at different phases of RA development. The production of autoantibodies is an early and asymptomatic event that precedes the clinical onset of RA by several years [215,216]. The presence of a chronic and amplifying immune response against bacterial-induced RA autoantigens, in particular citrullinated antigens is, therefore, one of the most attractive hypothesis to explain disease initiation and potentially a causal association. In this context, this model explains why there is so much interest in establishing a causal relationship between *P. gingivalis* and the production of ACPAs in either experimental arthritis or RA. Although the current evidence neither demonstrate nor exclude the possibility that PPAD generates citrullinated autoantigens, other possibilities may explain a potential role of *P. gingivalis* in RA pathogenesis. Interestingly, protein citrullination is a process that is increased during inflammation [217]. However, while transient inflammation may not be sufficient to initiate an immune response to citrullinated proteins, periodontitis is a chronic non-fatal illnesses that can start during adolescence and progress over decades [218]. During this time, it is possible that some individuals at risk may develop autoantibodies to citrullinated proteins. *P. gingivalis*, a keystone microorganism in periodontitis, is certainly a strong candidate for promoting chronic inflammation [100], which may indirectly drive the production of autoantibodies in susceptible individuals.

In contrast to *P. gingivalis*, a potential role of *Aa* in the lack of tolerance to RA-associated autoantigens involves the induction of lytic hypercitrullination [92]. In this regard, different factors such as *Aa* virulence (i.e., LtxA production) and bacterial load may define the risk of developing autoantibodies in the context of *Aa* infection in susceptible individuals [92,211]. Importantly, as other bacterial species also produce pore-forming toxins [219], it is possible that other pathogens may induce hypercitrullination and ACPAs at other mucosal sites, including the lung and gut [1,209]. LTH as a mechanism of autoantigen production by different pathogens may explain why every patient with seropositive RA does not have exposure to *Aa* and/or PD.

Interestingly, patients with RA show abnormalities in central and peripheral B cell tolerance checkpoints [220–222], likely due to an intrinsic genetic predisposition [223,224]. This results in the accumulation of autoreactive and polyreactive B cells that can recognize immunoglobulins and citrullinated peptides [220,221]. Depending on genetic and environmental risk factors, autoreactive or polyreactive naïve B cells may have a selective advantage to develop into high affinity autoreactive memory B cells through somatic mutations and affinity maturation. In this scenario, autoantigens generated by arthritogenic bacteria may promote the expansion and maturation of already existing autoreactive cells, rather than initiating the loss of tolerance to host antigens. A prerequisite of having autoreactive/polyreactive B cells to induce pathogenic autoantibodies by *P. gingivalis* or *Aa* may explain why only a limited number of individuals with PD may develop RA.

Although the hypothesis that periodontal pathogens (e.g., *P. gingivalis* or *Aa*) are causal agents of RA is an attractive idea, it is also possible that these bacteria may only be relevant as risk factors for the development of ACPA-positive RA. Alternatively, once RA has been established, persistent low-grade inflammation associated with PD may modulate RA progression and severity. Lastly, despite the enormous enthusiasm of demonstrating that periodontitis is relevant for RA pathogenesis, it cannot yet be excluded that patients with RA may have a higher risk of developing PD (even during the pre-clinical phase of RA), but neither periodontitis, *P. gingivalis*, nor *Aa* may play a pathogenic role in the disease.

8. Therapeutic Implications

The possibility of identifying a factor that triggers a multifactorial disease, such as RA, has critical implications for treatment and preventive interventions. The success of any therapy, however, may depend on targeting such a factor at the correct time during the evolution of the disease [225]. In this regard, although a systematic review and meta-analysis suggested that periodontal treatment may decrease some markers of disease activity in RA [226], these findings remain controversial [227]. The lack of an efficient response to PD treatment on RA disease activity may suggest that periodontitis has no pathogenic role in RA, or that it is most important for disease initiation, during the pre-clinical phase, and that treatment during established disease is no longer effective. If a periodontal pathogen is relevant for the initial breech of tolerance to arthritogenic autoantigens, aiming to treat asymptomatic autoantibody positive (e.g., anti-CCP, RF, or any other autoantibody) individuals may still be too late to stop the progression to symptomatic RA. In this scenario, preventive therapies (e.g., oral hygiene and potentially vaccines against periodontal pathogens) should be initiated in at-risk individuals prior to the development of these serologies. In contrast, if periodontitis is important for the amplification of the autoimmune response in preclinical RA, there is a window of opportunity to target seropositive asymptomatic individuals. Indeed, to date, this is the most feasible hypothesis that could be therapeutically addressed. However, if periodontal pathogens only play a role in the induction of specific subtypes of autoantibodies (e.g., ACPAs), eradication of these agents during the pre-clinical phase of the disease may only decrease the risk of developing certain autoantibodies (and potentially further RA severity), but may not change the course of the disease, including the production of antibodies to other autoantigens. Interestingly, recent evidence suggest that periodontitis is a potential source of proteins modified by malondialdehyde-acetaldehyde adducts and carbamylation [228], which are also common targets of autoantibodies in RA. [229] Thus, independent of the periodontal pathogen, preventing, or targeting periodontitis may be the best exploratory option to prevent RA.

9. Conclusions

Although some epidemiological and mechanistic data supports a role for *P. gingivalis* and *Aa* in the pathogenic model of RA, it is important to underscore that these oral pathobionts do not fulfill the Henle-Koch's postulates of causation [230–232]. These microbial agents neither occur in every case of the disease, nor are specific for patients with RA. In the context of inducing ACPA production in vivo to satisfy the third postulate, it will require the use of animal models that can truly reproduce the autoantibody response observed in RA. Considering these shortcomings, demonstrating or discarding a role of *P. gingivalis* and *Aa* in the pathogenesis of RA may require a different view of how to define disease causality by these microbial agents [212].

In the case of *P. gingivalis*, it is imperative to recognize that its potential role in RA involves elucidation of at least three different questions. The first is whether *P. gingivalis* is relevant for RA pathogenesis, either by initiating or exacerbating the disease. The second is whether *P. gingivalis* is important for RA because of the production of PPAD or because it plays a critical role in the induction of periodontitis by inciting inflammation. Indeed, it appears that ligation-induced periodontitis (without additional infection with *P. gingivalis*) is sufficient to exacerbate CIA in Wistar rats [233]. The third is whether PPAD drives RA due to the production of citrullinated antigens and the induction of ACPAs in the host or because this enzyme is a virulence factor that facilitates bacterial growth and the establishment of PD. Although these questions have been somewhat addressed, definitive conclusions cannot be reached from the available data. Defining the role of PPAD in the production of citrullinated antigens and whether C-terminal deimination offers an advantage for peptide immunogenicity remains a high priority. Importantly, other potential arthritogenic mechanisms induced by *P. gingivalis*, besides autoantigen citrullination, should be kept in consideration.

In the case of *Aa*, this model offers an advantage over other periodontal bacteria because of its capacity to induce neutrophil hypercitrullination and the release of citrullinated autoantigens through osmotic lysis [92]. However, the number of studies linking *Aa* with RA are too limited to truly determine its pathogenic significance for the disease. Similar to *P. gingivalis*, rigorous studies are necessary to support or refute the role of *Aa* in the etiology of RA. Together, these oral pathobionts pose an opportunity to understand whether bacterial-associated citrullination is a mechanism involved in RA pathogenesis. This has important implications for the implementation of preventive interventions in RA.

Author Contributions: Conceptualization and writing—original draft preparation: F.A.; writing—review and editing: E.G.-B., A.M., and E.D.

References

1. Darrah, E.; Andrade, F. Rheumatoid arthritis and citrullination. *Curr. Opin. Rheumatol.* **2018**, *30*, 72–78. [CrossRef]
2. Carmona, L.; Cross, M.; Williams, B.; Lassere, M.; March, L. Rheumatoid arthritis. *Best Pract. Res. Clin. Rheumatol.* **2010**, *24*, 733–745. [CrossRef] [PubMed]
3. Mantle, A. The etiology of rheumatism considered from a bacterial point of view. *Br. Med. J.* **1887**, *1*, 1381–1384. [CrossRef] [PubMed]
4. Bannatyne, G.A.; Wohlmann, A.S.; Blaxall, F.R. Rheumatoid arthritis: Its clinical history, etiology, and pathology. *Lancet* **1896**, *147*, 1120–1125. [CrossRef]
5. Schuller, M. The relation of chronic villous polyarthritis to the dumb-bell shaped bacilli. *Am. J. Med. Sci.* **1906**, *132*, 231–239. [CrossRef]

6. Schuller, M. Chirurgische Mittheilungen über die Chronisch-Rheumatischen Glenkentzündungen. In *Archiv Fur Klinische Chirurgie*; Bergman, E.V., Billroth, T., Gurlt, E., Eds.; Verlag Von August Hirschwald: Berlin, Germany, 1893; pp. 153–185.
7. McInnes, I.B.; Schett, G. The Pathogenesis of Rheumatoid Arthritis. *N. Engl. J. Med.* **2011**, *365*, 2205–2219. [CrossRef] [PubMed]
8. Deane, K.D.; Demoruelle, M.K.; Kelmenson, L.B.; Kuhn, K.A.; Norris, J.M.; Holers, V.M. Genetic and environmental risk factors for rheumatoid arthritis. *Best Pract. Res. Clin. Rheumatol.* **2017**, *31*, 3–18. [CrossRef] [PubMed]
9. Svendsen, A.J.; Kyvik, K.O.; Houen, G.; Junker, P.; Christensen, K.; Christiansen, L.; Nielsen, C.; Skytthe, A.; Hjelmborg, J.V. On the Origin of Rheumatoid Arthritis: The Impact of Environment and Genes—A Population Based Twin Study. *PLoS ONE* **2013**, *8*, e57304. [CrossRef] [PubMed]
10. Frisell, T.; Saevarsdottir, S.; Askling, J.; Frisell, T. Family history of rheumatoid arthritis: An old concept with new developments. *Nat. Rev. Rheumatol.* **2016**, *12*, 335–343. [CrossRef] [PubMed]
11. Silman, A.J.; MacGregor, A.J.; Thomson, W.; Holligan, S.; Carthy, D.; Farhan, A.; Ollier, W.E.R. Twin concordance rates for rheumatoid arthritis: Results from a nationwide study. *Br. J. Rheumatol.* **1993**, *32*, 903–907. [CrossRef] [PubMed]
12. Svendsen, A.J.; Holm, N.V.; Kyvik, K.; Petersen, P.H.; Junker, P. Relative importance of genetic effects in rheumatoid arthritis: Historical cohort study of Danish nationwide twin population. *BMJ* **2002**, *324*, 264. [CrossRef] [PubMed]
13. Caminer, A.C.; Haberman, R.; Scher, J.U. Human microbiome, infections, and rheumatic disease. *Clin. Rheumatol.* **2017**, *36*, 2645–2653. [CrossRef] [PubMed]
14. Potempa, J.; Mydel, P.; Koziel, J. The case for periodontitis in the pathogenesis of rheumatoid arthritis. *Nat. Rev. Rheumatol.* **2017**, *13*, 606–620. [CrossRef] [PubMed]
15. Scher, J.U.; Littman, D.R.; Abramson, S.B. Microbiome in Inflammatory Arthritis and Human Rheumatic Diseases. *Arthritis Rheumatol.* **2016**, *68*, 35–45. [CrossRef] [PubMed]
16. Dunbar, L.L. Oral manifestations in arthritic and gouty conditions. *JAMA* **1895**, *24*, 75–77. [CrossRef]
17. Landré-Beauvais, A.J. The first description of rheumatoid arthritis. Unabridged text of the doctoral dissertation presented in 1800. *Jt. Bone Spine* **2001**, *68*, 130–143.
18. Garrod, A.B. Rheumatic Gout. In *The Nature and Treatment of Gout and Rheumatic Gout*; Garrod, A.B., Ed.; Walton and Maberly: London, UK, 1859; pp. 526–556.
19. Richards, J.H. Bacteriologic Studies in Chronic Arthritis and Chorea. *J. Bacteriol.* **1920**, *5*, 511–525. [PubMed]
20. Swett, P.P. Synovectomy in chronic infectious arthritis. *J. Bone Jt. Surg.* **1923**, *5*, 110–121.
21. Kinsella, R.A. Chronic infectious arthritis. *J. Am. Med. Assoc.* **1923**, *80*, 0671–0674. [CrossRef]
22. Margolis, M.H.; Dorsey, A.H.E. Chronic arthritis—Bacteriology of affected tissues. *Arch. Intern. Med.* **1930**, *46*, 121–136. [CrossRef]
23. Goadby, K.W. The Hunterian Lecture on the Association of Disease of the Mouth with Rheumatoid Arthritis and Certain other Forms of Rheumatism. Delivered at the Royal College of Surgeons of England on March 6th, 1911. *Lancet* **1911**, *1*, 639–649.
24. Lane, S.A. A Lecture on Tertiary Syphilis, or Syphilitic Cachexia. *Br. Med. J.* **1873**, *2*, 421–423. [CrossRef] [PubMed]
25. Billings, I.K. Focal infection—Its broader application in the etiology of general disease. *J. Am. Med. Assoc.* **1914**, *63*, 899–903. [CrossRef]
26. Lambert, J. A report of some points in the etiology and onset of 195 cases of rheumatoid arthritis. *Bull. Comm. Study Spec. Dis.* **1908**, *2*, 83–94.
27. Lindsay, J. The relation of infective foci to rheumatoid arthritis. *Bull. Comm. Study Spec. Dis.* **1908**, *2*, 106–116.
28. Billings, F. Chronic focal infections and their etiologic relations to arthritis and nephritis. *Arch. Intern. Med.* **1912**, *9*, 484–498. [CrossRef]
29. Billings, F. Chronic focal infection as a causative factor in chronic arthritis. *J. Am. Med. Assoc.* **1913**, *61*, 819–822. [CrossRef]
30. Billings, F. Mouth infection as a source of systemic disease. *J. Am. Med. Assoc.* **1914**, *63*, 2024–2025. [CrossRef]
31. Bywaters, E.G.L. Historical Aspects of the Aetiology of Rheumatoid Arthritis. *Br. J. Rheumatol.* **1988**, 110–115. [CrossRef]

32. Hughes, R.A. Focal infection revisited. *Br. J. Rheumatol.* **1994**, *33*, 370–377. [CrossRef]
33. Miller, W.D. The Human Mouth as a Focus of Infection. *Dent. Cosmos.* **1891**, *33*, 689–713. [CrossRef]
34. Miller, W.D. Diseases of the Human Body Which Have Been Traced to the Action of Mouth-Bacteria. *Am. J. Dent. Sci.* **1891**, *25*, 311–319. [PubMed]
35. Hunter, W. Oral Sepsis as a Cause of Disease. *Br. Med. J.* **1900**, *2*, 215–216. [CrossRef] [PubMed]
36. Hunter, W. A Case of Pernicious Anæmia; with Observations regarding Mode of Onset, Clinical Features, Infective Nature, Prognosis, and Antiseptic and Serum Treatment of the Disease. *J. R. Soc. Med.* **1901**, *84*, 205–249.
37. Hunter, W. Further observations on pernicious anaemia (seven cases): A chronic infective disease; its relation to infection from the mouth and stomach; suggested serum treatment. *Lancet* **1900**, *155*, 296–299. [CrossRef]
38. Hunter, W. Further investigations regarding the infective nature and etiology of pernicius anaemia. *Lancet* **1903**, *161*, 367–371. [CrossRef]
39. Roberts, H.L. Focal infection. *Br. J. Derm. Syph.* **1921**, *33*, 319–334. [CrossRef]
40. Roberts, H.L. Focal infection. *Br. J. Derm. Syph.* **1921**, *33*, 353–373. [CrossRef]
41. Rush, B. An Account of the Cure of Several Diseases by the Extraction of Decayed Teeth. In *Medical Inquiries and Observations*, 5th ed.; Rush, B., Ed.; Printed by M. Carey & Son; B. Warner; A. Finley; S. W. Conrad; T. & W. Bradford; B. & T. Kite, and Bennett and Walton; National Library of Medicine: Philadelphia, PA, USA, 1818; Volume 1, pp. 197–201. Available online: https://collections.nlm.nih.gov/catalog/nlm:nlmuid-2569006RX1-mvpart (accessed on 26 August 2019).
42. Miltner, L.J.; Kulowski, J. The effect of treatment and erradication of foci on infection in chronic rheumatoid arthritis. *J. Bone Jt. Surg.* **1933**, *15*, 383–396.
43. Cecil, R.; Angevine, A. Clinical and experimental observations on focal infection. *Ann. Intern. Med.* **1938**, *12*, 577–584.
44. Vaizey, J.M.; Clark-Kennedy, A.E. Dental Sepsis: Anaemia, Dyspepsia, and Rheumatism. *Br. Med. J.* **1939**, *1*, 1269–1273. [CrossRef]
45. Riggs, J.W. Suppurative Inflammation of the Gums and Absorption of the Gums and the Alveolar Process. *Am. J. Dent. Sci.* **1999**, *32*, 401–407.
46. Hajishengallis, G. Immunomicrobial pathogenesis of periodontitis: Keystones, pathobionts, and host response. *Trends Immunol.* **2014**, *35*, 3–11. [CrossRef]
47. Brandtzaeg, P.; Kraus, F.W. Autoimmunity and periodontal disease. *Odontol. Tidskr.* **1965**, *73*, 281.
48. Snyderman, R.; McCarty, G.A. Analogous Mechanisms of Tissue Destruction in Rheumatoid Arthritis and Periodontal Disease. In *Host-Parasite Interactions in Periodontal Diseases*; Genco, R.J., Mergenhagen, S.E., Eds.; American Society of Microbiology: Washington, DC, USA, 1982; pp. 354–362.
49. Seymour, G.J.; Powell, R.N.; Davies, W.I.R. The immunopathogenesis of progressive chronic inflammatory periodontal disease. *J. Oral. Pathol. Med.* **1979**, *8*, 249–265. [CrossRef]
50. Greenwald, R.A.; Kirkwood, K. Adult periodontitis as a model for rheumatoid arthritis (with emphasis on treatment strategies). *J. Rheumatol.* **1999**, *26*, 1650–1653.
51. Katz, J.; Goultschin, J.; Benoliel, R.; Brautbar, C. Human leukocyte antigen (HLA) DR4. Positive association with rapidly progressing periodontitis. *J. Periodontol.* **1987**, *58*, 607–610. [CrossRef]
52. Bonfil, J.J.; Dillier, F.L.; Mercier, P.; Reviron, D.; Foti, B.; Sambuc, R.; Brodeur, J.M.; Sedarat, C. A "case control" study on the role of HLA DR4 in severe periodontitis and rapidly progressive periodontitis. Identification of types and subtypes using molecular biology (PCR.SSO). *J. Clin. Periodontol.* **1999**, *26*, 77–84. [CrossRef]
53. Rizzo, A.A.; Mitchell, C.T. Chronic allergic inflammation induced by repeated deposition of antigen in rabbit gingival pockets. *Periodontics* **1966**, *4*, 5.
54. McHugh, W.D. Some aspects of the development of gingival epithelium. *Periodontics* **1963**, *1*, 239–244.
55. Schroeder, H. Quantitative parameters of early human gingival inflammation. *Arch. Oral Biol.* **1970**, *15*, 383–IN4. [CrossRef]
56. Sugawara, M.; Yamashita, K.; Yoshie, H.; Hara, K. Detection of, and anti-collagen antibody produced by, CD5-positive B cells in inflamed gingival tissues. *J. Periodontal Res.* **1992**, *27*, 489–498. [CrossRef]
57. Kristoffersen, T.; Tonder, O. Anti-immunoglobulin activity in inflamed human gingiva. *J. Dent. Res.* **1973**, *52*, 991.

58. Gargiulo, A.V.; Robinson, J.; Toto, P.D.; Gargiulo, A.W. Identification of Rheumatoid Factor in Periodontal Disease. *J. Periodontol.* **1982**, *53*, 568–577. [CrossRef]
59. Gargiulo, A.V., Jr.; Toto, P.D.; Robinson, J.A.; Gargiulo, A.W. Latex slide agglutination vs. ELISA system: Rheumatoid factor detection in inflamed human gingiva. *J. Periodontal Res.* **1985**, *20*, 31–34. [CrossRef]
60. Malmström, M.; Natvig, J.B. IgG Rheumatoid Factor in Dental Periapical Lesions of Patients with Rheumatoid Disease. *Scand. J. Rheumatol.* **1975**, *4*, 177–185. [CrossRef]
61. McGraw, W.T.; Potempa, J.; Farley, D.; Travis, J. Purification, Characterization, and Sequence Analysis of a Potential Virulence Factor from Porphyromonas gingivalis, Peptidylarginine Deiminase. *Infect. Immun.* **1999**, *67*, 3248–3256.
62. Rosenstein, E.D.; Greenwald, R.A.; Kushner, L.J.; Weissmann, G. Hypothesis: The Humoral Immune Response to Oral Bacteria Provides a Stimulus for the Development of Rheumatoid Arthritis. *Inflammation* **2004**, *28*, 311–318. [CrossRef]
63. Schellekens, G.A.; De Jong, B.A.; Hoogen, F.H.V.D.; Van De Putte, L.B.; Van Venrooij, W.J. Citrulline is an essential constituent of antigenic determinants recognized by rheumatoid arthritis-specific autoantibodies. *J. Clin. Investig.* **1998**, *101*, 273–281. [CrossRef]
64. Kaur, S.; White, S.; Bartold, P.M. Periodontal disease and rheumatoid arthritis: A systematic review. *J. Dent. Res.* **2013**, *92*, 399–408. [CrossRef]
65. Fuggle, N.R.; Smith, T.O.; Kaul, A.; Sofat, N. Hand to Mouth: A Systematic Review and Meta-Analysis of the Association between Rheumatoid Arthritis and Periodontitis. *Front. Immunol.* **2016**, *7*, 80. [CrossRef]
66. Araujo, V.M.; Melo, I.M.; Lima, V. Relationship between Periodontitis and Rheumatoid Arthritis: Review of the Literature. *Med.iat. Inflamm.* **2015**, *2015*, 259074. [CrossRef]
67. Kindstedt, E.; Johansson, L.; Palmqvist, P.; Holm, C.K.; Kokkonen, H.; Johansson, I.; Dahlqvist, S.R.; Lundberg, P. Association Between Marginal Jawbone Loss and Onset of Rheumatoid Arthritis and Relationship to Plasma Levels of RANKL. *Arthritis Rheumatol.* **2018**, *70*, 508–515. [CrossRef]
68. Eriksson, K.; Nise, L.; Kats, A.; Luttropp, E.; Catrina, A.I.; Askling, J.; Jansson, L.; Alfredsson, L.; Klareskog, L.; Lundberg, K.; et al. Prevalence of Periodontitis in Patients with Established Rheumatoid Arthritis: A Swedish Population Based Case-Control Study. *PLoS ONE* **2016**, *11*, e0155956. [CrossRef]
69. Sjöström, L.; Laurell, L.; Hugoson, A.; Håkansson, J.P. Periodontal conditions in adults with rheumatoid arthritis. *Community Dent. Oral Epidemiol.* **1989**, *17*, 234–236. [CrossRef]
70. Eke, P.I.; Dye, B.A.; Wei, L.; Thornton-Evans, G.O.; Genco, R.J. CDC Periodontal Disease Surveillance workgroup: James Beck GDRP. Prevalence of periodontitis in adults in the United States: 2009 and 2010. *J. Dent. Res.* **2012**, *91*, 914–920. [CrossRef]
71. Kassebaum, N.J.; Bernabe, E.; Dahiya, M.; Bhandari, B.; Murray, C.J.; Marcenes, W. Global burden of severe periodontitis in 1990-2010, a systematic review and meta-regression. *J. Dent. Res.* **2014**, *93*, 1045–1053. [CrossRef]
72. dos Anjos, L.M.; Pereira, I.A.; 'Orsi, E.; Seaman, A.P.; Burlingame, R.W.; Morato, E.F. A comparative study of IgG second- and third-generation anti-cyclic citrullinated peptide (CCP) ELISAs and their combination with IgA third-generation CCP ELISA for the diagnosis of rheumatoid arthritis. *Clin. Rheumatol.* **2009**, *28*, 153–158. [CrossRef]
73. Lutteri, L.; Malaise, M.; Chapelle, J.P. Comparison of second- and third-generation anti-cyclic citrullinated peptide antibodies assays for detecting rheumatoid arthritis. *Clin. Chim. Acta* **2007**, *386*, 76–81. [CrossRef]
74. Sugawara, K.; Fujisaki, M. Properties of Peptidylarginine Deiminase from the Epidermis of Newborn Rats. *J. Biochem.* **1981**, *89*, 257–263.
75. Raijmakers, R.; Zendman, A.J.; Egberts, W.V.; Vossenaar, E.R.; Raats, J.; Soede-Huijbregts, C.; Rutjes, F.P.; Van Veelen, P.A.; Drijfhout, J.W.; Pruijn, G.J. Methylation of Arginine Residues Interferes with Citrullination by Peptidylarginine Deiminases in vitro. *J. Mol. Biol.* **2007**, *367*, 1118–1129. [CrossRef]
76. Kinloch, A.; Lundberg, K.; Wait, R.; Wegner, N.; Lim, N.H.; Zendman, A.J.W.; Saxne, T.; Malmstr, V.; Venables, P.J.; Kinloch, A. Synovial fluid is a site of citrullination of autoantigens in inflammatory arthritis. *Arthritis Rheum.* **2008**, *58*, 2287–2295. [CrossRef]
77. Foulquier, C.; Sebbag, M.; Clavel, C.; Chapuy-Regaud, S.; Al Badine, R.; Méchin, M.C.; Vincent, C.; Nachat, R.; Yamada, M.; Takahara, H.; et al. Peptidyl arginine deiminase type 2 (PAD-2) and PAD-4 but not PAD-1, PAD-3, and PAD-6 are expressed in rheumatoid arthritis synovium in close association with tissue inflammation. *Arthritis Rheum.* **2007**, *56*, 3541–3553. [CrossRef]

78. Chang, X.; Yamada, R.; Suzuki, A.; Sawada, T.; Yoshino, S.; Tokuhiro, S.; Yamamoto, K. Localization of peptidylarginine deiminase 4 (PADI4) and citrullinated protein in synovial tissue of rheumatoid arthritis. *Rheumatology (Oxf.)* **2005**, *44*, 40–50. [CrossRef]
79. Arita, K.; Hashimoto, H.; Shimizu, T.; Nakashima, K.; Yamada, M.; Sato, M. Structural basis for Ca^{2+}-induced activation of human PAD4. *Nat. Struct. Mol. Biol.* **2004**, *11*, 777–783. [CrossRef]
80. Slade, D.J.; Fang, P.; Dreyton, C.J.; Zhang, Y.; Fuhrmann, J.; Rempel, D.; Bax, B.D.; Coonrod, S.A.; Lewis, H.D.; Guo, M.; et al. Protein Arginine Deiminase 2 Binds Calcium in an Ordered Fashion: Implications for Inhibitor Design. *ACS Chem. Biol.* **2015**, *10*, 1043–1053. [CrossRef]
81. Saijo, S.; Nagai, A.; Kinjo, S.; Mashimo, R.; Akimoto, M.; Kizawa, K.; Yabe-Wada, T.; Shimizu, N.; Takahara, H.; Unno, M. Monomeric Form of Peptidylarginine Deiminase Type I Revealed by X-ray Crystallography and Small-Angle X-ray Scattering. *J. Mol. Biol.* **2016**, *428*, 3058–3073. [CrossRef]
82. Kearney, P.L.; Bhatia, M.; Jones, N.G.; Yuan, L.; Glascock, M.C.; Catchings, K.L.; Yamada, M.; Thompson, P.R. Kinetic Characterization of Protein Arginine Deiminase 4: A Transcriptional Corepressor Implicated in the Onset and Progression of Rheumatoid Arthritis. *Biochemistry* **2005**, *44*, 10570–10582. [CrossRef]
83. Vossenaar, E.R.; Zendman, A.J.; Van Venrooij, W.J.; Pruijn, G.J. PAD, a growing family of citrullinating enzymes: Genes, features and involvement in disease. *BioEssays* **2003**, *25*, 1106–1118. [CrossRef]
84. Witalison, E.E.; Thompson, P.R.; Hofseth, L.J. Protein Arginine Deiminases and Associated Citrullination: Physiological Functions and Diseases Associated with Dysregulation. *Curr. Drug Targets* **2015**, *16*, 700–710. [CrossRef]
85. Lee, C.Y.; Wang, D.; Wilhelm, M.; Zolg, D.P.; Schmidt, T.; Schnatbaum, K.; Reimer, U.; Ponten, F.; Uhlen, M.; Hahne, H.; et al. Mining the Human Tissue Proteome for Protein Citrullination. *Mol. Cell. Proteom.* **2018**, *17*, 1378–1391. [CrossRef]
86. van Beers, J.J.; Schwarte, C.M.; Stammen-Vogelzangs, J.; Oosterink, E.; Bozic, B.; Pruijn, G.J. The rheumatoid arthritis synovial fluid citrullinome reveals novel citrullinated epitopes in apolipoprotein E, myeloid nuclear differentiation antigen, and beta-actin. *Arthritis Rheum.* **2013**, *65*, 69–80. [CrossRef]
87. Romero, V.; Fert-Bober, J.; Nigrovic, P.A.; Darrah, E.; Haque, U.J.; Lee, D.M.; Van Eyk, J.; Rosen, A.; Andrade, F. Immune-Mediated Pore-Forming Pathways Induce Cellular Hypercitrullination and Generate Citrullinated Autoantigens in Rheumatoid Arthritis. *Sci. Transl. Med.* **2013**, *5*, 209ra150. [CrossRef]
88. Tutturen, A.E.V.; Fleckenstein, B.; De Souza, G.A. Assessing the Citrullinome in Rheumatoid Arthritis Synovial Fluid with and without Enrichment of Citrullinated Peptides. *J. Proteome Res.* **2014**, *13*, 2867–2873. [CrossRef]
89. Wang, F.; Chen, F.F.; Gao, W.B.; Wang, H.Y.; Zhao, N.W.; Xu, M.; Gao, D.Y.; Yu, W.; Yan, X.L.; Zhao, J.N.; et al. Identification of citrullinated peptides in the synovial fluid of patients with rheumatoid arthritis using LC-MALDI-TOF/TOF. *Clin. Rheumatol.* **2016**, *35*, 2185–2194. [CrossRef]
90. Tilvawala, R.; Nguyen, S.H.; Maurais, A.J.; Nemmara, V.V.; Nagar, M.; Salinger, A.J.; Nagpal, S.; Weerapana, E.; Thompson, P.R. The Rheumatoid Arthritis-Associated Citrullinome. *Cell Chem. Biol.* **2018**, *25*, 691–704.e6. [CrossRef]
91. Bennike, T.B.; Ellingsen, T.; Glerup, H.; Bonderup, O.K.; Carlsen, T.G.; Meyer, M.K.; Bøgsted, M.; Christiansen, G.; Birkelund, S.; Andersen, V.; et al. Proteome Analysis of Rheumatoid Arthritis Gut Mucosa. *J. Proteome Res.* **2017**, *16*, 346–354. [CrossRef]
92. Konig, M.F.; Abusleme, L.; Reinholdt, J.; Palmer, R.J.; Teles, R.P.; Sampson, K.; Rosen, A.; Nigrovic, P.A.; Sokolove, J.; Giles, J.T.; et al. Aggregatibacter actinomycetemcomitans-induced hypercitrullination links periodontal infection to autoimmunity in rheumatoid arthritis. *Sci. Transl. Med.* **2016**, *8*, 369ra176. [CrossRef]
93. Schwenzer, A.; Quirke, A.M.; Marzeda, A.M.; Wong, A.; Montgomery, A.B.; Sayles, H.R.; Eick, S.; Gawron, K.; Chomyszyn-Gajewska, M.; et al. Association of Distinct Fine Specificities of Anti-Citrullinated Peptide Antibodies with Elevated Immune Responses to Prevotella intermedia in a Subgroup of Patients With Rheumatoid Arthritis and Periodontitis. *Arthritis Rheumatol.* **2017**, *69*, 2303–2313. [CrossRef]
94. Macdonald, J.B.; Gibbons, R.J.; Socransky, S.S. Bacterial mechanisms in periodontal disease. *Ann. N. Y. Acad. Sci.* **1960**, *85*, 467–478. [CrossRef]
95. Finegold, S.M.; Barnes, E.M. Report of Icsb Taxonomic Subcommittee on Gram-Negative Anaerobic Rods. *Int. J. Syst. Bacteriol.* **1977**, *27*, 388–391. [CrossRef]

96. Reed, M.J.; Slots, J.; Mouton, C.; Genco, R.J. Antigenic Studies of Oral and Non-Oral Black-Pigmented Bacteroides Strains. *Infect. Immun.* **1980**, *29*, 564–574.
97. Kaczmarek, F.S.; Coykendall, A.L. Production of phenylacetic acid by strains of *Bacteroides asaccharolyticus* and *Bacteroides gingivalis* (sp. nov). *J. Clin. Microbiol.* **1980**, *12*, 288–290.
98. Shah, H.N.; Collins, M.D. Proposal for Reclassification of Bacteroides asaccharolyticus, Bacteroides gingivalis, and Bacteroides endodontalis in a New Genus, Porphyromonas. *Int. J. Syst. Bacteriol.* **1988**, *38*, 128–131. [CrossRef]
99. Lamont, R.J.; Koo, H.; Hajishengallis, G. The oral microbiota: Dynamic communities and host interactions. *Nat. Rev. Genet.* **2018**, *16*, 745–759. [CrossRef]
100. Hajishengallis, G.; Darveau, R.P.; Curtis, M.A. The keystone-pathogen hypothesis. *Nat. Rev. Microbiol.* **2012**, *10*, 717–725. [CrossRef]
101. de Smit, M.; Westra, J.; Vissink, A.; Doornbos-van der Meer, B.; Brouwer, E.; van Winkelhoff, A.J. Periodontitis in established rheumatoid arthritis patients: A cross-sectional clinical, microbiological and serological study. *Arthritis Res. Ther.* **2012**, *14*, R222. [CrossRef]
102. Engström, M.; Eriksson, K.; Lee, L.; Hermansson, M.; Johansson, A.; Nicholas, A.P.; Gerasimcik, N.; Lundberg, K.; Klareskog, L.; Catrina, A.I.; et al. Increased citrullination and expression of peptidylarginine deiminases independently of *P. gingivalis* and *A. actinomycetemcomitans* in gingival tissue of patients with periodontitis. *J. Transl. Med.* **2018**, *16*, 214. [CrossRef]
103. Eriksson, K.; Fei, G.; Lundmark, A.; Benchimol, D.; Lee, L.; Hu, Y.O.O.; Kats, A.; Saevarsdottir, S.; Catrina, A.I.; Klinge, B.; et al. Periodontal Health and Oral Microbiota in Patients with Rheumatoid Arthritis. *J. Clin. Med.* **2019**, *8*, 630. [CrossRef]
104. Schmickler, J.; Rupprecht, A.; Patschan, S.; Patschan, D.; Müller, G.A.; Haak, R.; Mausberg, R.F.; Schmalz, G.; Kottmann, T.; Ziebolz, D.; et al. Cross-Sectional Evaluation of Periodontal Status and Microbiologic and Rheumatoid Parameters in a Large Cohort of Patients with Rheumatoid Arthritis. *J. Periodontol.* **2017**, *88*, 368–379. [CrossRef]
105. Ziebolz, D.; Pabel, S.O.; Lange, K.; Krohn-Grimberghe, B.; Hornecker, E.; Mausberg, R.F. Clinical Periodontal and Microbiologic Parameters in Patients with Rheumatoid Arthritis. *J. Periodontol.* **2011**, *82*, 1424–1432. [CrossRef]
106. Beyer, K.; Zaura, E.; Brandt, B.W.; Buijs, M.J.; Brun, J.G.; Crielaard, W.; Bolstad, A.I. Subgingival microbiome of rheumatoid arthritis patients in relation to their disease status and periodontal health. *PLoS ONE* **2018**, *13*, e0202278. [CrossRef]
107. Laugisch, O.; Wong, A.; Sroka, A.; Kantyka, T.; Koziel, J.; Neuhaus, K.; Sculean, A.; Venables, P.J.; Potempa, J.; Möller, B.; et al. Citrullination in the periodontium—A possible link between periodontitis and rheumatoid arthritis. *Clin. Oral Investig.* **2015**, *20*, 675–683. [CrossRef]
108. Lopez-Oliva, I.; Paropkari, A.D.; Saraswat, S.; Serban, S.; Yonel, Z.; Sharma, P.; De Pablo, P.; Raza, K.; Filer, A.; Chapple, I.; et al. Dysbiotic Subgingival Microbial Communities in Periodontally Healthy Patients with Rheumatoid Arthritis. *Arthritis Rheumatol.* **2018**, *70*, 1008–1013. [CrossRef]
109. Zhang, X.; Zhang, D.; Jia, H.; Feng, Q.; Wang, D.; Liang, D.; Wu, X.; Li, J.; Tang, L.; Li, Y.; et al. The oral and gut microbiomes are perturbed in rheumatoid arthritis and partly normalized after treatment. *Nat. Med.* **2015**, *21*, 895–905. [CrossRef]
110. Mikuls, T.R.; Walker, C.; Qiu, F.; Yu, F.; Thiele, G.M.; Alfant, B.; Li, E.C.; Zhao, L.Y.; Wang, G.P.; Datta, S.; et al. The subgingival microbiome in patients with established rheumatoid arthritis. *Rheumatology* **2018**, *57*, 1162–1172. [CrossRef]
111. Scher, J.U.; Ubeda, C.; Equinda, M.; Khanin, R.; Buischi, Y.; Viale, A.; Lipuma, L.; Attur, M.; Pillinger, M.H.; Weissmann, G.; et al. Periodontal Disease and the Oral Microbiota in New-Onset Rheumatoid Arthritis. *Arthritis Rheum.* **2012**, *64*, 3083–3094. [CrossRef]
112. Mankia, K.; Cheng, Z.; Do, T.; Hunt, L.; Meade, J.; Kang, J.; Clerehugh, V.; Speirs, A.; Tugnait, A.; Hensor, E.M.A.; et al. Prevalence of Periodontal Disease and Periodontopathic Bacteria in Anti–Cyclic Citrullinated Protein Antibody–Positive At-Risk Adults Without Arthritis. *JAMA Netw. Open* **2019**, *2*, e195394. [CrossRef]

113. Arvikar, S.L.; Collier, D.S.; Fisher, M.C.; Unizony, S.; Cohen, G.L.; McHugh, G.; Kawai, T.; Strle, K.; Steere, A.C. Clinical correlations with Porphyromonas gingivalis antibody responses in patients with early rheumatoid arthritis. *Arthritis Res. Ther.* **2013**, *15*, R109. [CrossRef]
114. Okada, M.; Kobayashi, T.; Ito, S.; Yokoyama, T.; Komatsu, Y.; Abe, A.; Murasawa, A.; Yoshie, H. Antibody Responses to Periodontopathic Bacteria in Relation to Rheumatoid Arthritis in Japanese Adults. *J. Periodontol.* **2011**, *82*, 1433–1441. [CrossRef]
115. Mikuls, T.R.; Payne, J.B.; Reinhardt, R.A.; Thiele, G.M.; Maziarz, E.; Cannella, A.C.; Holers, V.M.; Kuhn, K.A.; O'Dell, J.R. Antibody responses to Porphyromonas gingivalis (P. gingivalis) in subjects with rheumatoid arthritis and periodontitis. *Int. Immunopharmacol.* **2009**, *9*, 38–42. [CrossRef]
116. Ogrendik, M.; Kokino, S.; Ozdemir, F.; Bird, P.S.; Hamlet, S. Serum Antibodies to Oral Anaerobic Bacteria in Patients with Rheumatoid Arthritis. *MedGenMed Medscape Gen. Med.* **2005**, *7*, 2.
117. Yusof, Z.R.; Porter, S.; Greenman, J.; Scully, C. Levels of Serum IgG against Porphyromonas gingivalis in Patients with Rapidly Progressive Periodontitis, Rheumatoid Arthritis and Adult Periodontitis. *J. Nihon Univ. Sch. Dent.* **1995**, *37*, 197–200. [CrossRef]
118. Moen, K.; Brun, J.G.; Madland, T.M.; Tynning, T.; Jonsson, R. Immunoglobulin G and a Antibody Responses to Bacteroides forsythus and Prevotella intermedia in Sera and Synovial Fluids of Arthritis Patients. *Clin. Diagn. Lab. Immunol.* **2003**, *10*, 1043–1050. [CrossRef]
119. de Smit, M.; van de Stadt, L.A.; Janssen, K.M.; Doornbos-van der Meer, B.; Vissink, A.; van Winkelhoff, A.J.; Brouwer, E.; Westra, J.; van Schaardenburg, D. Antibodies against Porphyromonas gingivalis in seropositive arthralgia patients do not predict development of rheumatoid arthritis. *Ann. Rheum. Dis.* **2014**, *73*, 1277–1279. [CrossRef]
120. Konig, M.F.; Paracha, A.S.; Moni, M.; Bingham, C.O., III; Andrade, F. Defining the role of Porphyromonas gingivalis peptidylarginine deiminase (PPAD) in rheumatoid arthritis through the study of PPAD biology. *Ann. Rheum. Dis.* **2015**, *74*, 2054–2061. [CrossRef]
121. Quirke, A.M.; Lugli, E.B.; Wegner, N.; Hamilton, B.C.; Charles, P.; Chowdhury, M.; Ytterberg, A.J.; Zubarev, R.A.; Potempa, J.; Culshaw, S.; et al. Heightened immune response to autocitrullinated Porphyromonas gingivalis peptidylarginine deiminase: A potential mechanism for breaching immunologic tolerance in rheumatoid arthritis. *Ann. Rheum. Dis.* **2014**, *73*, 263–269. [CrossRef]
122. Fisher, B.A.; Cartwright, A.J.; Quirke, A.M.; de Pablo, P.; Romaguera, D.; Panico, S.; Mattiello, A.; Gavrila, D.; Navarro, C.; Sacerdote, C.; et al. Smoking, Porphyromonas gingivalis and the immune response to citrullinated autoantigens before the clinical onset of rheumatoid arthritis in a Southern European nested case-control study. *BMC Musculoskelet. Disord.* **2015**, *16*, 331. [CrossRef]
123. Johansson, L.; Sherina, N.; Kharlamova, N.; Potempa, B.; Larsson, B.; Israelsson, L.; Potempa, J.; Rantapää-Dahlqvist, S.; Lundberg, K. Concentration of antibodies against Porphyromonas gingivalis is increased before the onset of symptoms of rheumatoid arthritis. *Arthritis Res. Ther.* **2016**, *18*, 201. [CrossRef]
124. Kharlamova, N.; Jiang, X.; Sherina, N.; Potempa, B.; Israelsson, L.; Quirke, A.-M.; Eriksson, K.; Yucel-Lindberg, T.; Venables, P.J.; Potempa, J.; et al. Antibodies to Porphyromonas gingivalis indicate interaction between oral infection, smoking and risk genes in rheumatoid arthritis etiology. *Arthritis Rheumatol.* **2016**, *68*, 604–613. [CrossRef]
125. Mikuls, T.R.; Payne, J.B.; Yu, F.; Thiele, G.M.; Reynolds, R.J.; Cannon, G.W.; Markt, J.; McGowan, D.; Kerr, G.S.; Redman, R.S.; et al. Periodontitis and Porphyromonas gingivalis in Patients with Rheumatoid Arthritis. *Arthritis Rheumatol.* **2014**, *66*, 1090–1100. [CrossRef]
126. Okada, M.; Kobayashi, T.; Ito, S.; Yokoyama, T.; Abe, A.; Murasawa, A.; Yoshie, H. Periodontal Treatment Decreases Levels of Antibodies to Porphyromonas gingivalis and Citrulline in Patients with Rheumatoid Arthritis and Periodontitis. *J. Periodontol.* **2013**, *84*, e74–e84. [CrossRef]
127. Rinaudo-Gaujous, M.; Blasco-Baque, V.; Miossec, P.; Gaudin, P.; Farge, P.; Roblin, X.; Thomas, T.; Paul, S.; Marotte, H. Infliximab Induced a Dissociated Response of Severe Periodontal Biomarkers in Rheumatoid Arthritis Patients. *J. Clin. Med.* **2019**, *8*, 751. [CrossRef]

128. Stobernack, T.; Glasner, C.; Junker, S.; Gabarrini, G.; De Smit, M.; Van Winkelhoff, A.J.; De Jong, A.; Otto, A.; Becher, D.; Van Dijl, J.M. Extracellular Proteome and Citrullinome of the Oral Pathogen Porphyromonas gingivalis. *J. Proteome Res.* **2016**, *15*, 4532–4543. [CrossRef]
129. Bae, S.C.; Lee, Y.H. Association between anti-Porphyromonas gingivalis antibody, anti-citrullinated protein antibodies, and rheumatoid arthritis a meta-analysis. *Z. Für Rheumatol.* **2018**, *77*, 522–532. [CrossRef]
130. Bender, P.; Burgin, W.B.; Sculean, A.; Eick, S. Serum antibody levels against Porphyromonas gingivalis in patients with and without rheumatoid arthritis - a systematic review and meta-analysis. *Clin. Oral Investig.* **2017**, *21*, 33–42. [CrossRef]
131. Maresz, K.J.; Hellvard, A.; Sroka, A.; Adamowicz, K.; Bielecka, E.; Koziel, J.; Gawron, K.; Mizgalska, D.; Marcinska, K.A.; Benedyk, M.; et al. Porphyromonas gingivalis Facilitates the Development and Progression of Destructive Arthritis through Its Unique Bacterial Peptidylarginine Deiminase (PAD). *PLoS Pathog.* **2013**, *9*, e1003627. [CrossRef]
132. de Aquino, S.G.; Abdollahi-Roodsaz, S.; Koenders, M.I.; van de Loo, F.A.; Pruijn, G.J.; Marijnissen, R.J.; Walgreen, B.; Helsen, M.M.; van den Bersselaar, L.A.; de Molon, R.S.; et al. Periodontal pathogens directly promote autoimmune experimental arthritis by inducing a TLR2- and IL-1-driven Th17 response. *J. Immunol.* **2014**, *192*, 4103–4111. [CrossRef]
133. de Aquino, S.G.; Talbot, J.; Sônego, F.; Turato, W.M.; Grespan, R.; Avila-Campos, M.J.; Cunha, F.Q.; Cirelli, J.A. The aggravation of arthritis by periodontitis is dependent of IL-17 receptor a activation. *J. Clin. Periodontol.* **2017**, *44*, 881–891. [CrossRef]
134. Marchesan, J.T.; Gerow, E.A.; Schaff, R.; Taut, A.D.; Shin, S.Y.; Sugai, J.; Brand, D.; Burberry, A.; Jorns, J.; Lundy, S.K.; et al. Porphyromonas gingivalis oral infection exacerbates the development and severity of collagen-induced arthritis. *Arthritis Res. Ther.* **2013**, *15*, R186. [CrossRef]
135. Jung, H.; Jung, S.M.; Rim, Y.A.; Park, N.; Nam, Y.; Lee, J.; Park, S.H.; Ju, J.H. Arthritic role of Porphyromonas gingivalis in collagen-induced arthritis mice. *PLoS ONE* **2017**, *12*, e0188698. [CrossRef]
136. Chukkapalli, S.; Rivera-Kweh, M.; Gehlot, P.; Velsko, I.; Bhattacharyya, I.; Calise, S.J.; Satoh, M.; Chan, E.K.L.; Holoshitz, J.; Kesavalu, L. Periodontal bacterial colonization in synovial tissues exacerbates collagen-induced arthritis in B10.RIII mice. *Arthritis Res. Ther.* **2016**, *18*, 161. [CrossRef]
137. Sato, K.; Takahashi, N.; Kato, T.; Matsuda, Y.; Yokoji, M.; Yamada, M.; Nakajima, T.; Kondo, N.; Endo, N.; Yamamoto, R.; et al. Aggravation of collagen-induced arthritis by orally administered Porphyromonas gingivalis through modulation of the gut microbiota and gut immune system. *Sci. Rep.* **2017**, *7*, 6955. [CrossRef]
138. Yamakawa, M.; Ouhara, K.; Kajiya, M.; Munenaga, S.; Kittaka, M.; Yamasaki, S.; Takeda, K.; Takeshita, K.; Mizuno, N.; Fujita, T.; et al. Porphyromonas gingivalis infection exacerbates the onset of rheumatoid arthritis in SKG mice. *Clin. Exp. Immunol.* **2016**, *186*, 177–189. [CrossRef]
139. Sandal, I.; Karydis, A.; Luo, J.; Prislovsky, A.; Whittington, K.B.; Rosloniec, E.F.; Dong, C.; Novack, D.V.; Mydel, P.; Zheng, S.G.; et al. Bone loss and aggravated autoimmune arthritis in HLA-DR beta 1-bearing humanized mice following oral challenge with Porphyromonas gingivalis. *Arthritis Res. Ther.* **2016**, *18*, 249. [CrossRef]
140. Gully, N.; Bright, R.; Marino, V.; Marchant, C.; Cantley, M.; Haynes, D.; Butler, C.; Dashper, S.; Reynolds, E.; Bartold, M. Porphyromonas gingivalis Peptidylarginine Deiminase, a Key Contributor in the Pathogenesis of Experimental Periodontal Disease and Experimental Arthritis. *PLoS ONE* **2014**, *9*, e100838. [CrossRef]
141. Munenaga, S.; Ouhara, K.; Hamamoto, Y.; Kajiya, M.; Takeda, K.; Yamasaki, S.; Kawai, T.; Mizuno, N.; Fujita, T.; Sugiyama, E.; et al. The involvement of C5a in the progression of experimental arthritis with Porphyromonas gingivalis infection in SKG mice. *Arthritis Res. Ther.* **2018**, *20*, 247. [CrossRef]
142. Ebbers, M.; Lübcke, P.M.; Volzke, J.; Kriebel, K.; Hieke, C.; Engelmann, R.; Lang, H.; Kreikemeyer, B.; Müller-Hilke, B.; et al. Interplay between P. gingivalis, F. nucleatum and A. actinomycetemcomitans in murine alveolar bone loss, arthritis onset and progression. *Sci. Rep.* **2018**, *8*, 15129. [CrossRef]
143. Eriksson, K.; Lönnblom, E.; Tour, G.; Kats, A.; Mydel, P.; Georgsson, P.; Hultgren, C.; Kharlamova, N.; Norin, U.; Jönsson, J.; et al. Effects by periodontitis on pristane-induced arthritis in rats. *J. Transl. Med.* **2016**, *14*, 311. [CrossRef]
144. Courbon, G.; Rinaudo-Gaujous, M.; Blasco-Baque, V.; Auger, I.; Caire, R.; Mijola, L.; Vico, L.; Paul, S.; Marotte, H. Porphyromonas gingivalis experimentally induces periodontis and an anti-CCP2-associated arthritis in the rat. *Ann. Rheum. Dis.* **2019**, *78*, 594–599. [CrossRef]

145. Kinloch, A.J.; Alzabin, S.; Brintnell, W.; Wilson, E.; Barra, L.; Wegner, N.; Bell, D.A.; Cairns, E.; Venables, P.J. Immunization with Porphyromonas gingivalis enolase induces autoimmunity to mammalian alpha-enolase and arthritis in DR4-IE-transgenic mice. *Arthritis Rheum.* **2011**, *63*, 3818–3823. [CrossRef]
146. Mangat, P.; Wegner, N.; Venables, P.J.; Potempa, J. Bacterial and human peptidylarginine deiminases: Targets for inhibiting the autoimmune response in rheumatoid arthritis? *Arthritis Res. Ther.* **2010**, *12*, 209. [CrossRef]
147. Hayashi, H.; Morioka, M.; Ichimiya, S.; Yamato, K.; Hinode, D.; Nagata, A.; Nakamura, R. Participation of an arginyl residue of insulin chain B in the inhibition of hemagglutination by Porphyromonas gingivalis. *Oral Microbiol. Immunol.* **1993**, *8*, 386–389. [CrossRef]
148. Goulas, T.; Mizgalska, D.; Garcia-Ferrer, I.; Kantyka, T.; Guevara, T.; Szmigielski, B.; Sroka, A.; Millán, C.; Usón, I.; Veillard, F.; et al. Structure and mechanism of a bacterial host-protein citrullinating virulence factor, Porphyromonas gingivalis peptidylarginine deiminase. *Sci. Rep.* **2015**, *5*, 11969. [CrossRef]
149. Montgomery, A.B.; Kopec, J.; Shrestha, L.; Thezenas, M.L.; Burgess-Brown, N.A.; Fischer, R.; Yue, W.W.; Venables, P.J. Crystal structure of Porphyromonas gingivalis peptidylarginine deiminase: Implications for autoimmunity in rheumatoid arthritis. *Ann. Rheum. Dis.* **2016**, *75*, 1255–1261. [CrossRef]
150. Bereta, G.; Goulas, T.; Madej, M.; Bielecka, E.; Solà, M.; Potempa, J.; Gomis-Rüth, F.X. Structure, function, and inhibition of a genomic/clinical variant of Porphyromonas gingivalis peptidylarginine deiminase. *Protein Sci.* **2019**, *28*, 478–486. [CrossRef]
151. Gabarrini, G.; Heida, R.; Van Ieperen, N.; Curtis, M.A.; Van Winkelhoff, A.J.; Van Dijl, J.M. Dropping anchor: Attachment of peptidylarginine deiminase via A-LPS to secreted outer membrane vesicles of Porphyromonas gingivalis. *Sci. Rep.* **2018**, *8*, 8949. [CrossRef]
152. Gabarrini, G.; Medina, L.M.P.; Stobernack, T.; Prins, R.C.; Espina, M.D.T.; Kuipers, J.; Chlebowicz, M.A.; Rossen, J.W.A.; Van Winkelhoff, A.J.; Van Dijl, J.M. There's no place like OM: Vesicular sorting and secretion of the peptidylarginine deiminase of Porphyromonas gingivalis. *Virulence* **2018**, *9*, 456–464. [CrossRef]
153. Casiano-Colón, A.; Marquis, R.E. Role of the arginine deiminase system in protecting oral bacteria and an enzymatic basis for acid tolerance. *Appl. Environ. Microbiol.* **1988**, *54*, 1318–1324.
154. Niederman, R.; Brunkhorst, B.; Smith, S.; Weinreb, R.; Ryder, M. Ammonia as a potential mediator of adult human periodontal infection: Inhibition of neutrophil function. *Arch. Oral Biol.* **1990**, *35*, S205–S209. [CrossRef]
155. Shawcross, D.L.; Wright, G.A.K.; Stadlbauer, V.; Hodges, S.J.; Davies, N.A.; Wheeler-Jones, C.; Pitsillides, A.A.; Jalan, R. Ammonia impairs neutrophil phagocytic function in liver disease. *Hepatology* **2008**, *48*, 1202–1212. [CrossRef]
156. Wegner, N.; Wait, R.; Sroka, A.; Eick, S.; Nguyen, K.A.; Lundberg, K.; Kinloch, A.; Culshaw, S.; Potempa, J.; Venables, P.J. Peptidylarginine deiminase from Porphyromonas gingivalis citrullinates human fibrinogen and alpha-enolase: Implications for autoimmunity in rheumatoid arthritis. *Arthritis Rheum.* **2010**, *62*, 2662–2672. [CrossRef]
157. Li, S.; Yu, Y.; Yue, Y.; Liao, H.; Xie, W.; Thai, J.; Mikuls, T.R.; Thiele, G.M.; Duryee, M.J.; Sayles, H.; et al. Autoantibodies from Single Circulating Plasmablasts React With Citrullinated Antigens and Porphyromonas gingivalis in Rheumatoid Arthritis. *Arthritis Rheumatol.* **2016**, *68*, 614–626. [CrossRef]
158. Rodríguez, S.B.; Stitt, B.L.; Ash, D.E. Expression of Peptidylarginine Deiminase from Porphyromonas gingivalis in Escherichia coli: Enzyme Purification and Characterization. *Arch. Biochem. Biophys.* **2009**, *488*, 14–22. [CrossRef]
159. Sato, K.; Yukitake, H.; Narita, Y.; Shoji, M.; Naito, M.; Nakayama, K. Identification of Porphyromonas gingivalis proteins secreted by the Por secretion system. *FEMS Microbiol. Lett.* **2013**, *338*, 68–76. [CrossRef]
160. Shoji, M.; Sato, K.; Yukitake, H.; Kondo, Y.; Narita, Y.; Kadowaki, T.; Naito, M.; Nakayama, K. Por Secretion System-Dependent Secretion and Glycosylation of Porphyromonas gingivalis Hemin-Binding Protein 35. *PLoS ONE* **2011**, *6*, e21372. [CrossRef]
161. Konig, M.F.; Bingham, C.O., III; Andrade, F. PPAD is not targeted as a citrullinated protein in rheumatoid arthritis, but remains a candidate for inducing autoimmunity. *Ann. Rheum. Dis.* **2015**, *74*, e8. [CrossRef]
162. Quirke, A.-M.; Lundberg, K.; Potempa, J.; Mikuls, T.R.; Venables, P.J. PPAD remains a credible candidate for inducing autoimmunity in rheumatoid arthritis: Comment on the article by Konig et al. *Ann. Rheum. Dis.* **2014**, *74*, e7. [CrossRef]
163. Kobayashi, T.; Ito, S.; Kobayashi, D.; Shimada, A.; Narita, I.; Murasawa, A.; Nakazono, K.; Yoshie, H. Serum Immunoglobulin G Levels to Porphyromonas gingivalis Peptidylarginine Deiminase Affect Clinical Response

to Biological Disease-Modifying Antirheumatic Drug in Rheumatoid Arthritis. *PLoS ONE* **2016**, *11*, e0154182. [CrossRef]

164. Shimada, A.; Kobayashi, T.; Ito, S.; Okada, M.; Murasawa, A.; Nakazono, K.; Yoshie, H. Expression of anti-Porphyromonas gingivalis peptidylarginine deiminase immunoglobulin G and peptidylarginine deiminase-4 in patients with rheumatoid arthritis and periodontitis. *J. Periodontal Res.* **2016**, *51*, 103–111. [CrossRef]
165. Vossenaar, E.R.; Nijenhuis, S.; Helsen, M.M.A.; Van Der Heijden, A.; Senshu, T.; Berg, W.B.V.D.; Van Venrooij, W.J.; Joosten, L.A.B. Citrullination of synovial proteins in murine models of rheumatoid arthritis. *Arthritis Rheum.* **2003**, *48*, 2489–2500. [CrossRef]
166. Cantaert, T.; Teitsma, C.; Tak, P.P.; Baeten, D. Presence and Role of Anti-Citrullinated Protein Antibodies in Experimental Arthritis Models. *Arthritis Rheum.* **2013**, *65*, 939–948. [CrossRef]
167. Konig, M.F.; Darrah, E.; Andrade, F. Insights into the significance of peptidylarginine deiminase 4 and antibodies against citrullinated antigens in the absence of "true ACPAs" in an experimental model of arthritis: Comment on the article by Shelef et al. *Arthritis Rheumatol.* **2014**, *66*, 2642–2644. [CrossRef]
168. Shelef, M.A.; Sokolove, J.; Robinson, W.H.; Huttenlocher, A. Insights into the significance of peptidylarginine deiminase 4 and antibodies against citrullinated antigens in the absence of "true ACPAs" in an experimental model of arthritis: Comment on the article by Shelef et al Reply. *Arthritis Rheumatol.* **2014**, *66*, 2644–2645. [CrossRef]
169. Vossenaar, E.R.; Van Boekel, M.A.M.; Van Venrooij, W.J.; López-Hoyoz, M.; Merino, J.; Merino, R.; Joosten, L.A.B. Absence of citrulline-specific autoantibodies in animal models of autoimmunity. *Arthritis Rheum.* **2004**, *50*, 2370–2372. [CrossRef]
170. Kingler, R. Untersuchungen über menschliche Aktinomycose. *Zent. Bakteriol* **1912**, *62*, 191–200.
171. Potts, T.V.; Zambon, J.J.; Genco, R.J. Reassignment of Actinobacillus-Actinomycetemcomitans to the Genus Hemophilus as Haemophilus-Actinomycetemcomitans Comb-Nov. *Int. J. Syst. Bacteriol.* **1985**, *35*, 337–341. [CrossRef]
172. Norskov-Lauritsen, N.; Kilian, M. Reclassification of *Actinobacillus actinomycetemcomitans*, Haemophilus aphrophilus, Haemophilus paraphrophilus and Haemophilus segnis as *Aggregatibacter actinomycetemcomitans* gen. nov., comb. nov., *Aggregatibacter aphrophilus* comb. nov. and Aggregatibacter segnis comb. nov., and emended description of Aggregatibacter aphrophilus to include V factor-dependent and V factor-independent isolates. *Int. J. Syst. Evol. Microbiol.* **2006**, *56*, 2135–2146.
173. Heinrich, S.; Pulverer, G. Zur Ätiologie und Mikrobiologie der Aktinomykose III. Die pathogene Bedeutung des Actinobacillus actinomycetem-comitans unter den "Begleitbakterien" des Actinomyces israeli. *Zent. Bakteriol* **1959**, *176*, 91–101.
174. Colebrook, L. The mycelial and other micro-organisms associated with human actinomycosis. *Br. J. Exp. Pathol.* **1920**, *1*, 197–212.
175. King, E.O.; Tatum, H.W. Actinobacillus Actinomycetemcomitans and Hemophilus Aphrophilus. *J. Infect. Dis.* **1962**, *111*, 85–94. [CrossRef]
176. Mitchell, R.G.; Gillespie, W.A. Bacterial endocarditis due to an actinobacillus. *J. Clin. Pathol.* **1964**, *17*, 511–512. [CrossRef]
177. Page, M.I.; King, E.O. Infection Due to Actinobacillus Actinomycetemcomitans and Haemophilus Aphrophilus. *N. Engl. J. Med.* **1966**, *275*, 181–188. [CrossRef]
178. Geraci, J.E.; Wilson, W.R. Symposium on infective endocarditis. III. Endocarditis due to gram-negative bacteria. Report of 56 cases. *Mayo Clin. Proc.* **1982**, *57*, 145–148.
179. Kaplan, A.H.; Weber, D.J.; Oddone, E.Z.; Perfect, J.R. Infection Due to Actinobacillus-Actinomycetemcomitans - 15 Cases and Review. *Rev. Infect. Dis.* **1989**, *11*, 46–63. [CrossRef]
180. van Winkelhoff, A.J.; Slots, J. Actinobacillus actinomycetemcomitans and Porphyromonas gingivalis in nonoral infections. *Periodontol. 2000.* **1999**, *20*, 122–135. [CrossRef]
181. Tanner, A.C.R.; Haffer, C.; Bratthall, G.T.; Visconti, R.A.; Socransky, S.S. A study of the bacteria associated with advancing periodontitis in man. *J. Clin. Periodontol.* **1979**, *6*, 278–307. [CrossRef]
182. Slots, J.; Reynolds, H.S.; Genco, R.J. Actinobacillus actinomycetemcomitans in Human Periodontal Disease: A Cross-Sectional Microbiological Investigation. *Infect. Immun.* **1980**, *29*, 1013–1020.

183. Zambon, J.J.; Christersson, L.A.; Slots, J. Actinobacillus actinomycetemcomitans in human periodontal disease. Prevalence in patient groups and distribution of biotypes and serotypes within families. *J. Periodontol.* **1983**, *54*, 707–711. [CrossRef]
184. Zambon, J.J.; Slots, J.; Genco, R.J. Serology of oral Actinobacillus actinomycetemcomitans and serotype distribution in human periodontal disease. *Infect. Immun.* **1983**, *41*, 19–27.
185. Slots, J.; Bragd, L.; Wikström, M.; Dahlén, G. The occurrence of Actinobacillus actinomycetemcomitans, Bacteroides gingivalis and Bacteroides intermedius in destructive periodontal disease in adults. *J. Clin. Periodontol.* **1986**, *13*, 570–577. [CrossRef]
186. Johansson, A. Aggregatibacter actinomycetemcomitans leukotoxin: A powerful tool with capacity to cause imbalance in the host inflammatory response. *Toxins (Basel)* **2011**, *3*, 242–259. [CrossRef]
187. Claesson, R.; Höglund-Åberg, C.; Haubek, D.; Johansson, A. Age-related prevalence and characteristics of Aggregatibacter actinomycetemcomitans in periodontitis patients living in Sweden. *J. Oral Microbiol.* **2017**, *9*, 1334504. [CrossRef]
188. Zambon, J.J. Actinobacillus actinomycetemcomitans in human periodontal disease. *J. Clin. Periodontol.* **1985**, *12*, 1–20. [CrossRef]
189. Chen, C.; Wang, T.; Chen, W. Occurrence of Aggregatibacter actinomycetemcomitans serotypes in subgingival plaque from United States subjects. *Mol. Oral Microbiol.* **2010**, *25*, 207–214. [CrossRef]
190. Pahumunto, N.; Ruangsri, P.; Wongsuwanlert, M.; Piwat, S.; Dahlén, G.; Teanpaisan, R. Aggregatibacter actinomycetemcomitans serotypes and DGGE subtypes in Thai adults with chronic periodontitis. *Arch. Oral Biol.* **2015**, *60*, 1789–1796. [CrossRef]
191. Kim, T.S.; Frank, P.; Eickholz, P.; Eick, S.; Kim, C.K. Serotypes of Aggregatibacter actinomycetemcomitans in patients with different ethnic backgrounds. *J. Periodontol.* **2009**, *80*, 2020–2027. [CrossRef]
192. Mínguez, M.; Pousa, X.; Herrera, D.; Blasi, A.; Sánchez, M.C.; León, R.; Sanz, M. Characterization and serotype distribution of Aggregatibacter actinomycetemcomitans isolated from a population of periodontitis patients in Spain. *Arch. Oral Biol.* **2014**, *59*, 1359–1367. [CrossRef]
193. Yang, H.W.; Huang, Y.F.; Chan, Y.; Chou, M.Y. Relationship of Actinobacillus actinomycetemcomitans serotypes to periodontal condition: Prevalence and proportions in subgingival plaque. *Eur. J. Oral Sci.* **2005**, *113*, 28–33. [CrossRef]
194. Arenas Rodrigues, V.A.; de Avila, E.D.; Nakano, V.; Avila-Campos, M.J. Qualitative, quantitative and genotypic evaluation of Aggregatibacter actinomycetemcomitans and Fusobacterium nucleatum isolated from individuals with different periodontal clinical conditions. *Anaerobe* **2018**, *52*, 50–58. [CrossRef]
195. Åberg, C.H.; Haubek, D.; Kwamin, F.; Johansson, A.; Claesson, R. Leukotoxic Activity of Aggregatibacter actinomycetemcomitans and Periodontal Attachment Loss. *PLoS ONE* **2014**, *9*, e104095.
196. Aberg, C.H.; Kelk, P.; Johansson, A. Aggregatibacter actinomycetemcomitans: Virulence of its leukotoxin and association with aggressive periodontitis. *Virulence* **2015**, *6*, 188–195. [CrossRef]
197. Linhartová, I.; Bumba, L.; Mašín, J.; Basler, M.; Osička, R.; Kamanová, J.; Procházková, K.; Adkins, I.; Hejnová-Holubová, J.; Sadílková, L.; et al. RTX proteins: A highly diverse family secreted by a common mechanism. *FEMS Microbiol. Rev.* **2010**, *34*, 1076–1112. [CrossRef]
198. Reinholdt, J.; Poulsen, K.; Brinkmann, C.R.; Hoffmann, S.V.; Stapulionis, R.; Enghild, J.J.; Jensen, U.B.; Boesen, T.; Vorup-Jensen, T. Monodisperse and LPS-free Aggregatibacter actinomycetemcomitans leukotoxin: Interactions with human beta2 integrins and erythrocytes. *Biochim. Biophys. Acta* **2013**, *1834*, 546–558. [CrossRef]
199. Brogan, J.M.; Lally, E.T.; Poulsen, K.; Kilian, M.; DeMuth, D.R. Regulation of Actinobacillus actinomycetemcomitans leukotoxin expression: Analysis of the promoter regions of leukotoxic and minimally leukotoxic strains. *Infect. Immun.* **1994**, *62*, 501–508.
200. Zambon, J.J.; Haraszthy, V.I.; Hariharan, G.; Lally, E.T.; DeMuth, D.R. The Microbiology of early-onset periodontitis: Association of highly toxic Actinobacillus actinomycetemcomitans strains with localized juvenile periodontitis. *J. Periodontol.* **1996**, *67*, 282–290. [CrossRef]
201. Sampathkumar, V.; Velusamy, S.K.; Godboley, D.; Fine, D.H. Increased leukotoxin production: Characterization of 100 base pairs within the 530 base pair leukotoxin promoter region of Aggregatibacter actinomycetemcomitans. *Sci. Rep.* **2017**, *7*, 1887. [CrossRef]

202. Burgess, D.; Huang, H.; Harrison, P.; Aukhil, I.; Shaddox, L. Aggregatibacter actinomycetemcomitans in African Americans with Localized Aggressive Periodontitis. *JDR Clin. Transl. Res.* **2017**, *2*, 249–257. [CrossRef]
203. Oscarsson, J.; Claesson, R.; Lindholm, M.; Höglund Åberg, C.; Johansson, A. Tools of Aggregatibacter actinomycetemcomitans to Evade the Host Response. *J. Clin. Med.* **2019**, *8*, 1079. [CrossRef]
204. Harvey, G.P.; Fitzsimmons, T.R.; Dhamarpatni, A.A.; Marchant, C.; Haynes, D.R.; Bartold, P.M. Expression of peptidylarginine deiminase-2 and -4, citrullinated proteins and anti-citrullinated protein antibodies in human gingiva. *J. Periodontal Res.* **2013**, *48*, 252–261. [CrossRef]
205. Nesse, W.; Westra, J.; van der Wal, J.E.; Abbas, F.; Nicholas, A.P.; Vissink, A.; Brouwer, E. The periodontium of periodontitis patients contains citrullinated proteins which may play a role in ACPA (anti-citrullinated protein antibody) formation. *J. Clin. Periodontol.* **2012**, *39*, 599–607. [CrossRef]
206. Malinin, T.I.; Pekin, T.J.; Zvaifler, N.J. Cytology of Synovial Fluid in Rheumatoid Arthritis. *Am. J. Clin. Pathol.* **1967**, *47*, 203–208. [CrossRef]
207. Darrah, E.; Rosen, A.; Giles, J.T.; Andrade, F. Peptidylarginine deiminase 2, 3 and 4 have distinct specificities against cellular substrates: Novel insights into autoantigen selection in rheumatoid arthritis. *Ann. Rheum. Dis.* **2012**, *71*, 92–98. [CrossRef]
208. Delima, A.J.; Van Dyke, T.E. Origin and function of the cellular components in gingival crevice fluid. *Periodontol 2000* **2003**, *31*, 55–76. [CrossRef]
209. Konig, M.F.; Andrade, F. A critical reappraisal of neutrophil extracellular traps (NETs) and NETosis mimics based on differential requirements for protein citrullination. *Front. Immunol.* **2016**, *7*, 461. [CrossRef]
210. Volkov, M.; Dekkers, J.; Loos, B.G.; Bizzarro, S.; Huizinga, T.W.J.; Praetorius, H.A.; Toes, R.E.M.; Van Der Woude, D. Comment on Aggregatibacter actinomycetemcomitans—Induced hypercitrullination links periodontal infection to autoimmunity in rheumatoid arthritis. *Sci. Transl. Med.* **2018**, *10*, eaan8349. [CrossRef]
211. Mukherjee, A.; Jantsch, V.; Khan, R.; Hartung, W.; Fischer, R.; Jantsch, J.; Ehrenstein, B.; Konig, M.F.; Andrade, F. Rheumatoid Arthritis-Associated Autoimmunity Due to Aggregatibacter actinomycetemcomitans and Its Resolution with Antibiotic Therapy. *Front. Immunol.* **2018**, *9*, 2352. [CrossRef]
212. Konig, M.F.; Giles, J.T.; Teles, R.P.; Moutsopoulos, N.M.; Andrade, F. Response to comment on "Aggregatibacter actinomycetemcomitans–induced hypercitrullination links periodontal infection to autoimmunity in rheumatoid arthritis". *Sci. Transl. Med.* **2018**, *10*, eaao3031. [CrossRef]
213. Queiroz-Junior, C.M.; Madeira, M.F.M.; Coelho, F.M.; Oliveira, C.R.; Cândido, L.C.M.; Garlet, G.P.; Teixeira, M.M.; Souza, D.D.G.; Da Silva, T.A.; Queiroz-Junior, C.M. Experimental arthritis exacerbates Aggregatibacter actinomycetemcomitans-induced periodontitis in mice. *J. Clin. Periodontol.* **2012**, *39*, 608–616. [CrossRef]
214. Taichman, N.S.; Shenker, B.J.; Tsai, C.C.; Glickman, L.T.; Baehni, P.C.; Stevens, R.; Hammond, B.F. Cytopathic effects of Actinobacillus actinomycetemcomitans on monkey blood leukocytes. *J. Periodontal Res.* **1984**, *19*, 133–145. [CrossRef]
215. Rantapää-Dahlqvist, S.; De Jong, B.A.W.; Berglin, E.; Hallmans, G.; Wadell, G.; Stenlund, H.; Sundin, U.; Van Venrooij, W.J. Antibodies against cyclic citrullinated peptide and IgA rheumatoid factor predict the development of rheumatoid arthritis. *Arthritis Rheum.* **2003**, *48*, 2741–2749. [CrossRef]
216. Nielen, M.M.J.; Van Schaardenburg, D.; Reesink, H.W.; Van De Stadt, R.J.; Van Der Horst-Bruinsma, I.E.; De Koning, M.H.M.T.; Habibuw, M.R.; Vandenbroucke, J.P.; Dijkmans, B.A.C.; Van Der Horst-Bruinsma, I.E. Specific autoantibodies precede the symptoms of rheumatoid arthritis: A study of serial measurements in blood donors. *Arthritis Rheum.* **2004**, *50*, 380–386. [CrossRef]
217. Makrygiannakis, D.; Klint, E.A.; Lundberg, I.E.; Lofberg, R.; Ulfgren, A.K.; Klareskog, L.; Catrina, A.I. Citrullination is an inflammation-dependent process. *Ann. Rheum. Dis.* **2006**, *65*, 1219–1222. [CrossRef]
218. Ramseier, C.A.; Anerud, A.; Dulac, M.; Lulic, M.; Cullinan, M.P.; Seymour, G.J.; Faddy, M.J.; Bürgin, W.; Schätzle, M.; Lang, N.P. Natural history of periodontitis: Disease progression and tooth loss over 40 years. *J. Clin. Periodontol.* **2017**, *44*, 1182–1191. [CrossRef]
219. Dal, P.M.; van der Goot, F.G. Pore-forming toxins: Ancient, but never really out of fashion. *Nat. Rev. Microbiol.* **2016**, *14*, 77–92.
220. Samuels, J.; Ng, Y.-S.; Coupillaud, C.; Paget, D.; Meffre, E. Impaired early B cell tolerance in patients with rheumatoid arthritis. *J. Exp. Med.* **2005**, *201*, 1659–1667. [CrossRef]

221. Samuels, J.; Ng, Y.S.; Coupillaud, C.; Paget, D.; Meffre, E. Human B cell tolerance and its failure in rheumatoid arthritis. *Ann. N. Y. Acad. Sci.* **2005**, *1062*, 116–126. [CrossRef]
222. Meffre, E.; Wardemann, H. B-cell tolerance checkpoints in health and autoimmunity. *Curr. Opin. Immunol.* **2008**, *20*, 632–638. [CrossRef]
223. Menard, L.; Samuels, J.; Ng, Y.S.; Meffre, E. Inflammation-independent defective early B cell tolerance checkpoints in rheumatoid arthritis. *Arthritis Rheum.* **2011**, *63*, 1237–1245. [CrossRef]
224. Borsotti, C.; Danzl, N.M.; Nauman, G.; Hölzl, M.A.; French, C.; Chavez, E.; Khosravi-Maharlooei, M.; Glauzy, S.; Delmotte, F.R.; Meffre, E.; et al. HSC extrinsic sex-related and intrinsic autoimmune disease–related human B-cell variation is recapitulated in humanized mice. *Blood Adv.* **2017**, *1*, 2007–2018. [CrossRef]
225. Marotte, H. Determining the Right Time for the Right Treatment—Application to Preclinical Rheumatoid Arthritis. *JAMA Netw. Open* **2019**, *2*, e195358. [CrossRef]
226. Kaur, S.; Bright, R.; Proudman, S.M.; Bartold, P.M. Does periodontal treatment influence clinical and biochemical measures for rheumatoid arthritis? A systematic review and meta-analysis. *Semin. Arthritis Rheum.* **2014**, *44*, 113–122. [CrossRef]
227. Monsarrat, P.; De Grado, G.F.; Constantin, A.; Willmann, C.; Nabet, C.; Sixou, M.; Cantagrel, A.; Barnetche, T.; Mehsen-Cetre, N.; Schaeverbeke, T.; et al. The effect of periodontal treatment on patients with rheumatoid arthritis: The ESPERA randomised controlled trial. *Jt. Bone Spine* **2019**, in press. [CrossRef]
228. Bright, R.; Thiele, G.M.; Manavis, J.; Mikuls, T.R.; Payne, J.B.; Bartold, P.M. Gingival tissue, an extrasynovial source of malondialdehyde-acetaldehyde adducts, citrullinated and carbamylated proteins. *J. Periodontal Res.* **2018**, *53*, 139–143. [CrossRef]
229. Darrah, E.; Andrade, F. Editorial: citrullination, and carbamylation, and malondialdehyde-acetaldehyde! Oh my! Entering the forest of autoantigen modifications in rheumatoid arthritis. *Arthritis Rheumatol.* **2015**, *67*, 604–608. [CrossRef]
230. Henle, J. *Von den Miasmen und Kontagien: Und Von den Miasmatisch-Kontagiösen Krankheiten (1840)*; Verlag von J. A. Barth: Leipzig, Germany, 1910.
231. Koch, R. Über Bakteriologische Forschung. In *Verhandlungen des X*; Internationalen Medicinischen Congresses: Berlin, Germany, 1890; Volume 1.
232. Rivers, T.M. Viruses and Koch's postulates. *J. Bacteriol.* **1937**, *33*, 1–12.
233. Correa, M.G.; Sacchetti, S.B.; Ribeiro, F.V.; Pimentel, S.P.; Casarin, R.C.V.; Cirano, F.R.; Casati, M.Z. Periodontitis increases rheumatic factor serum levels and citrullinated proteins in gingival tissues and alter cytokine balance in arthritic rats. *PLoS ONE* **2017**, *12*, e0174442. [CrossRef]

15

Porphyromonas gingivalis Mfa1 Induces Chemokine and Cell Adhesion Molecules in Mouse Gingival Fibroblasts via Toll-Like Receptors

Yuhei Takayanagi [1], Takeshi Kikuchi [1,*], Yoshiaki Hasegawa [2], Yoshikazu Naiki [2], Hisashi Goto [1], Kousuke Okada [1], Iichiro Okabe [1], Yosuke Kamiya [1], Yuki Suzuki [1], Noritaka Sawada [1], Teppei Okabe [1], Yuki Suzuki [1], Shun Kondo [1], Tasuku Ohno [1], Jun-Ichiro Hayashi [1] and Akio Mitani [1]

1 Department of Periodontology, School of Dentistry, Aichi Gakuin University, 2-11 Suemoridori, Chikusaku, Nagoya, Aichi 464-8651, Japan; ag173d14@dpc.agu.ac.jp (Y.T.); hisashi@dpc.agu.ac.jp (H.G.); okakou@dpc.agu.ac.jp (K.O.); iichiro@dpc.agu.ac.jp (I.O.); k-yosuke@dpc.agu.ac.jp (Y.K.); yukip@dpc.agu.ac.jp (Y.S); ag173d11@dpc.agu.ac.jp (N.S.); ag183d03@dpc.agu.ac.jp (T.O.); ag193d11@dpc.agu.ac.jp (Y.S.); ag193d07@dpc.agu.ac.jp (S.K.); tasuku@dpc.agu.ac.jp (T.O.); jun1row@dpc.agu.ac.jp (J.-I.H.); minita@dpc.agu.ac.jp (A.M.)

2 Department of Microbiology, School of Dentistry, Aichi Gakuin University, 1-100 Kusumoto-cho, Chikusaku, Nagoya, Aichi 464-8651, Japan; yhase@dpc.agu.ac.jp (Y.H.); naikiy@dpc.agu.ac.jp (Y.N.)

* Correspondence: tkikuchi@dpc.agu.ac.jp

Abstract: *Porphyromonas gingivalis* Mfa1 fimbriae are thought to act as adhesion factors and to direct periodontal tissue destruction but their immunomodulatory actions are poorly understood. Here, we investigated the effect of Mfa1 stimulation on the immune and metabolic mechanisms of gingival fibroblasts from periodontal connective tissue. We also determined the role of Toll-like receptor (TLR) 2 and TLR4 in Mfa1 recognition. Mfa1 increased the expression of genes encoding chemokine (C-X-C motif) ligand (CXCL) 1, CXCL3, intercellular adhesion molecule (ICAM) 1 and Selectin endothelium (E) in gingival fibroblasts, but did not have a significant effect on genes that regulate metabolism. Mfa1-stimulated up-regulation of genes was significantly suppressed in *Tlr4* siRNA-transfected cells compared with that in control siRNA-transfected cells, which indicates that recognition by TLR4 is essential for immunomodulation by Mfa1. Additionally, suppression of *Tlr2* expression partially attenuated the stimulatory effect of Mfa1. Overall, these results help explain the involvement of *P. gingivalis* Mfa1 fimbriae in the progression of periodontal disease.

Keywords: *Porphyromonas gingivalis*; Mfa1; Toll-like receptors; gingival fibroblast

1. Introduction

Periodontitis is a chronic inflammatory disease caused by multiple periodontal pathogenic bacterial species [1]. Socransky et al. indicated that three bacteria, *Porphyromonas gingivalis*, *Tannerella forsythia*, and *Treponema denticola*, are the main cause of the onset and progression of periodontitis and they suggested that these three species be called "red complexes" [2].

Among the three species, *P. gingivalis* is the major pathogen associated with periodontitis. Riviere et al. found that *P. gingivalis* was more prevalent at diseased sites than at healthy sites in diseased subjects [3]. The number of *P. gingivalis* in plaque samples was associated with the plaque score and clinical attachment level [4]. From the perspective of oral flora, *P. gingivalis* is considered to act as a keystone pathogen that creates a dysbiosis between the host and the dental biofilm. This altered oral commensal microbiota is responsible for initiating pathological bone loss [5]. *P. gingivalis* expresses a number of potential virulence factors, including lipopolysaccharides, gingipines, and fimbriae [6].

Fimbriae are filamentous proteinaceous appendages on the surface of *P. gingivalis* bacteria that play a pivotal role in colonization through association with other bacteria and host tissues [7,8]. *P. gingivalis* ATCC strain 33,277 has fimbriae consisting of either FimA (*fimA* gene product) or Mfa1 (*mfa1* gene product), with apparent molecular masses of approximately 38 and 75 kDa, respectively [9].

Mfa1, encoded by the *mfa1* gene, is a structural subunit of a protein complex whose length varies from 60 to 500 nm [10]. In addition to the primary Mfa1 protein, mature fimbriae also have affiliated Mfa2–5 proteins. Mfa2 plays an anchor role, while Mfa3 can bind with Mfa1/2/4/5 in vitro to connect with other fimbrial subunits [11]. Recent data indicate that the C-terminal domain of Mfa1, rather than Mfa3, affects the aggregation and maturation of downstream fimbrial proteins [12].

Several studies have demonstrated different roles for FimA and Mfa1 fimbriae. FimA fimbriae act as an adhesive that mediates periodontal tissue colonization and host cell invasion [8,13,14]. They also induce inflammatory processes in periodontal tissues through several mechanisms [15–17]. FimA fimbriae promote early biofilm formation in a single species of *P. gingivalis*, whereas Mfa1 plays an inhibitory role in the formation of a homotypic biofilm in *P. gingivalis* [18]. However, although there are few reports on the host immune response to Mfa1 fimbriae, an Mfa1-deficient strain causes almost no alveolar bone resorption in a mouse model of oral infection [19].

The present study aimed to examine the effect of *P. gingivalis* Mfa1 stimulation on the immune and metabolic mechanisms of mouse gingival fibroblasts (MGFs) and to examine the effects of Toll-like receptor (TLR) 2 and TLR4 knock down on *P. gingivalis* Mfa1-stimulated MGFs. Our results show that Mfa1 fimbriae had a large effect on immunomodulation exerted by gingival fibroblasts, but did not have a significant effect on metabolic regulation. Our results also indicate that recognition of Mfa1 by TLR4 on MGFs is essential for the expression of genes related to cell migration and cell adhesion. Overall, these results help to explain how *P. gingivalis* Mfa1 fimbriae are involved in the progression of periodontal disease.

2. Materials and Methods

2.1. Cell Culture

MGFs were isolated from healthy gingival tissue from the palate of BALB/c mice which were purchased from CLEA Japan, Inc. (Tokyo, Japan). The MGFs were cultured in Minimum Essential Medium α (Thermo Fisher Scientific, Wilmington, DE, USA) containing 10% fetal bovine serum (Hyclone Laboratories Inc, Logan, UT, USA), 100 U/mL penicillin, and 100 μg/mL streptomycin at 37 °C in a CO_2 incubator. When the cells reached confluency, they were separated by treatment with 0.25% trypsin-EDTA (Thermo Fisher Scientific) and collected by centrifugation. This study was approved by the Institutional Animal Care and Use Committees of Aichi Gakuin University (AGUD438; approved date 31 March 2019) and all animal experiments were conducted following the national guidelines and the relevant national laws on the protection of animals. Ultrapure lipopolysaccharide from *P. gingivalis* was purchased for experiments (InvivoGen, San Diego, CA, USA).

2.2. Purification of Mfa1 Fimbriae

In this study, we used *P. gingivalis* mutant strains derived from ATCC 33,277. Mfa1 fimbriae were purified from JI-1, in which *fimA* was deleted, as described previously [20,21]. Mfa1 fimbriae were also purified from *mfa5* mutant FMFA5, in which *mfa5* was disrupted by *ermF-B*, and genetic complementation strain FMFA5C, as described previously [21,22]. Briefly, *P. gingivalis* cells were collected from 2 L of culture, suspended in 40 mL of 20 mM Tris/HCl buffer at pH 8.0, supplemented with protease inhibitors (1 mM phenylmethylsulfonyl fluoride and 1 mM Nα-p-tosyl-L-lysine chloromethyl ketone). The cells were disrupted by a French press. Unbroken cells were removed by centrifugation. The supernatant was subjected to precipitation at 50% ammonium sulfate saturation.

The precipitate was dialyzed with 20 mM Tris/HCl buffer at pH 8.0, and then applied to DEAE Sepharose Fast Flow chromatography (GE Healthcare Bio-Sciences AB, Uppsala, Sweden) with 50 mL of bed volume. After washing thoroughly with the buffer, sample was fractionated by a linear gradient elution with 400 mL of NaCl (0 to 0.3 M) in the buffer. Purity and identity were verified by sodium dodecyl sulfate-polyacrylamide gel electrophoresis (Bio-Rad Laboratories, Hercules, CA, USA) and transmission electron microscopy. Details are described in the Supplementary Material.

2.3. RT2 Profiler PCR Array Analysis

MGF (1×10^6 cells/dish) were seeded onto 60-mm dishes. When the cells reached confluency, they were incubated for 2 hours in the presence or absence of 1 μg/mL Mfa1, FMFA5, FMFA5C, FimA, or LPS of *P. gingivalis*. Total RNA was then collected. Complementary deoxyribonucleic acid (cDNA) was synthesized using the RT^2 First Strand Kit (Qiagen, Germantown, MD, USA) according to the manufacturer's instructions and then applied to the Mouse Antibacterial Response RT^2Profile PCR Array (Qiagen) and the Mouse Extracellular Matrix & Adhesion Molecules RT^2Profile PCR Array (Qiagen). Amplification was performed using the RT^2 SYBR Green/ROX qPCR master mix (Qiagen) and the StepOnePlus™ Real-time PCR system (Thermo Fisher Scientific) with associated software (version 2.3; Thermo Fisher Scientific). CT values were transferred to an Excel file to build a table of CT values, which was then uploaded onto the data analysis web portal at http://www.qiagen.com/geneglobe.

2.4. Real-Time PCR

MGFs (1×10^6 cells/dish) were seeded onto 60-mm dishes. When the cells reached confluency, they were incubated for 2 hours in the presence or absence of 1 μg/mL JI-1, FMFA5, FMFA5C, FimA or LPS of *P. gingivalis*. Total RNA was then extracted with a Nucleospin RNA kit (Macherey-Nagel Inc., Bethlehem, PA, USA) according to the manufacturer's instructions, and purity and concentration were assessed by calculating the A230/A260 and A260/A280 ratios using a NanoDrop Lite (Thermo Fisher Scientific). To quantify mRNA, quantitative PCR was performed using the TaqMan gene expression assay (Thermo Fisher Scientific) for mouse *Cxcl1* (Mm04207460_m1), *Cxcl3* (Mm01701838), *Icam1* (Mm00516023_m1), *Sele* (Mm00441278_m1), *Tlr2* (Mm00442346_m1) and *Tlr4* (Mm00445273_m1) with the TaqMan Universal PCR Master Mix (Thermo Fisher Scientific). mRNA levels were normalized to the level of eukaryotic 18S rRNA (Hs99999901_s1). Quantitative PCR was performed using the StepOnePlus Real-Time System. PCR conditions were 10 minutes at 95 °C, followed by 40 cycles of 15 seconds at 95 °C and 1 minute at 60 °C. The relative amounts of target mRNAs were determined by subtracting the cycle threshold (CT) value for 18S rRNA from that for the gene (ΔCT). Then, the ΔCT value for the control group was subtracted from that for the experimental group (ΔΔCT). The results are expressed as the fold change (2-ΔΔCT) between the mRNA levels of control and experimental groups, where ΔΔCT was calculated as follows: ((CT for the target mRNA – CT for 18S rRNA) for the experimental group)–((CT for the target mRNA – CT for 18S rRNA) for the control group).

2.5. siRNA Transfection

MGFs were transfected with siRNA targeting TLR2 and TLR4 (Silencer Select Pre-designed siRNAs, Ambion, Austin, TX, USA) or non-targeting control siRNA (Ambion) using Lipofectamine RNAiMAX (Thermo Fisher Scientific) according to the manufacturer's protocol. Twenty-four hours after transfection, cells were stimulated with 1 μg/mL Mfa1, FMFA5, FMFA5C, FimA or LPS of *P. gingivalis* for 2 hours. The cells were then collected and TLR2 and TLR4 protein levels were determined by flow cytometry. Similarly, gene expression levels were determined by Real-Time PCR.

2.6. Flow Cytometry

MGFs (1×10^6 cells in 100 μL) were incubated with anti-mouse CD282 (TLR2) phycoerythrin (PE) (BioLegend, San Diego, CA, USA, Cat: 148604), anti-mouse CD284 (TLR4) phycoerythrin (PE) (BioLegend, Cat: 117605), or isotype control antibody phycoerythrin (PE) (BioLegend, Cat: 400508) and analyzed by flow cytometry using a MACSQuant analyzer and MACSQuantify software version 2.4 (Miltenyi Biotec, Tokyo, Japan).

2.7. Statistical Analysis

Data were analyzed using PASW Statistics software (version 18.0; SPSS Japan, Tokyo, Japan). Differences among groups were examined by one-factor analysis of variance (ANOVA) and Bonferroni's multiple comparison test. Comparisons of two independent groups were performed using Student's t-test. Data are expressed as the mean ± standard deviation (SD). Significance was accepted at $p < 0.05$.

3. Results

3.1. Analysis of Antibacterial Response-Associated Genes in Gingival Fibroblasts to Various Fimbriae

A mouse antibacterial response PCR array was used to investigate differences in the expression of 84 genes involved in bacteria-cell interactions. Figure 1 shows the fold changes in expression between control and 1 µg/mL various fimbriae or *P. gingivalis* LPS after stimulation for 2 hours. Among the 84 genes, *Cxcl1* and *Cxcl3* were upregulated in common by 4-fold in *JI-1, FMFA5* or *FMFA5C*-stimulated cells compared with non-stimulated cells (Figure 1A–C). Other genes that were elevated include *Nfkbia, Jun, Ccl5, Tlr6, Nod2* in *JI-1* stimulated cells, Nfkbia, Jun, Irf5, Birc3 in FMFA5-stimulated cells, and Hsp90aa1, Nfkb1, Nfkbia, Jun, Nod1, Slpi, Tirap, Rela, Ccl5, Tlr2, Irf5, Irf7, Nod2, Birc3, Lcn2 in FMFA5C-stimulated cells. Many genes (*Tnfrsf1a, Mapk1, Tollip, Irak1, Fadd, Map3k7, Map2k4, Slpi, Ripk2, Il18, Rela, Irak3, Card6, Camp, Irf5, Birc3, Slc11a1, Tlr9, Casp1, Crp*), including *Cxcl3* were up-regulated in FimA-stimulated cells compared with non-stimulated cells (Figure 1D). *P. gingivalis* LPS stimulation changed several genes expression (*Ccl5, Tlr6, Irf5, Nod2, Casp1*) compared with non-stimulated cells (Figure 1E).

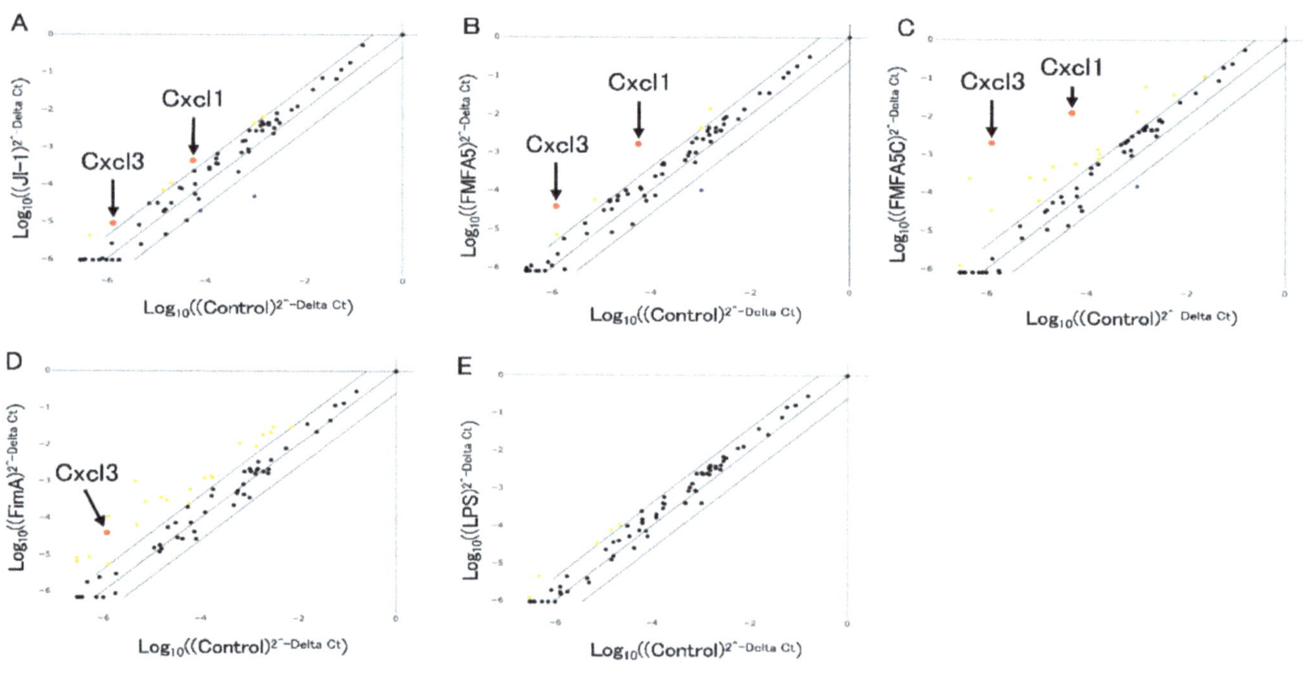

Figure 1. Analysis of antibacterial response-associated genes in mouse gingival fibroblasts in response to Mfa1, FimA, or *Porphyromonas gingivalis* LPS. Graphs show the fold changes of gene expression in cells stimulated with JI-1 (**A**), FMFA5 (**B**), FMFA5C (**C**), FimA (**D**), and LPS (**E**) compared with non-stimulated cells. *Cxcl1* and *Cxcl3* were up-regulated over 4-fold in JI-1, FMFA5 or FMFA5C-stimulated cells.

3.2. Confirmation of PCR Array Data for Selected Antibacterial Response-Associated Genes by Quantitative Real Time-PCR

To validate the PCR array data, Real Time-PCR showed that JI-1 stimulation increased the gene expression of the cell migration factors, *Cxcl1* and *Cxcl3*, compared with FimA stimulation (Figure 2). Furthermore, the highest increase in gene expression was observed with FMFA5 stimulation (Figure 2).

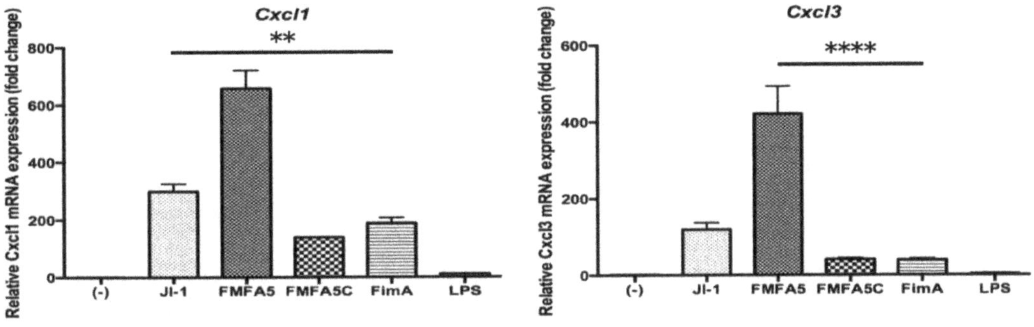

Figure 2. Mfa1 induces *Cxcl1* and *Cxcl3* in mouse gingival fibroblasts. Mouse gingival fibroblasts (MGFs) were cultured for 2 hours in the presence or absence of 1 μg/mL JI-1, FMFA5, FMFA5C, FimA, or LPS of *P. gingivalis* and then mRNA levels were examined using real-time PCR. Values are expressed as fold changes. Differences among groups were analyzed by one-way ANOVA. Data represent the mean + SD ($n = 3$). ** $p < 0.01$, **** $p < 0.0001$.

3.3. Analysis of Extracellular Matrix and Adhesion Molecule-Associated Genes in Gingival Fibroblasts in Response to Various Fimbriae

A mouse extracellular matrix and adhesion molecules PCR array was used to investigate differences in the expression of 84 genes involved in cell–cell and cell–matrix interactions. Figure 3 shows the fold changes in expression between control and 1 μg/mL various fimbriae or *P. gingivalis* LPS after stimulation for 2 hours. Among the 84 genes, *Icam1* expression was upregulated 4-fold in FMFA5-stimulated cells compared with non-stimulated cells (Figure 3B). FMFA5C stimulation similarly induced *Icam1* and also *Selectin E (Sele)* (Figure 3C). No obvious changes in gene expression were observed with JI-1, FimA or *P. gingivalis* LPS stimulation compared with unstimulated cells (Figure 3A,D,E).

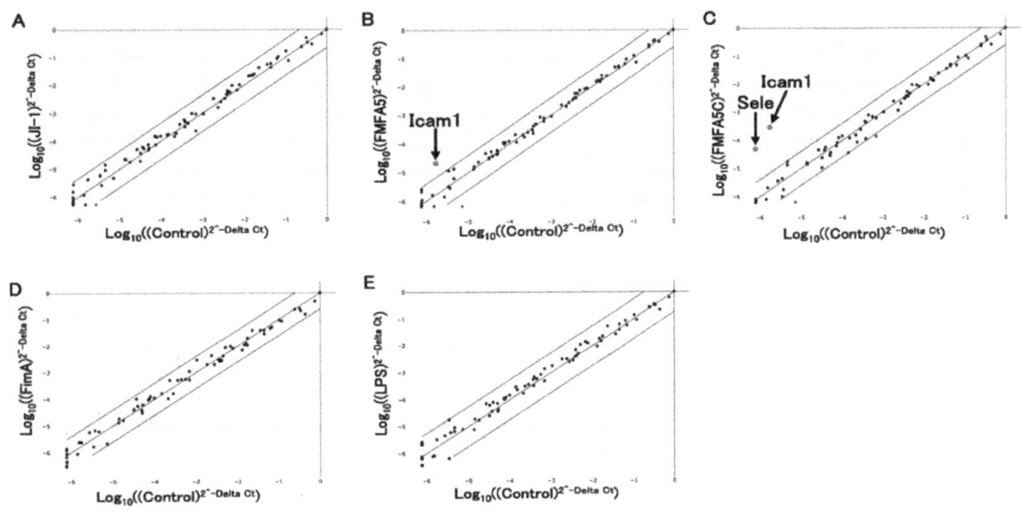

Figure 3. Analysis of extracellular matrix and adhesion molecule-associated genes in mouse gingival fibroblasts in response to Mfa1, FimA, or *P. gingivalis* LPS. Graphs show fold changes of gene expression in cells stimulated with JI-1 (**A**), FMFA5 (**B**), FMFA5C (**C**), FimA (**D**), and LPS (**E**) compared with non-stimulated cells. *Icam1* and *Sele* were up-regulated over 4-fold in FMFA5C-stimulated cells.

3.4. Confirmation of PCR Array Data for Selected Extracellular Matrix and Adhesion Molecule-Associated Genes by Quantitative RT-PCR

Expression of cell adhesion factors, *Icam1* and *Sele*, was increased to a greater extent by JI-1 stimulation compared with FimA stimulation (Figure 4). The highest increase in gene expression was observed with FMFA5 stimulation (Figure 4).

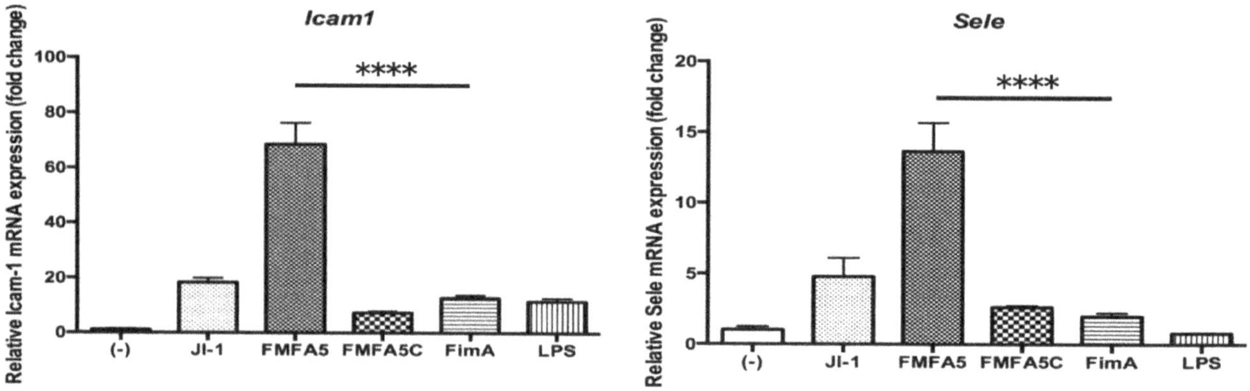

Figure 4. Mfa1 induces *Icam1* and *Sele* in mouse gingival fibroblasts. MGFs were cultured for 2 hours in the presence or absence of 1 μg/mL JI-1, FMFA5, FMFA5C, FimA, or LPS of *P. gingivalis* and then mRNA levels were examined using real-time PCR. Values are expressed as fold changes. Differences among groups were analyzed by one-way ANOVA. Data represent the mean + SD ($n = 3$). **** $p < 0.0001$.

3.5. Induction of Tlr2 and Tlr4 Gene Expression by Various Fimbriae and LPS Stimulation in Gingival Fibroblasts

Tlr2 showed the same change in expression as the other factors, such as *Cxcl1*, but *Tlr4*, the receptor for LPS, did not show any significant variation in gene expression in response to various stimulants (Figure 5).

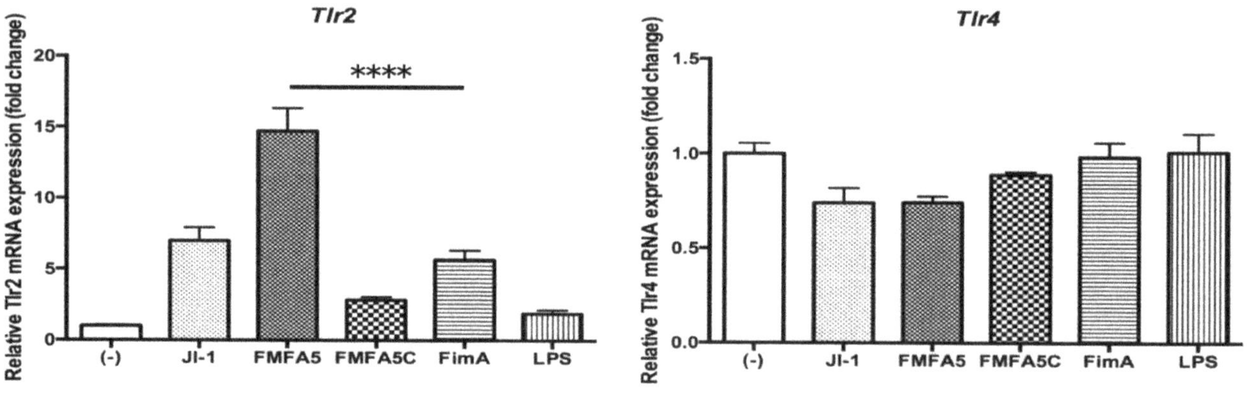

Figure 5. Mfa1 induces TLR2 but not TLR4 in mouse gingival fibroblasts. MGFs were cultured for 2 hours in the presence or absence of 1 μg/mL JI-1, FMFA5, FMFA5C, FimA or LPS of *P. gingivalis* and then mRNA levels were examined using real-time PCR. Values are expressed as fold changes. Differences among groups were analyzed by one-way ANOVA. Data represent the mean + SD ($n = 3$). **** $p < 0.0001$.

3.6. Transfection of *Tlr2* and *Tlr4* siRNA into Gingival Fibroblasts

Tlr2 and *Tlr4*siRNA-transfected gingival fibroblast cells showed obvious knockdown of *Tlr2* and *Tlr4*mRNA, respectively, compared with control siRNA-transfected gingival fibroblast cells (Figure 6A). FACS analysis confirmed a decrease in the surface expression of *Tlr2* and *Tlr4* in the respective siRNA-transfected gingival fibroblast cells compared with control cells (Figure 6B).

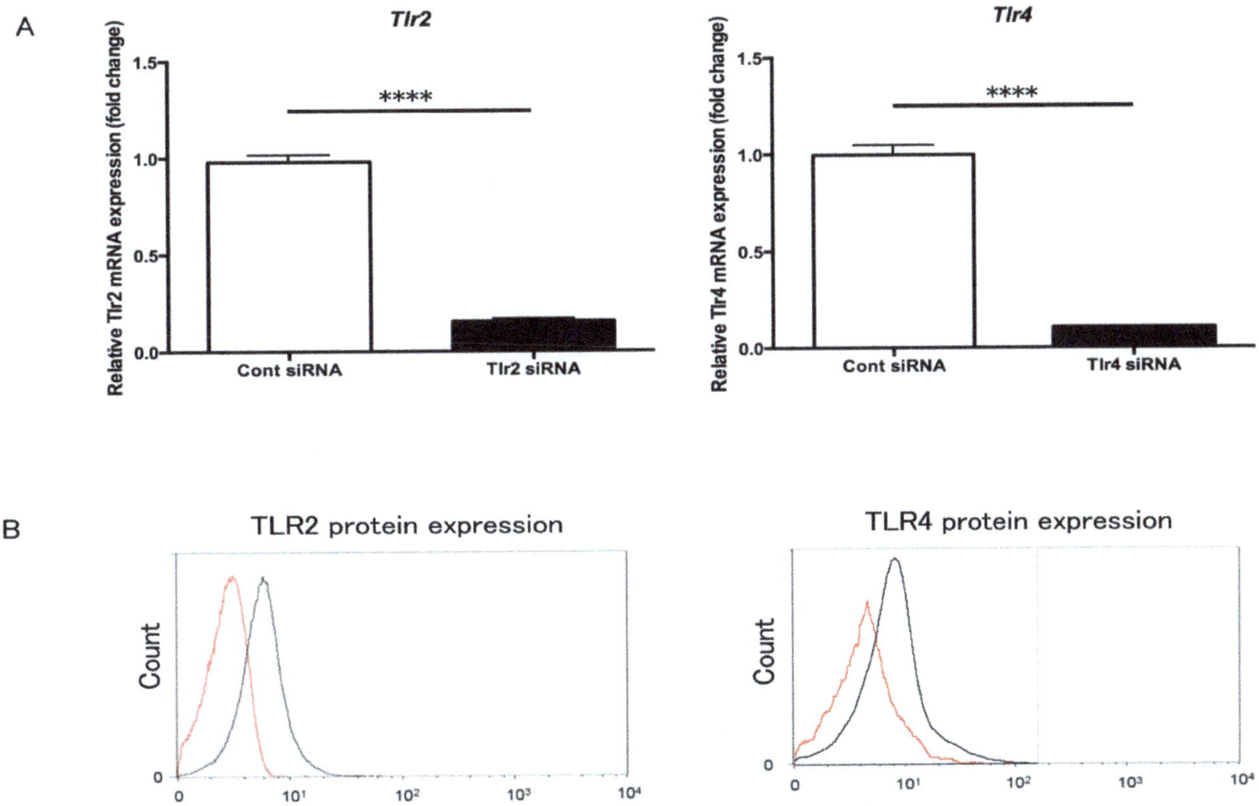

Figure 6. Suppression of *Tlr2* and *Tlr4* in mouse gingival fibroblasts using siRNA. (**A**) *Tlr2* (left) and *Tlr4* (right) mRNA levels were examined using real-time PCR. *Tlr2* and *Tlr4* siRNA-transfected cells showed clear knockdown of *Tlr2* and *Tlr4* mRNAs, respectively, compared with control siRNA-transfected cells. (**B**) TLR2 (left) and TLR4 (right) protein levels were examined using flow cytometry. *Tlr2* or *Tlr4* siRNA transfected cells (red line) showed decreased levels of the respective receptors compared with control siRNA-transfected cells (black line). **** $p < 0.0001$.

3.7. Expression of Selected Genes in *Tlr2* and *Tlr4* siRNA-Transfected Cells

Expression of the cell migration-related factor and cell adhesion factor genes in JI-1, FMFA5, and FMFA5C-stimulated *Tlr4* siRNA-transfected cells were significantly suppressed compared with control siRNA-transfected cells (Figure 7). Also, the suppression of *Tlr2* expression partially attenuated the stimulation effect (Figure 7).

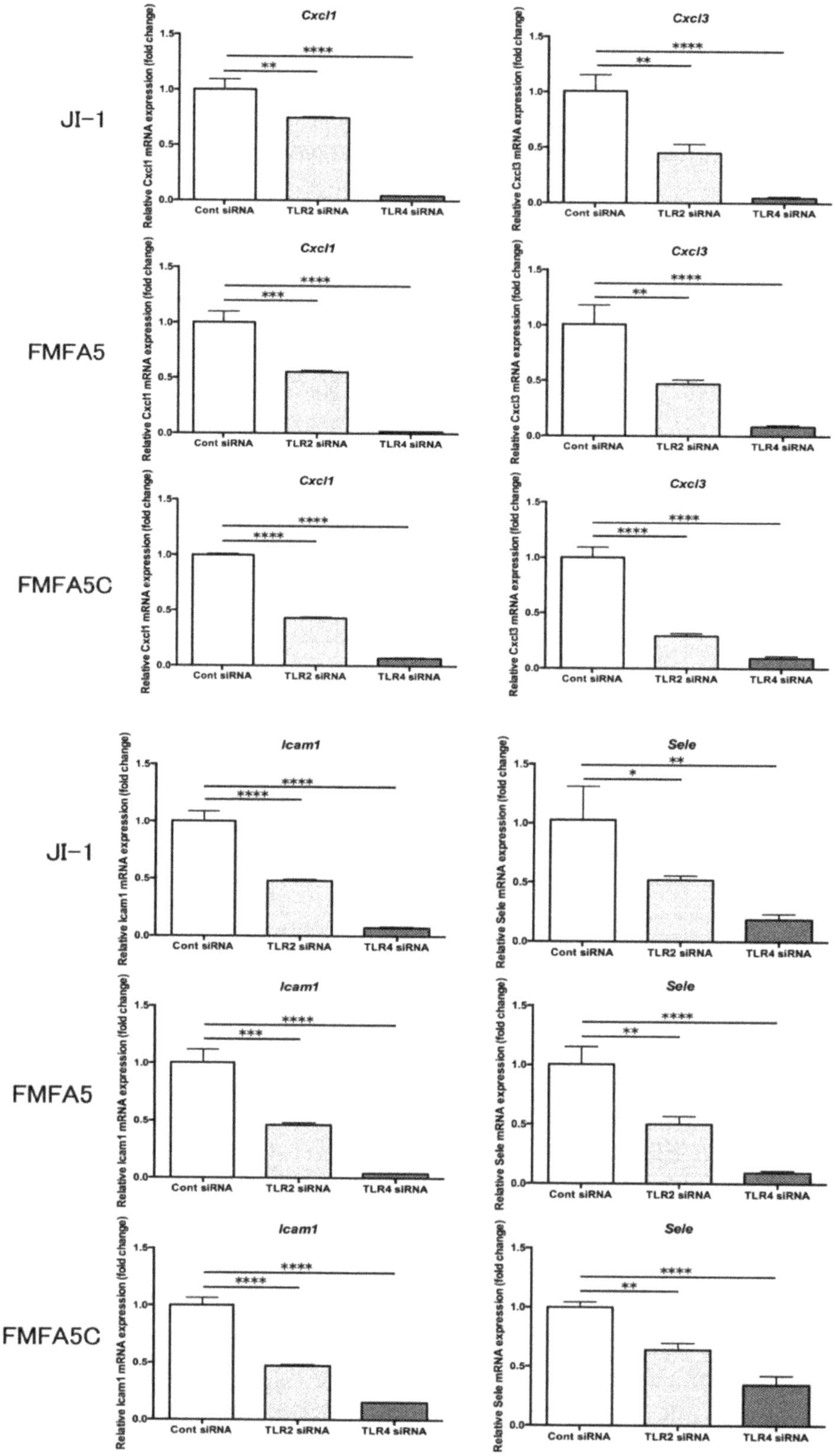

Figure 7. Involvement of TLR2 and TLR4 in the expression of Mfa1-induced cell migration and cell adhesion-related factors. *Tlr2* siRNA, *Tlr4* siRNA, or control siRNA-transfected mouse gingival fibroblasts were cultured for 2 hours in the presence or absence of 1 μg/mL JI-1, FMFA5, or FMFA5C and then mRNA levels were examined using real-time PCR. Values are expressed as fold changes. Differences among groups were analyzed by one-way ANOVA. Data represent the mean + SD ($n = 3$). * $p < 0.05$, ** $p < 0.01$, *** $p < 0.001$, **** $p < 0.0001$.

4. Discussion

In this study, we demonstrated that Mfa1 fimbriae stimulation markedly increased the expression of cell migration/cell adhesion-related genes in mouse gingival fibroblasts, and that the increase was more pronounced than with FimA stimulation. In addition, the ability of Mfa1 to regulate cell migration and cell adhesion was significantly attenuated in mouse gingival fibroblasts in which *Tlr4* expression was suppressed.

When the effect of JI-1 on gingival fibroblasts, which constitute the gingival connective tissue, was examined, a remarkable increase in the expression of *Cxcl1* and *Cxcl3*, which are involved in cell migration, was observed. Higher levels of CXCL1 were found in human and rat gingiva from periodontitis sites compared with periodontally healthy sites [23]. There was also a significant difference in the level of CXCL1 in gingival crevicular fluid between healthy and periodontitis subjects [24]. CXCL1 stimulates gingiva fibroblast migration [25] and it may be related to periodontal tissue healing. There is no literature reporting the relationship between CXCL3 and periodontitis, but its activity is similar to that of CXCL2, which may play an important role in the initiation of inflammation and subsequent periodontal tissue destruction [26], which suggests that it is involved in the progression of periodontitis. JI-1 stimulation produced a higher increase in *Cxcl1* and *Cxcl3* expression compared with FimA stimulation. FimA induces *Cxcl1* expression in mouse peritoneal macrophages [27]. It is possible that the immunomodulatory capacity of Mfa1 outperforms that of FimA for some factors in certain cell types.

Next, we investigated which part of the fimbriae structure is important for the immunomodulatory ability of Mfa1. FMFA5, with the Mfa3–5 tip structure of JI-1 removed, and FMFA5C, with the tip structure was complemented in FMFA5, were compared for their ability to induce immunomodulation. Compared with JI-1, a markedly higher increase in gene expression was observed with FMFA5 stimulation, while that of FMFA5C was significantly reduced. From this result, it is indicated that the incomplete fimbriae deficient in tip structure increase the stimulation ability.

When we confirmed the effects of Mfa1 on extracellular matrix and adhesion molecules, we found a marked increase in the expression of the cell adhesion factor genes, *Icam1* and *Sele*. ICAM1 deficiencies increase susceptibility to and severity of alveolar bone loss after *P. gingivalis* infection [28]. Selectin Platelet/Selectin E-deficient mice exhibit spontaneous early onset alveolar bone loss [29]. FimA and Mfa1 induce ICAM1 and Selectin E in human aortic endothelial cells [30]. These fimbriae appear to have similar effects on gingival fibroblasts. Similar to the results for cell migration factors, a markedly higher increase in cell adhesion factor gene expression was observed with FMFA5 stimulation and the stimulation ability of FMFA5C was significantly reduced compared with JI-1 stimulation. These results indicate that the regulation of cell adhesion factors by Mfa1 is also greatly influenced by the Mfa1 molecule in the shaft portion.

Cells use pattern recognition receptors, such as TLRs, to recognize pathogen-associated molecular patterns (PAMPs). Ten TLRs have been identified in humans and 12 in mice and the host innate immune response to pathogens is largely mediated via TLR signaling [31]. TLR2 and TLR4 are the most widely studied extracellular innate receptors that recognize various PAMPs and are likely to play a role in the pathogenesis of periodontitis [32]. TLR2 has been shown to be important for *P. gingivalis* to produce inflammatory cytokines [33,34]. TLR4 recognizes LPS (from *Escherichia coli*), which is a bacterial cell wall component [31]. Uniquely, *P. gingivalis* LPS is recognized by both TLR2 and TLR4 [35]. The $LPS_{1435/1449}$ and LPS_{1690} isoforms can produce opposite effects on TLR2 and TLR4 activation [36,37]. *P. gingivalis* LPS and *E. coli* LPS regulate cytokine production differently in human gingival fibroblasts [38]. The heterogeneity of *P. gingivalis* LPS might contribute to one of the strategies used by *P. gingivalis* to evade the innate host defense in gingival tissues [39]. FimA activates human peripheral blood monocytes via TLR2 and CD14 [40]. TLR2-dependent signaling leads to CD11b-CD18 activation in human monocytes upon recognition of FimA through CD14 [41]. However, the receptor for Mfa1 is still unclear. The gingival fibroblasts constitutively express TLR2 and TLR4 [42]. When we examined the expression of *Tlr2* and *Tlr4* genes in MGFs stimulated by various fimbriae and LPS,

Tlr2 showed the same changes in expression as the other factors, but *Tlr4* did not show any significant changes in expression in response to various fimbriae or LPS. Therefore, to clarify the receptor of Mfa1, MGFs in which *Tlr2* and *Tlr4* were knocked down were stimulated with Mfa1 and their reactivity was assessed. Control siRNA, *Tlr2* siRNA and *Tlr4* siRNA were introduced into MGFs, and cells were stimulated with JI-1, FMFA5, and FMFA5C. Gene expression of cell migration-related genes, *Cxcl1* and *Cxcl3*, and cell adhesion genes, *Icam1* and *Sele*, were analyzed. The suppression of TLR4 was significantly reduced by Mfa1 fimbriae stimulation. Also, suppression of *Tlr2* partially attenuated this stimulation. Recognition of Mfa1 by TLR4 is suggested to be essential for the expression of genes related to cell migration and cell adhesion. This result is different from previous reports in which anti-TLR2 antibody pretreatment significantly inhibited pro-inflammatory cytokines in mouse macrophages stimulated with Mfa1 fimbriae [43]. Conversely, Hajishengallis et al. reported that native Mfa1 induced proinflammatory cytokines in a CD14- and TLR2-dependent mode, which was likely due to a fimbriae-associated 12-kDa lipoprotein [44]. There is a similar report on FimA-like lipoproteins or lipopeptides associated with FimA that could, at least in part, account for signaling via TLR2 and subsequent TNF-α production in macrophages [45]. Furthermore, the following reports demonstrate the stimulation ability of LPS. A lipoprotein from *P. gingivalis* LPS was shown to be a principal component for TLR2-mediated cell activation [46]. A lipopolysaccharide preparation extracted from a *P. gingivalis* lipoprotein-deficient mutant showed a marked decrease in TLR2-mediated signaling [47]. Recombinant FimA stimulated cytokine release in THP-1 mononuclear cells via CD14 and TLR4 but not TLR2 [44], while recombinant FimA induced an inflammatory response via the TLR4/NF-kB signaling pathway in human peripheral blood mononuclear cells [48]. *P. gingivalis* lipid A and its synthetic counterpart activate cells through a TLR4-dependent pathway [46,49]. From our results, we speculate that wild-type purified Mfa1 is mainly recognized by TLR4, but TLR2 might recognize the lipoprotein of fimbriae and contributes to the overall action. In the future, it is necessary to confirm the reactivity of purified Mfa1 from which lipoprotein has been removed.

There are several reports on the importance of TLR4 in periodontitis. TLR4- but not TLR2-mediated stimulation, was positively associated with plaque score and bleeding on probing score of teeth from which the plaque samples were taken [4]. The ratio of TLR4/TLR2-mediated stimulation activity was also positively associated with probing depth and clinical attachment level [4]. TLR4- but not TLR2-stimulation of subgingival plaque is associated with plaque index [50]. Therefore, TLR4 may play an important role in the progression of periodontitis, in which stimulation by Mfa1 may play a role.

Recent reports suggest that intracellular DC-SIGN, an intracellularly expressed pattern recognition receptor, could be critical for recognition of Mfa1 by dendritic cells [51]. We assayed expression of DC-SIGN in MGFs after stimulation with various fimbriae, but we could not detect its expression. This may be because of differences between immunocompetent cells and periodontal tissue constituent cells.

In conclusion, Mfa1 fimbriae have a significant effect on immunomodulation in gingival fibroblasts of periodontal tissue. We also suggest that recognition of Mfa1 by TLR4 on MGFs is essential for the expression of genes related to cell migration and cell adhesion. More detailed analysis, such as using an animal infection model, is needed to assess the immunomodulatory capacity of Mfa1 fimbriae in the progression of periodontitis.

Author Contributions: Conceptualization, Y.T., T.K., Y.H., and A.M.; methodology, Y.T., T.K., Y.H., and A.M.; validation, Y.T., T.K., and A.M.; formal analysis, Y.T., H.G., I.O., Y.S. (0000-0002-7536-5931), N.S., and T.O. (Tasuku Ohno); investigation, Y.T., Y.N., H.G., K.O., I.O., Y.K., Y.S. (0000-0002-7536-5931), N.S., T.O. (Teppei Okabe), and Y.S.(0000-0003-3660-6867); data curation, Y.K., Y.S. (0000-0003-3660-6867), and S.K.; writing—original draft preparation, Y.T., T.K., and A.M.; writing—review and editing, Y.T., T.K., Y.H., J.-I.H., and A.M.; visualization, Y.T. and T.K.; supervision, T.K., Y.H., J.H., and A.M.; project administration, A.M.; funding acquisition, T.K., Y.H. All authors have read and agreed to the published version of the manuscript.

Acknowledgments: We thank Jeremy Allen, PhD, from Edanz Group (https://en-author-services.edanzgroup.com/) for editing a draft of this manuscript.

References

1. Pihlstrom, B.L.; Michalowicz, B.S.; Johnson, N.W. Periodontal diseases. *Lancet* **2005**, *366*, 1809–1820. [CrossRef]
2. Socransky, S.S.; Haffajee, A.D.; Cugini, M.A.; Smith, C.; Kent, R.L., Jr. Microbial complexes in subgingival plaque. *J. Clin. Periodontol.* **1998**, *25*, 134–144. [CrossRef] [PubMed]
3. Riviere, G.R.; Smith, K.S.; Tzagaroulaki, E.; Kay, S.L.; Zhu, X.; DeRouen, T.A.; Adams, D.F. Periodontal status and detection frequency of bacteria at sites of periodontal health and gingivitis. *J. Periodontol.* **1996**, *67*, 109–115. [CrossRef] [PubMed]
4. Yoshioka, H.; Yoshimura, A.; Kaneko, T.; Golenbock, D.T.; Hara, Y. Analysis of the activity to induce toll-like receptor (TLR)2- and TLR4-mediated stimulation of supragingival plaque. *J. Periodontol.* **2008**, *79*, 920–928. [CrossRef]
5. Darveau, R.P.; Hajishengallis, G.; Curtis, M.A. Porphyromonas gingivalis as a potential community activist for disease. *J. Dent. Res.* **2012**, *91*, 816–820. [CrossRef]
6. Lamont, R.J.; Jenkinson, H.F. Life below the gum line: Pathogenic mechanisms of Porphyromonas gingivalis. *Microbiol. Mol. Biol. Rev.* **1998**, *62*, 1244–1263. [CrossRef]
7. Hospenthal, M.K.; Costa, T.R.D.; Waksman, G. A comprehensive guide to pilus biogenesis in Gram-negative bacteria. *Nat. Rev. Microbiol.* **2017**, *15*, 365–379. [CrossRef]
8. Lamont, R.J.; Jenkinson, H.F. Subgingival colonization by Porphyromonas gingivalis. *Oral Microbiol. Immunol.* **2000**, *15*, 341–349. [CrossRef]
9. Yoshimura, F.; Murakami, Y.; Nishikawa, K.; Hasegawa, Y.; Kawaminami, S. Surface components of Porphyromonas gingivalis. *J. Periodontal. Res.* **2009**, *44*, 1–12. [CrossRef]
10. Enersen, M.; Nakano, K.; Amano, A. Porphyromonas gingivalis fimbriae. *J. Oral Microbiol.* **2013**, *5*, 20265. [CrossRef]
11. Ikai, R.; Hasegawa, Y.; Izumigawa, M.; Nagano, K.; Yoshida, Y.; Kitai, N.; Lamont, R.J.; Yoshimura, F.; Murakami, Y. Mfa4, an Accessory Protein of Mfa1 Fimbriae, Modulates Fimbrial Biogenesis, Cell Auto-Aggregation, and Biofilm Formation in Porphyromonas gingivalis. *PLoS ONE* **2015**, *10*, e0139454. [CrossRef] [PubMed]
12. Hall, M.; Hasegawa, Y.; Yoshimura, F.; Persson, K. Structural and functional characterization of shaft, anchor, and tip proteins of the Mfa1 fimbria from the periodontal pathogen Porphyromonas gingivalis. *Sci. Rep.* **2018**, *8*, 1793. [CrossRef] [PubMed]
13. Yilmaz, O.; Watanabe, K.; Lamont, R.J. Involvement of integrins in fimbriae-mediated binding and invasion by Porphyromonas gingivalis. *Cell Microbiol.* **2002**, *4*, 305–314. [CrossRef] [PubMed]
14. Amano, A.; Nakagawa, I.; Okahashi, N.; Hamada, N. Variations of Porphyromonas gingivalis fimbriae in relation to microbial pathogenesis. *J. Periodontol. Res.* **2004**, *39*, 136–142. [CrossRef] [PubMed]
15. Hajishengallis, G.; Wang, M.; Liang, S.; Shakhatreh, M.A.; James, D.; Nishiyama, S.; Yoshimura, F.; Demuth, D.R. Subversion of innate immunity by periodontopathic bacteria via exploitation of complement receptor-3. *Adv. Exp. Med. Biol.* **2008**, *632*, 203–219. [CrossRef] [PubMed]
16. Amano, A. Host-parasite interactions in periodontitis: Subgingival infection and host sensing. *Periodontology 2000* **2010**, *52*, 7–11. [CrossRef] [PubMed]
17. Amano, A. Host-parasite interactions in periodontitis: Microbial pathogenicity and innate immunity. *Periodontology 2000* **2010**, *54*, 9–14. [CrossRef]
18. Kuboniwa, M.; Amano, A.; Hashino, E.; Yamamoto, Y.; Inaba, H.; Hamada, N.; Nakayama, K.; Tribble, G.D.; Lamont, R.J.; Shizukuishi, S. Distinct roles of long/short fimbriae and gingipains in homotypic biofilm development by Porphyromonas gingivalis. *BMC Microbiol.* **2009**, *9*, 105. [CrossRef]
19. Umemoto, T.; Hamada, N. Characterization of biologically active cell surface components of a periodontal pathogen. The roles of major and minor fimbriae of Porphyromonas gingivalis. *J. Periodontol.* **2003**, *74*, 119–122. [CrossRef]
20. Hasegawa, Y.; Nagano, K.; Ikai, R.; Izumigawa, M.; Yoshida, Y.; Kitai, N.; Lamont, R.J.; Murakami, Y.; Yoshimura, F. Localization and function of the accessory protein Mfa3 in Porphyromonas gingivalis Mfa1 fimbriae. *Mol. Oral Microbiol.* **2013**, *28*, 467–480. [CrossRef]
21. Hasegawa, Y.; Nagano, K.; Murakami, Y.; Lamont, R.J. Purification of Native Mfa1 Fimbriae from Porphyromonas gingivalis. *Methods Mol. Biol.* **2021**, *2210*, 75–86. [CrossRef] [PubMed]

22. Hasegawa, Y.; Iijima, Y.; Persson, K.; Nagano, K.; Yoshida, Y.; Lamont, R.J.; Kikuchi, T.; Mitani, A.; Yoshimura, F. Role of Mfa5 in Expression of Mfa1 Fimbriae in Porphyromonas gingivalis. *J. Dent. Res.* **2016**, *95*, 1291–1297. [CrossRef] [PubMed]
23. Rath-Deschner, B.; Memmert, S.; Damanaki, A.; Nokhbehsaim, M.; Eick, S.; Cirelli, J.A.; Gotz, W.; Deschner, J.; Jager, A.; Nogueira, A.V.B. CXCL1, CCL2, and CCL5 modulation by microbial and biomechanical signals in periodontal cells and tissues-in vitro and in vivo studies. *Clin. Oral Investig.* **2020**, *24*, 3661–3670. [CrossRef] [PubMed]
24. Sakai, A.; Ohshima, M.; Sugano, N.; Otsuka, K.; Ito, K. Profiling the cytokines in gingival crevicular fluid using a cytokine antibody array. *J. Periodontol.* **2006**, *77*, 856–864. [CrossRef] [PubMed]
25. Buskermolen, J.K.; Roffel, S.; Gibbs, S. Stimulation of oral fibroblast chemokine receptors identifies CCR3 and CCR4 as potential wound healing targets. *J. Cell. Physiol.* **2017**, *232*, 2996–3005. [CrossRef] [PubMed]
26. Miyauchi, M.; Kitagawa, S.; Hiraoka, M.; Saito, A.; Sato, S.; Kudo, Y.; Ogawa, I.; Takata, T. Immunolocalization of CXC chemokine and recruitment of polymorphonuclear leukocytes in the rat molar periodontal tissue after topical application of lipopolysaccharide. *Histochem. Cell. Biol.* **2004**, *121*, 291–297. [CrossRef]
27. Hanazawa, S.; Murakami, Y.; Takeshita, A.; Kitami, H.; Ohta, K.; Amano, S.; Kitano, S. Porphyromonas gingivalis fimbriae induce expression of the neutrophil chemotactic factor KC gene of mouse peritoneal macrophages: Role of protein kinase C. *Infect. Immun.* **1992**, *60*, 1544–1549. [CrossRef]
28. Baker, P.J.; DuFour, L.; Dixon, M.; Roopenian, D.C. Adhesion molecule deficiencies increase Porphyromonas gingivalis-induced alveolar bone loss in mice. *Infect. Immun.* **2000**, *68*, 3103–3107. [CrossRef]
29. Niederman, R.; Westernoff, T.; Lee, C.; Mark, L.L.; Kawashima, N.; Ullman-Culler, M.; Dewhirst, F.E.; Paster, B.J.; Wagner, D.D.; Mayadas, T.; et al. Infection-mediated early-onset periodontal disease in P/E-selectin-deficient mice. *J. Clin. Periodontol.* **2001**, *28*, 569–575. [CrossRef]
30. Takahashi, Y.; Davey, M.; Yumoto, H.; Gibson, F.C., 3rd; Genco, C.A. Fimbria-dependent activation of pro-inflammatory molecules in Porphyromonas gingivalis infected human aortic endothelial cells. *Cell Microbiol.* **2006**, *8*, 738–757. [CrossRef]
31. Akira, S.; Takeda, K. Toll-like receptor signalling. *Nat. Rev. Immunol.* **2004**, *4*, 499–511. [CrossRef] [PubMed]
32. Hajishengallis, G.; Lambris, J.D. Microbial manipulation of receptor crosstalk in innate immunity. *Nat. Rev. Immunol.* **2011**, *11*, 187–200. [CrossRef] [PubMed]
33. Burns, E.; Bachrach, G.; Shapira, L.; Nussbaum, G. Cutting Edge: TLR2 is required for the innate response to Porphyromonas gingivalis: Activation leads to bacterial persistence and TLR2 deficiency attenuates induced alveolar bone resorption. *J. Immunol.* **2006**, *177*, 8296–8300. [CrossRef] [PubMed]
34. Watanabe, N.; Yokoe, S.; Ogata, Y.; Sato, S.; Imai, K. Exposure to Porphyromonas gingivalis Induces Production of Proinflammatory Cytokine via TLR2 from Human Respiratory Epithelial Cells. *J. Clin. Med.* **2020**, *9*, 3433. [CrossRef]
35. Darveau, R.P.; Pham, T.T.; Lemley, K.; Reife, R.A.; Bainbridge, B.W.; Coats, S.R.; Howald, W.N.; Way, S.S.; Hajjar, A.M. Porphyromonas gingivalis lipopolysaccharide contains multiple lipid A species that functionally interact with both toll-like receptors 2 and 4. *Infect. Immun.* **2004**, *72*, 5041–5051. [CrossRef]
36. Olsen, I.; Singhrao, S.K. Importance of heterogeneity in Porhyromonas gingivalis lipopolysaccharide lipid A in tissue specific inflammatory signalling. *J. Oral Microbiol.* **2018**, *10*, 1440128. [CrossRef]
37. Herath, T.D.K.; Darveau, R.P.; Seneviratne, C.J.; Wang, C.Y.; Wang, Y.; Jin, L. Heterogeneous Porphyromonas gingivalis LPS modulates immuno-inflammatory response, antioxidant defense and cytoskeletal dynamics in human gingival fibroblasts. *Sci Rep.* **2016**, *6*, 29829. [CrossRef]
38. Andrukhov, O.; Ertlschweiger, S.; Moritz, A.; Bantleon, H.P.; Rausch-Fan, X. Different effects of P. gingivalis LPS and E. coli LPS on the expression of interleukin-6 in human gingival fibroblasts. *Acta Odontol. Scand.* **2014**, *72*, 337–345. [CrossRef]
39. Herath, T.D.; Darveau, R.P.; Seneviratne, C.J.; Wang, C.Y.; Wang, Y.; Jin, L. Tetra- and penta-acylated lipid A structures of Porphyromonas gingivalis LPS differentially activate TLR4-mediated NF-kappaB signal transduction cascade and immuno-inflammatory response in human gingival fibroblasts. *PLoS ONE* **2013**, *8*, e58496. [CrossRef]
40. Ogawa, T.; Asai, Y.; Hashimoto, M.; Uchida, H. Bacterial fimbriae activate human peripheral blood monocytes utilizing TLR2, CD14 and CD11a/CD18 as cellular receptors. *Eur. J. Immunol.* **2002**, *32*, 2543–2550. [CrossRef]
41. Harokopakis, E.; Hajishengallis, G. Integrin activation by bacterial fimbriae through a pathway involving CD14, Toll-like receptor 2, and phosphatidylinositol-3-kinase. *Eur. J. Immunol.* **2005**, *35*, 1201–1210. [CrossRef]

42. Tabeta, K.; Yamazaki, K.; Akashi, S.; Miyake, K.; Kumada, H.; Umemoto, T.; Yoshie, H. Toll-like receptors confer responsiveness to lipopolysaccharide from Porphyromonas gingivalis in human gingival fibroblasts. *Infect. Immun.* **2000**, *68*, 3731–3735. [CrossRef] [PubMed]
43. Hiramine, H.; Watanabe, K.; Hamada, N.; Umemoto, T. Porphyromonas gingivalis 67-kDa fimbriae induced cytokine production and osteoclast differentiation utilizing TLR2. *FEMS Microbiol. Lett.* **2003**, *229*, 49–55. [CrossRef]
44. Hajishengallis, G.; Martin, M.; Sojar, H.T.; Sharma, A.; Schifferle, R.E.; DeNardin, E.; Russell, M.W.; Genco, R.J. Dependence of bacterial protein adhesins on toll-like receptors for proinflammatory cytokine induction. *Clin. Diagn. Lab. Immunol.* **2002**, *9*, 403–411. [CrossRef]
45. Aoki, Y.; Tabeta, K.; Murakami, Y.; Yoshimura, F.; Yamazaki, K. Analysis of immunostimulatory activity of Porphyromonas gingivalis fimbriae conferred by Toll-like receptor 2. *Biochem. Biophys. Res. Commun.* **2010**, *398*, 86–91. [CrossRef]
46. Hashimoto, M.; Asai, Y.; Ogawa, T. Separation and structural analysis of lipoprotein in a lipopolysaccharide preparation from Porphyromonas gingivalis. *Int. Immunol.* **2004**, *16*, 1431–1437. [CrossRef]
47. Asai, Y.; Hashimoto, M.; Fletcher, H.M.; Miyake, K.; Akira, S.; Ogawa, T. Lipopolysaccharide preparation extracted from Porphyromonas gingivalis lipoprotein-deficient mutant shows a marked decrease in toll-like receptor 2-mediated signaling. *Infect. Immun.* **2005**, *73*, 2157–2163. [CrossRef]
48. Cai, J.; Chen, J.; Guo, H.; Pan, Y.; Zhang, Y.; Zhao, W.; Li, X.; Li, Y. Recombinant fimbriae protein of Porphyromonas gingivalis induces an inflammatory response via the TLR4/NFkappaB signaling pathway in human peripheral blood mononuclear cells. *Int. J. Mol. Med.* **2019**, *43*, 1430–1440. [CrossRef] [PubMed]
49. Reife, R.A.; Coats, S.R.; Al-Qutub, M.; Dixon, D.M.; Braham, P.A.; Billharz, R.J.; Howald, W.N.; Darveau, R.P. Porphyromonas gingivalis lipopolysaccharide lipid A heterogeneity: Differential activities of tetra- and penta-acylated lipid A structures on E-selectin expression and TLR4 recognition. *Cell Microbiol.* **2006**, *8*, 857–868. [CrossRef] [PubMed]
50. Ziauddin, S.M.; Montenegro Raudales, J.L.; Sato, K.; Yoshioka, H.; Ozaki, Y.; Kaneko, T.; Yoshimura, A.; Hara, Y. Analysis of Subgingival Plaque Ability to Stimulate Toll-Like Receptor 2 and 4. *J. Periodontol.* **2016**, *87*, 1083–1091. [CrossRef]
51. El-Awady, A.R.; Miles, B.; Scisci, E.; Kurago, Z.B.; Palani, C.D.; Arce, R.M.; Waller, J.L.; Genco, C.A.; Slocum, C.; Manning, M.; et al. Porphyromonas gingivalis evasion of autophagy and intracellular killing by human myeloid dendritic cells involves DC-SIGN-TLR2 crosstalk. *PLoS Pathog.* **2015**, *10*, e1004647. [CrossRef] [PubMed]

16

Next Generation Sequencing Discoveries of the Nitrate-Responsive Oral Microbiome and its Effect on Vascular Responses

Melissa M. Grant [1] and Daniel Jönsson [2,3,*]

[1] School of Dentistry, Institute of Clinical Sciences, University of Birmingham and Birmingham Community Healthcare Foundation Trust, Birmingham B5 7EG, UK
[2] Swedish Dental Service of Skåne, 222 37 Lund, Sweden
[3] Department of Periodontology, Faculty of Odontology, Malmö University, 214 21 Malmö, Sweden
* Correspondence: daniel.jonsson@mau.se

Abstract: Cardiovascular disease is a worldwide human condition which has multiple underlying contributing factors: one of these is long-term increased blood pressure—hypertension. Nitric oxide (NO) is a small nitrogenous radical species that has a number of physiological functions including vasodilation. It can be produced enzymatically through host nitric oxide synthases and by an alternative nitrate–nitrite–NO pathway from ingested inorganic nitrate. It was discovered that this route relies on the ability of the oral microbiota to reduce nitrate to nitrite and NO. Next generation sequencing has been used over the past two decades to gain deeper insight into the microbes involved, their location and the effect of their removal from the oral cavity. This review article presents this research and comments briefly on future directions.

Keywords: oral microbiome; saliva; nitric oxide; nitrate; nitrite

---

1. Introduction

Oral microbiota are the second most complex niche of the human microbiome [1]; they have been associated with several non-communicative diseases, including cancer [2], Alzheimer's disease [3] and cardiovascular disease (CVD) [4,5]. The current review will focus on the association between the oral microbiota and the most well established mechanistic pathway through which the oral microbiota may modify CVD, namely via the nitric oxide (NO) synthesis pathway.

In Europe, 3.9 million people die yearly from CVD, costing about 210 billion Euros per year in healthcare costs, productivity losses and informal care [6]. Hypertension is an important subclinical parameter for cardiovascular disease—about 54% of all stroke and 47% of ischemic heart disease are attributed to hypertension [7]. Hypertension is defined by WHO as systolic blood pressure ≥140 mm Hg and diastolic pressure ≥90, however it was recently reported that the definition of hypertension needs to be re-visited as lowering systolic blood pressure not to under 140 mm Hg, but to 120 mm Hg causes less fatal and non-fatal cardiovascular events. This also suggests that hypertension may be more important in CVD than previously described [8].

There are several important mechanisms behind hypertension, but one key underpinning is the L-arginine/NO synthesis pathway. In addition to hypertension, the NO synthesis pathway is important in the pathobiology of CVD via inflammation and platelet activation and aggregation [9].

2. The L-Arginine/NO Synthesis Pathway

In 1998, Robert F. Furchgott, Louis J. Ignarro and Ferid Murad were awarded the Nobel Prize for detecting and describing L-arginine/NO synthesis in cardiovascular physiology and disease. Furchgott described the accidental finding that acethylcholine, bradykinin, histamine and 5-hydroxytryptamine relax isolated preparations of blood vessels, but only when the endothelium is intact. In rabbit thoracic aorta prepared as a transverse ring, acetylcholine stimulation with muscarinic agonists caused dilatation, but not in aorta prepared as a helical strip. Later, it was noted that gently rubbing the endothelium of the transverse ring preparations similarly caused loss of smooth muscle cell relaxation. The endothelium-derived factor relaxing the smooth muscle cells lining the arteries was named endothelium-derived relaxing factor (EDRF) [10,11].

Following the discovery of EDRF, there was a wave of research inhibiting EDRF. What these inhibitors all had in common was their redox potency, except hemoglobin which inactivated EDRF by binding to it. This led to the suggestion that EDRF might be a free radical [12,13], and eventually Ignarro et al. [14] suggested that EDRF may in fact be NO, which at that time was not known to be synthesized in humans.

Then the question was where NO originates from, and in macrophages it was shown that NO originates from L-arginine [15,16]. Later, the enzyme responsible for the conversion of L-arginine to NO was identified as NO synthase. In addition to macrophages, NO was discovered in the central nervous system [17]. Depending on the system, different isoforms of NO synthase were identified, namely eNOS in endothelial cells, nNOS in the nervous system, and iNOS in the inflammatory system.

The inhibition of L-arginine and knockdown of eNOS in animal models led to the paradigm shift that hypertension is not due to increased resistance, but due to decreased conductance in the vascular system. The eNOS knockout mice also had increased endothelial-leucocyte interaction, platelet aggregation and thrombosis [18]. When knocking down eNOS in hypercholesterolemic ApoE mice, the eNOS-deficient mice had accelerated atherosclerosis [19]. Taken together, this work showed that the importance of eNOS and the L-arginine/NO synthesis pathway goes far beyond hypertension. In fact, NO from the eNOS activity of endothelial cells not only causes less contractility of the smooth muscle cells, but also results in inhibition of activation, adhesion and aggregation of platelets, less adhesivity of leucocytes and enhanced oxygen delivery from erythrocytes [20].

In 1986, Ludmer and coworkers [21] published a now classical study showing that in subjects with known CVD, acetylcholine resulted in a paradoxical NO-mediated vasoconstriction, in contrast to vasodilation in healthy subjects. Importantly, subjects with minimal CVD (angiographically) also displayed vasoconstriction. All three groups dilated in response to nitroglycerine. What this study suggested was that dysfunctional endothelial NO production and availability might precede the formation of clinically significant atherosclerotic lesions—today known as endothelial dysfunction. The clinical evaluation of endothelial function is through flow-mediated dilatation (FMD), today known as a subclinical predictor of CVD events [22] which is impaired in known CVD high risk groups, such as smokers and subjects with hypocholesteremia [23].

Endothelial dysfunction affects the L-arginine/NO-synthesis in two important ways—on a cellular level and on a molecular level. Endothelial cells can undergo phenotypical changes from healthy to a pro-inflammatory cell type. Healthy conditions, such as laminar blood flow, cause upregulation of transcription factors, such as Kruppel-like factors (KLF) 2 and 4, whereas athero-promoting flow and pro-inflammatory content of the blood cause upregulation of NFkB, eliciting a pro-inflammatory cell phenotype [24,25]. KLF2 promotes anti-CVD mechanisms, such as anti-inflammation by inhibiting the NFkB pathway [26,27], and anti-thrombogenic by inducing eNOS and thrombomodulin and reducing plasminogen activator inhibitor (PAI-1) [28]. Interestingly, KLF2 can be induced pharmacologically, via statins that exert atheroprotective effects via KLF2 [29]. NFkB is a pro-inflammatory transcription factor causing recruitment and activation of leucocytes at the site and subsequent endothelial dysfunction [24,25]. On a molecular level, the inflammatory micro-environment at an atherosclerotic lesion causes a net excess of reactive oxygen species (ROS), including superoxide which inactivates NO by forming peroxynitrite which could result in DNA damage and protein modification, but also through uncoupling of eNOS [30].

3. Microbiome Contributions to NO Synthesis

Research in the mid-1990s showed that NO production can be independent of NOS [31–33]. This production was linked directly to diet as, for example, nitrate-rich vegetable consumption could increase systemic nitrate and result in lowering of systolic blood pressure [34]. However, the activation of nitrate and transformation ultimately to NO requires its conversion to nitrite and mammals lack the enzymes required for this bioactivation. Termed the entero-salivary circulation, this requires consumption of nitrate which is absorbed by the upper gastrointestinal tract (Figure 1). Nitrate in circulation (approximately 25%, the remainder being secreted by the kidneys) is then selectively acquired by the sialin protein in the salivary glands and thus a high concentration of nitrate (1500 μM) is returned to the oral cavity [35]. There, the conversion of nitrate to nitrite is carried out by the oral microbiota [36]. Upon entering the stomach, the nitrite is protonated to nitrous acid (HNO_2) which can then decompose to NO and other oxides. The following section reviews the results from next generation sequencing approaches to understanding more about the bacteria involved in the conversion of nitrate to nitrite in the oral cavity.

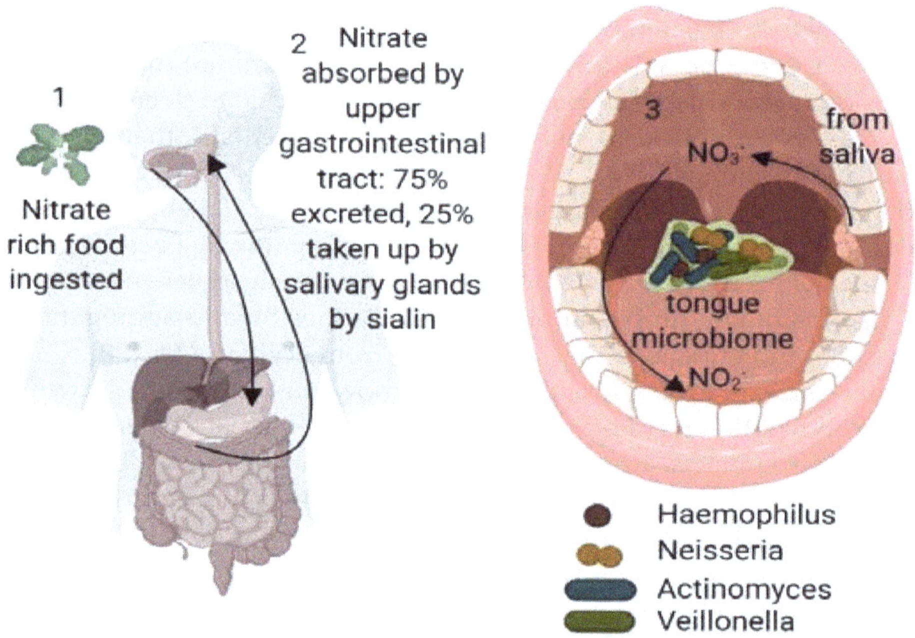

Figure 1. Enterosalivary nitrate production and the role of the oral microbiome. 1. Nitrate-rich food, such as leafy green vegetables, is ingested. 2. Nitrate is absorbed in the upper gastrointestinal tract and 25% is then found in saliva due to the action of the sialin anion transporter. 3. The oral microflora, particularly nitrate-reducing bacteria, such as *Actinomyces, Haemophilus, Neisseria* and *Veillonella*, residing in the dorsal tongue biofilm convert nitrate to nitrite, and also to nitric oxide (NO) which can be absorbed through the vascularized tongue or through swallowing back in to the gastrointestinal system for absorption. Image created in Biorender.

The first study examining the oral microbiota and the constituent microbes involved in nitrate and nitrite reduction was published in 2005 [36]. By mapping nitrate reduction across the mouth, Doel et al. could demonstrate that the majority of nitrate reductase activity was associated with the dorsum of the tongue. Indeed, the tongue dorsum has a distinct microbiome which is related to the other oral niches. It is more similar to the saliva microbiome than to the oral plaque microbiomes (Human microbiome project consortium 2012 [37]). They went further by isolating and culturing species associated within this site and verifying nitrate reductase activity. More species were found to have this activity under anaerobic conditions than aerobic conditions. Isolates of interest were 16S rRNA sequenced to gain their identity. The highest levels of nitrate reduction were found with

Actinomyces odontolytica which was the second most common tongue isolate, though the authors also detected *Veillonella atypica, Veillonella dispar, Veillonella parvula, Actinomyces naeslundii, Actinomyces viscosus, Rothia dentocariosa, Rothia mucilaginosa, Staphylococcus epidermidis, Staphylococcus hemolyticus, Corynebacterium matruchotii, Corynebacterium durum, Haemophilus parainfluenzae, Haemophilus segnis, Propionibacterium acnes, Granulicatella adiacens, Selenomonas noxia, Capnocytophaga sputigena, Eikinella corrodens* and *Microbacterium oxydans*. The next report showing the microbiome associated with nitrate reduction was published a decade later, once the metagenomics analysis tools had matured more fully. Hyde et al. [4] used 16S rRNA and whole genome analysis of whole tongue scrapings and of biofilms originated from the scrapings matured on polymethacrylate (PMMA) discs for up to 4 days. The change in technique from Doel et al. [36] allowed for a larger number of operational taxonomic units (OTUs) to be discovered and a wider range of genera: *Streptococcus, Veillonella, Prevotella, Neisseria* and *Haemophilus*. The authors noted that there was a wide variation between different donors. With the samples that were used to inoculate biofilms, it was also noted that the number of OTUs dropped dramatically within the first 24 h and that by 4 days the biofilms were dominated by the *Streptococcal* species. Koopman et al. [38] also demonstrated this loss of diversity when growing saliva samples in a nitrate-reducing bacteria discovery study. This is of interest in light of the report by Doel et al. where culturing was used to find the nitrate-reducing bacteria before sequencing as this may have resulted in under-estimation of the discoveries. With the whole genome sequencing and pathway analysis, by Hyde et al., the pathways associated with the samples were more consistent with a match across the top eight pathways, such as various amino acid metabolic or synthetic pathways and nitrogen metabolism. Hyde et al. also split their results into samples with high, intermediate and low nitrate reductase activity: these samples were derived from the inoculated biofilms and were derived from individual donors creating a dataset of 30. Using principal coordinate analysis (PCoA), they showed that the samples with high nitrate reduction capacity were more likely to contain *Granulicatella, Veillonella, Neisseria, Actinomyces, Prevotella, Haemophilus, Fusobacterium* and some unclassified species of the *Gemellaceae* family. Some of these were already known whilst others were novel. Of note was the fact that *Lactobacillus* was associated with the least nitrate-reducing samples and the authors speculated that these genera may have an inhibitory role through production of some unknown byproduct that may inhibit nitrate reduction in those communities. Last, these authors also grew four microorganisms with putative nitrate and/or nitrite reduction capacity: *A. odontolyticus, V. dispar, F. nucleatum* and *S. mutans*. This last aspect of their study showed that these species could work independently or in a consortium to effectively remove nitrate and/or nitrite from growth medium. This is an important illustration of the complex interdependent networks in which biofilms exist. This paper not only confirmed previous findings but took them a step further, however both studies relied on discoveries from only 10 and 6 tongue scraping donors.

Hyde et al. [39] also published an article characterizing the tongue microbiome of rats, in comparison to human tongue scrapings, with a focus on the effect of dietary nitrate. One of the main findings was that the rat tongue microbiome was less diverse and appeared to be missing or had a greatly decreased amount of *Veillonella, Prevotella, Neisseria* and *Porphyromonas* in comparison to human samples. However, one of the limitations of the study was that different methodologies were used between the rat and human samples. Nevertheless, they could also examine the effect of administration of sodium nitrate via drinking water and chlorhexidine via oral rinse. The supplementation by sodium nitrate significantly decreased diastolic blood pressure and heart rate and made non-significant decreases in systolic blood pressure and mean arterial pressure. These changes were associated with relative increases in tongue *Haemophilus* species and *Streptococcus* species, which are nitrate and nitrite reducers, respectively. The change in the microbiome had not previously been demonstrated but later Koopman et al. [38] used a saliva inoculum from two human donors to create microcosms in the multiplaque artificial mouth (MAM) biofilm model system and to examine the effect of nitrate supplementation on the resultant microcosms. For one donor, *Neisseria* were associated with the nitrate-treated microcosms whereas *Veillonella* was more associated with nitrate treatment in the microcosms from the other donor. As both these genera seem to be missing from the rat tongue microbiome and this human study used saliva, it is difficult to draw a conclusion from a comparison of these experiments.

Chlorhexidine can abolish the effect of sodium nitrate supplementation [34,40–42] and Hyde et al. [39,43] showed that its use as a mouth rinse in rats decreased *Haemophilus, Aggregaterbacter,* and *Micrococcaceae* but increased *Enterobacteriaceae, Corynebacterium* and *Morganella* with the overall effect being an increase in diversity through a change in low abundance taxa in the baseline samples. Unfortunately, the chlorhexidine oral rinse did not change the blood pressure or heart rate measures as expected and the authors concluded that it did not remain in the mouth for long enough to exert the intended effect.

Recently, attention has turned towards responses in a wider range of donors. Vanhatalo et al. [43] examined the oral microbiome in young and old healthy donors and the response of these microbiomes to supplementation using a crossover design with either a high nitrate beetroot drink or placebo nitrate depleted over 10 days each. The supplementation of the high nitrate beetroot juice increased plasma nitrate to a similar extent whereas nitrite increases were greater for older participants. Mean arterial pressure, systolic blood pressure and diastolic blood pressure all showed a greater decrease with age and nitrite dose. Overall, they showed high quantities of *Fusobacterium nucleatum nucleatum, Prevotella melaninogenica, Campylobacter concisus, Leptotrichia buccalis, Veillonella parvula, Prevotella intermedia, Fusobacterium nucleatum vincentii* and *Neisseria meningitidis* in the tongue swabs. Changes in the oral microbiome were assessed in saliva samples before and after nitrate supplementation: supplementation changed the oral microbial communities but age did not and diversity was similar across the categories. Fifty-two taxonomic units were significantly changed with supplementation: *Veillonella* and *Prevotella* decreased, whereas *Neisseria* increased and there was no observed change in *Campylobacter* or *Haemophilus*. Burleigh et al. [44] studied the effect of nitrate-rich beetroot juice or nitrate-depleted placebo supplementation on the tongue microbiome and how the altered microbiome responded to an acute dose of nitrate. As seen before, there were decreases in *Prevotella, Streptococcus* and *Actinomyces* and an increase in *Neisseria* with supplementation. For the acute dose, saliva and plasma nitrate and nitrite were measured 1.5 h and 2.5 h, respectively, after nitrate consumption both before and after 7 days of supplementation. At both time points, there was an increase in nitrate and nitrite in both compartments but the alteration of the microbiome by 7 days of beetroot juice consumption did not alter the maximal nitrite and nitrate concentrations after the acute dose. The authors suggest that excess nitrite may be rapidly excreted to prevent excessive drops in blood pressure, or that the change in the nitrate/nitrite-reducing genera (*Prevotella* and *Actinomyces*) may balance the overall capacity of the system.

Kapil et al. [45] explored the influence of gender on nitrate reduction and the oral microbiota. Female participants had higher saliva, plasma and urine nitrite levels than males, and after supplementation with inorganic nitrate they showed a greater increase in plasma nitrate. However, there was no difference between the composition of the salivary microbiota of male and female participants. Ashworth et al. [46] considered the difference in the oral microbiome and dietary intake of inorganic nitrate between vegetarians and omnivores, as previously it was suggested that vegetarian diets are associated with lower blood pressure [47] and this is associated with higher nitrate intake [48]. By using dietary questionnaires, they demonstrated no difference in the consumption of nitrate and that saliva and plasma levels of nitrate and nitrite were similar between the two groups. The oral microbiome was similar between the two groups. The authors also administered a chlorhexidine mouth rinse intervention for 7 days and this caused a decrease in diversity in both groups and a drop in nitrate-reducing bacteria in both groups. Thus, this study suggested no differences in macrodiet and oral microbiome. This is in contrast to previous studies [49–51] which could be due to differences in the individuals examined across studies.

Tribble et al. [52] described the effect of tongue cleaning on the tongue microbiome and nitrate levels. Tongue cleaning is a technique that has been used for the removal of oral malodor or halitosis that is often ascribed to the tongue coating [53]. In this study, orally and systemically healthy oral health professionals were followed over the course of eleven days during which samples (tongue scrapings and saliva) were taken at baseline, at 7 days after use of the chlorhexidine mouth rinse and after a further 3 and 7 days after recovery from use of the mouth rinse. Chlorhexidine caused an increase in systolic blood pressure in the range of 5 mm/Hg which is equivalent to manipulation of dietary salt intake [54], however the donors were also stratified by the frequency of tongue cleaning as either none, once or twice per day. For those participants cleaning their tongue twice per day, there was the greatest increase in systolic blood pressure after the use of chlorhexidine. When examining the tongue microflora, the most common operational taxonomic unit was *Haemophilus parainfluenzae* and the second *Neisseria subflava*. However, the most common genus changed between individuals with groups of *Neisseria*, *Prevotella* and *Leptotrichia* as the most common. The frequency of tongue cleaning changed the abundance of species found: for example, *Leptotrichia spp* were detected in higher abundance on tongues that were not cleaned and daily cleaning (either once or twice) increased the abundance of *H. parainfluenzae* found. This showed that the tongue microbiome when tongue cleaning was implemented has a greater nitrate reductase capability. However, chlorhexidine treatment did not cause large-scale changes in the microbiome community. Further exploration suggested that any changes that occur are transient, with the recovery phase being associated with an increase in bacterial metabolic activity.

Box 1: Definitions:

- 16S rRNA is part of the bacterial ribosome, assigning structural scaffolding, and is of interest in the phylogenetic assignment of bacteria due to its slow rate of evolution.
- OTUs (operational taxonomic units) group together closely related individuals when individuals cannot be distinguished by the data available.
- Biofilms are embedded collections of microorganisms growing together in a matrix of extracellular polymeric substances on a surface.
- Next generation sequencing describes a wide range of DNA sequencing technologies capable of sequencing millions of fragments of DNA in parallel.
- Whole genome analysis sequences the whole of one or more genomes rather than a single gene, as with 16S rRNA analysis.
- Microbiome defines all of the microbial genomes in a given sample or environment.
- Microbiota defines the entire microbial flora in a given sample or environment.
- Principal coordinate analysis (PCoA) is a multivariate statistical technique used to reduce dimensions in data analysis and allowed for representation of the data visually.

4. Concluding Remarks

Overall, these next generation sequencing studies have demonstrated that there are nitrate and nitrite-reducing bacteria found in the mouth and that their removal through mouth rinsing with chlorhexidine will cause a temporary increase in blood pressure. The microbes most often found in the studies were from *Actinomyces*, *Haemophilus*, *Neisseria* and *Veillonella* genera. Samples have been from the tongue dorsum, where nitrate-reducing species were first identified, and also in saliva which may be easier to collect. The microbiomes of these two compartments are distinct but closely related. Furthermore, saliva indeed bathes the tongue, thereby enabling that microbiome to be sampled. More recent studies are just beginning to report [43–46,52] on how the microbiota in both the tongue dorsum and saliva change with different conditions, as previously only samples from homogeneous and healthy donors have been described. The number of donors in each study is also rising, helped by decreases in the costs of these types of experiments, which will help to gain more generalizable data and data that may reveal more subtle nuances between diseases types, ethnicities and other characteristics. This review has highlighted the role of the oral microbiota in the conversion of nitrate to nitrite and its importance to systemic balance. Understanding more about the role that the oral microbiota can play will enable future interventions that may aid with a stratified medicine approach that may rely more on bolstering the useful oral microflora and potentially reduce the use of antimicrobials.

Author Contributions: M.M.G. and D.J. Writing—Original draft, review and editing.

References

1. Deo, PN.; Deshmukh, R. Oral microbiome: Unveiling the fundamentals. *J. Oral Maxillofac. Pathol.* **2019**, *23*, 122–128. [PubMed]
2. Chen, J.; Domingue, J.C.; Sears, C.L. Microbiota dysbiosis in select human cancers: Evidence of association and causality. *Semin. Immunol.* **2017**, *32*, 25–34. [CrossRef] [PubMed]
3. Dominy, S.S.; Lynch, C.; Ermini, F.; Benedyk, M.; Marczyk, A.; Konradi, A.; Nguyen, M.; Haditsch, U.; Raha, D.; Griffin, C.; et al. Porphyromonas gingivalis in Alzheimer's disease brains: Evidence for disease causation and treatment with small-molecule inhibitors. *Sci. Adv.* **2019**, *5*, eaau3333. [CrossRef] [PubMed]
4. Hyde, E.R.; Andrade, F.; Vaksman, Z.; Parthasarathy, K.; Jiang, H.; Parthasarathy, D.K.; Torregrossa, A.C.; Tribble, G.; Kaplan, H.B.; Petrosino, J.F.; et al. Metagenomic analysis of nitrate-reducing bacteria in the oral cavity: Implications for nitric oxide homeostasis. *PLoS ONE* **2014**, *9*, e88645. [CrossRef] [PubMed]
5. Desvarieux, M.; Demmer, R.T.; Rundek, T.; Boden-Albala, B.; Jacobs, D.R., Jr.; Sacco, R.L.; Papapanou, P.N. Periodontal microbiota and carotid intima-media thickness: The Oral Infections and Vascular Disease Epidemiology Study (INVEST). *Circulation* **2005**, *111*, 576–582. [CrossRef] [PubMed]
6. Timmis, A.; Townsend, N.; Gale, C.; Grobbee, R.; Maniadakis, N.; Flather, M.; Wilkins, E.; Wright, L.; Vos, R.; Bax, J.; et al. European Society of Cardiology: Cardiovascular Disease Statistics 2017. *Eur. Heart J.* **2018**, *39*, 508–579. [CrossRef]
7. Lawes, C.M.; Vander Hoorn, S.; Rodgers, A.; for the International Society of Hypertension. Global burden of blood-pressure-related disease, 2001. *Lancet* **2008**, *371*, 1513–1518. [CrossRef]
8. Group, S.R.; Wright, J.T., Jr.; Williamson, J.D.; Whelton, P.K.; Snyder, J.K.; Sink, K.M.; Rocco, M.V.; Reboussin, D.M.; Rahman, M.; Oparil, S.; et al. A Randomized Trial of Intensive versus Standard Blood-Pressure Control. *N. Engl. J. Med.* **2015**, *373*, 2103–2116. [CrossRef]
9. Radomski, M.W.; Palmer, R.M.; Moncada, S. An L-arginine/nitric oxide pathway present in human platelets regulates aggregation. *Proc. Natl. Acad. Sci. USA* **1990**, *87*, 5193–5197. [CrossRef]
10. Furchgott, R.F. The 1996 Albert Lasker Medical Research Awards. The discovery of endothelium-derived relaxing factor and its importance in the identification of nitric oxide. *JAMA* **1996**, *276*, 1186–1188. [CrossRef]
11. Furchgott, R.F.; Zawadzki, J.V. The obligatory role of endothelial cells in the relaxation of arterial smooth muscle by acetylcholine. *Nature* **1980**, *288*, 373–376. [CrossRef] [PubMed]
12. Gryglewski, R.J.; Palmer, R.M.; Moncada, S. Superoxide anion is involved in the breakdown of endothelium-derived vascular relaxing factor. *Nature* **1986**, *320*, 454–456. [CrossRef] [PubMed]
13. Moncada, S.; Palmer, R.M.; Gryglewski, R.J. Mechanism of action of some inhibitors of endothelium-derived relaxing factor. *Proc. Natl. Acad. Sci. USA* **1986**, *83*, 9164–9168. [CrossRef] [PubMed]
14. Ignarro, L.J.; Buga, G.M.; Wood, K.S.; Byrns, R.E.; Chaudhuri, G. Endothelium-derived relaxing factor produced and released from artery and vein is nitric oxide. *Proc. Natl. Acad. Sci. USA* **1987**, *84*, 9265–9269. [CrossRef] [PubMed]
15. Hibbs, J.B., Jr.; Taintor, R.R.; Vavrin, Z. Macrophage cytotoxicity: Role for L-arginine deiminase and imino nitrogen oxidation to nitrite. *Science* **1987**, *235*, 473–476. [CrossRef] [PubMed]
16. Iyengar, R.; Stuehr, D.J.; Marletta, M.A. Macrophage synthesis of nitrite, nitrate, and N-nitrosamines: Precursors and role of the respiratory burst. *Proc. Natl. Acad. Sci. USA* **1987**, *84*, 6369–6373. [CrossRef]
17. Moncada, S.; Palmer, R.M.; Higgs, E.A. Nitric oxide: Physiology, pathophysiology, and pharmacology. *Pharmacol. Rev.* **1991**, *43*, 109–142.
18. Moncada, S.; Higgs, E.A. The discovery of nitric oxide and its role in vascular biology. *Br. J. Pharmacol.* **2006**, *147* (Suppl. 1), S193–S201. [CrossRef]
19. Kuhlencordt, P.J.; Gyurko, R.; Han, F.; Scherrer-Crosbie, M.; Aretz, T.H.; Hajjar, R.; Picard, M.H.; Huang, P.L. Accelerated atherosclerosis, aortic aneurysm formation, and ischemic heart disease in apolipoprotein E/endothelial nitric oxide synthase double-knockout mice. *Circulation* **2001**, *104*, 448–454. [CrossRef]
20. Gimbrone, M.A., Jr.; Garcia-Cardena, G. Endothelial Cell Dysfunction and the Pathobiology of Atherosclerosis. *Circ. Res.* **2016**, *118*, 620–636. [CrossRef]

21. Ludmer, P.L.; Selwyn, A.P.; Shook, T.L.; Wayne, R.R.; Mudge, G.H.; Alexander, R.W.; Ganz, P. Paradoxical vasoconstriction induced by acetylcholine in atherosclerotic coronary arteries. *N. Engl. J. Med.* **1986**, *315*, 1046–1051. [CrossRef] [PubMed]
22. Yeboah, J.; Crouse, J.R.; Hsu, F.C.; Burke, G.L.; Herrington, D.M. Brachial flow-mediated dilation predicts incident cardiovascular events in older adults: The Cardiovascular Health Study. *Circulation* **2007**, *115*, 2390–2397. [CrossRef] [PubMed]
23. Celermajer, D.S.; Sorensen, K.E.; Gooch, V.M.; Spiegelhalter, D.J.; Miller, O.I.; Sullivan, I.D.; Lloyd, J.K.; Deanfield, J.E. Non-invasive detection of endothelial dysfunction in children and adults at risk of atherosclerosis. *Lancet* **1992**, *340*, 1111–1115. [CrossRef]
24. Atkins, G.B.; Simon, D.I. Interplay between NF-kappaB and Kruppel-like factors in vascular inflammation and atherosclerosis: Location, location, location. *J. Am. Heart Assoc.* **2013**, *2*, e000290. [CrossRef] [PubMed]
25. Davies, P.F.; Civelek, M.; Fang, Y.; Fleming, I. The atherosusceptible endothelium: Endothelial phenotypes in complex haemodynamic shear stress regions in vivo. *Cardiovasc. Res.* **2013**, *99*, 315–327. [CrossRef]
26. SenBanerjee, S.; Lin, Z.; Atkins, G.B.; Greif, D.M.; Rao, R.M.; Kumar, A.; Feinberg, M.W.; Chen, Z.; Simon, D.I.; Luscinskas, F.W.; et al. KLF2 Is a novel transcriptional regulator of endothelial proinflammatory activation. *J. Exp. Med.* **2004**, *199*, 1305–1315. [CrossRef]
27. Hamik, A.; Lin, Z.; Kumar, A.; Balcells, M.; Sinha, S.; Katz, J.; Feinberg, M.W.; Gerzsten, R.E.; Edelman, E.R.; Jain, M.K. Kruppel-like factor 4 regulates endothelial inflammation. *J. Biol. Chem.* **2007**, *282*, 13769–13779. [CrossRef]
28. Lin, Z.; Kumar, A.; SenBanerjee, S.; Staniszewski, K.; Parmar, K.; Vaughan, D.E.; Gimbrone, M.A., Jr.; Balasubramanian, V.; Garcia-Cardena, G.; Jain, M.K. Kruppel-like factor 2 (KLF2) regulates endothelial thrombotic function. *Circ. Res.* **2005**, *96*, e48–e57. [CrossRef]
29. Parmar, K.M.; Nambudiri, V.; Dai, G.; Larman, H.B.; Gimbrone, M.A., Jr.; Garcia-Cardena, G. Statins exert endothelial atheroprotective effects via the KLF2 transcription factor. *J. Biol. Chem.* **2005**, *280*, 26714–26719. [CrossRef]
30. Forstermann, U.; Xia, N.; Li, H. Roles of Vascular Oxidative Stress and Nitric Oxide in the Pathogenesis of Atherosclerosis. *Circ. Res.* **2017**, *120*, 713–735. [CrossRef]
31. Benjamin, N.; O'Driscoll, F.; Dougall, H.; Duncan, C.; Smith, L.; Golden, M.; McKenzie, H. Stomach NO synthesis. *Nature* **1994**, *368*, 502. [CrossRef] [PubMed]
32. Lundberg, J.O.; Weitzberg, E.; Lundberg, J.M.; Alving, K. Intragastric nitric oxide production in humans: Measurements in expelled air. *Gut* **1994**, *35*, 1543–1546. [CrossRef] [PubMed]
33. Zweier, J.L.; Wang, P.; Samouilov, A.; Kuppusamy, P. Enzyme-independent formation of nitric oxide in biological tissues. *Nat. Med.* **1995**, *1*, 804–809. [CrossRef] [PubMed]
34. Webb, A.J.; Patel, N.; Loukogeorgakis, S.; Okorie, M.; Aboud, Z.; Misra, S.; Rashid, R.; Miall, P.; Deanfield, J.; Benjamin, N.; et al. Acute blood pressure lowering, vasoprotective, and antiplatelet properties of dietary nitrate via bioconversion to nitrite. *Hypertension* **2008**, *51*, 784–790. [CrossRef] [PubMed]
35. Reimer, R.J. SLC17: A functionally diverse family of organic anion transporters. *Mol. Aspects Med.* **2013**, *34*, 350–359. [CrossRef] [PubMed]
36. Doel, J.J.; Benjamin, N.; Hector, M.P.; Rogers, M.; Allaker, R.P. Evaluation of bacterial nitrate reduction in the human oral cavity. *Eur. J. Oral Sci.* **2005**, *113*, 14–19. [CrossRef]
37. The Human Microbiome Project Consortium. Structure, function and diversity of the healthy human microbiome. *Nature* **2012**, *486*, 207–214. [CrossRef]
38. Koopman, J.E.; Buijs, M.J.; Brandt, B.W.; Keijser, B.J.; Crielaard, W.; Zaura, E. Nitrate and the Origin of Saliva Influence Composition and Short Chain Fatty Acid Production of Oral Microcosms. *Microb. Ecol.* **2016**, *72*, 479–492. [CrossRef]
39. Hyde, E.R.; Luk, B.; Cron, S.; Kusic, L.; McCue, T.; Bauch, T.; Kaplan, H.; Tribble, G.; Petrosino, J.F.; Bryan, N.S. Characterization of the rat oral microbiome and the effects of dietary nitrate. *Free Radic. Biol. Med.* **2014**, *77*, 249–257. [CrossRef]
40. Kapil, V.; Haydar, S.M.; Pearl, V.; Lundberg, J.O.; Weitzberg, E.; Ahluwalia, A. Physiological role for nitrate-reducing oral bacteria in blood pressure control. *Free Radic. Biol. Med.* **2013**, *55*, 93–100. [CrossRef]
41. Bondonno, C.P.; Liu, A.H.; Croft, K.D.; Considine, M.J.; Puddey, I.B.; Woodman, R.J.; Hodgson, J.M. Antibacterial mouthwash blunts oral nitrate reduction and increases blood pressure in treated hypertensive men and women. *Am. J. Hypertens.* **2015**, *28*, 572–575. [CrossRef] [PubMed]

42. Govoni, M.; Jansson, E.A.; Weitzberg, E.; Lundberg, J.O. The increase in plasma nitrite after a dietary nitrate load is markedly attenuated by an antibacterial mouthwash. *Nitric Oxide* **2008**, *19*, 333–337. [CrossRef] [PubMed]
43. Vanhatalo, A.; Blackwell, J.R.; L'Heureux, J.E.; Williams, D.W.; Smith, A.; van der Giezen, M.; Winyard, P.G.; Kelly, J.; Jones, A.M. Nitrate-responsive oral microbiome modulates nitric oxide homeostasis and blood pressure in humans. *Free Radic. Biol. Med.* **2018**, *124*, 21–30. [CrossRef] [PubMed]
44. Burleigh, M.; Liddle, L.; Muggeridge, D.J.; Monaghan, C.; Sculthorpe, N.; Butcher, J.; Henriquez, F.; Easton, C. Dietary nitrate supplementation alters the oral microbiome but does not improve the vascular responses to an acute nitrate dose. *Nitric Oxide* **2019**, *89*, 54–63. [CrossRef] [PubMed]
45. Kapil, V.; Rathod, K.S.; Khambata, R.S.; Bahra, M.; Velmurugan, S.; Purba, A.; Watson, D.S.; Barnes, M.R.; Wade, W.G.; Ahluwalia, A. Sex differences in the nitrate-nitrite-NO(*) pathway: Role of oral nitrate-reducing bacteria. *Free Radic. Biol. Med.* **2018**, *126*, 113–121. [CrossRef] [PubMed]
46. Ashworth, A.; Cutler, C.; Farnham, G.; Liddle, L.; Burleigh, M.; Rodiles, A.; Sillitti, C.; Kiernan, M.; Moore, M.; Hickson, M.; et al. Dietary intake of inorganic nitrate in vegetarians and omnivores and its impact on blood pressure, resting metabolic rate and the oral microbiome. *Free Radic. Biol. Med.* **2019**, *138*, 63–72. [CrossRef] [PubMed]
47. Yokoyama, Y.; Nishimura, K.; Barnard, N.D.; Takegami, M.; Watanabe, M.; Sekikawa, A.; Okamura, T.; Miyamoto, Y. Vegetarian diets and blood pressure: A meta-analysis. *JAMA Intern. Med.* **2014**, *174*, 577–587. [CrossRef]
48. Hord, N.G.; Tang, Y.; Bryan, N.S. Food sources of nitrates and nitrites: The physiologic context for potential health benefits. *Am. J. Clin. Nutr.* **2009**, *90*, 1–10. [CrossRef]
49. Mitek, M.; Anyzewska, A.; Wawrzyniak, A. Estimated dietary intakes of nitrates in vegetarians compared to a traditional diet in Poland and acceptable daily intakes: Is there a risk? *Rocz. Panstw. Zakl. Hig.* **2013**, *64*, 105–109.
50. De Filippis, F.; Vannini, L.; La Storia, A.; Laghi, L.; Piombino, P.; Stellato, G.; Serrazanetti, D.I.; Gozzi, G.; Turroni, S.; Ferrocino, I.; et al. The same microbiota and a potentially discriminant metabolome in the saliva of omnivore, ovo-lacto-vegetarian and Vegan individuals. *PLoS ONE* **2014**, *9*, e112373. [CrossRef]
51. Hansen, T.H.; Kern, T.; Bak, E.G.; Kashani, A.; Allin, K.H.; Nielsen, T.; Hansen, T.; Pedersen, O. Impact of a vegan diet on the human salivary microbiota. *Sci. Rep.* **2018**, *8*, 5847. [CrossRef] [PubMed]
52. Tribble, G.D.; Angelov, N.; Weltman, R.; Wang, B.Y.; Eswaran, S.V.; Gay, I.C.; Parthasarathy, K.; Dao, D.V.; Richardson, K.N.; Ismail, N.M.; et al. Frequency of Tongue Cleaning Impacts the Human Tongue Microbiome Composition and Enterosalivary Circulation of Nitrate. *Front. Cell. Infect. Microbiol.* **2019**, *9*, 39. [CrossRef] [PubMed]
53. Quirynen, M.; Dadamio, J.; Van den Velde, S.; De Smit, M.; Dekeyser, C.; Van Tornout, M.; Vandekerckhove, B. Characteristics of 2000 patients who visited a halitosis clinic. *J. Clin. Periodontol.* **2009**, *36*, 970–975. [CrossRef] [PubMed]
54. Graudal, N.A.; Hubeck-Graudal, T.; Jurgens, G. Effects of low sodium diet versus high sodium diet on blood pressure, renin, aldosterone, catecholamines, cholesterol, and triglyceride. *Cochrane Database Syst. Rev.* **2017**, *4*, CD004022. [CrossRef] [PubMed]

17

Tools of *Aggregatibacter actinomycetemcomitans* to Evade the Host Response

Jan Oscarsson [1], Rolf Claesson [1], Mark Lindholm [1], Carola Höglund Åberg [2] and Anders Johansson [2,*]

1 Department of Odontology, Oral Microbiology, Umeå University, S-90187 Umeå, Sweden
2 Department of Odontology, Molecular Periodontology, Umeå University, S-901 87 Umeå, Sweden
* Correspondence: anders.p.johansson@umu.se

Abstract: Periodontitis is an infection-induced inflammatory disease that affects the tooth supporting tissues, i.e., bone and connective tissues. The initiation and progression of this disease depend on dysbiotic ecological changes in the oral microbiome, thereby affecting the severity of disease through multiple immune-inflammatory responses. *Aggregatibacter actinomycetemcomitans* is a facultative anaerobic Gram-negative bacterium associated with such cellular and molecular mechanisms associated with the pathogenesis of periodontitis. In the present review, we outline virulence mechanisms that help the bacterium to escape the host response. These properties include invasiveness, secretion of exotoxins, serum resistance, and release of outer membrane vesicles. Virulence properties of *A. actinomycetemcomitans* that can contribute to treatment resistance in the infected individuals and upon translocation to the circulation, also induce pathogenic mechanisms associated with several systemic diseases.

Keywords: *Aggregatibacter actinomycetemcomitans*; invasiveness; leukotoxin; cytolethal distending toxin; serum resistance; outer membrane vesicles

---

1. Introduction

Aggregatibacter actinomycetemcomitans is an opportunistic pathogen associated with aggressive forms of periodontitis that affect young individuals [1,2]. The bacterium colonizes the oral mucosa early in life and is inherited by vertical transmission from close relatives [3]. Colonization of *A. actinomycetemcomitans* on the mucosa is not associated with disease but is considered as a risk factor for translocation of the organism to the gingival margin [4]. Bacteria that colonize this ecological niche have the potential to initiate periodontal diseases if they are allowed to stay, proliferate, and express virulence factors [5,6]. *A. actinomycetemcomitans* is a facultative anaerobic Gram-negative bacterium with the capacity to produce a number of virulence factors, and it exhibits a large genetic diversity [2,7]. This bacterium is an early colonizer in the disease process, and resists oxygen and hydrogen peroxide, but is later often replaced by more strict anaerobes in the deep periodontal pocket [1]. In addition to colonizing the oral cavity, systemic translocation of this bacterium is frequently reported [8,9]. *A. actinomycetemcomitans* expresses adhesins that allow colonization of to the tooth surface and the oral epithelium, as well as to mature supragingival plaque [2]. The bacterium is described as an organism that utilizes the other inhabitants in the biofilm for its survival and utilizes metabolic products from other inhabitants of the biofilm for survival and growth [1]. In addition, it is suggested that *A. actinomycetemcomitans* can promote the overgrowth of other bacterial species, which can result in local host dysbiosis and susceptibility to infection [1]. The association of *A. actinomycetemcomitans* to systemic diseases includes endocarditis, cardiovascular diseases, diabetes, Alzheimer´s disease, and rheumatoid arthritis [10–15]. The mechanisms behind these associations are not known, but several virulence properties of *A. actinomycetemcomitans*, such as tissue invasiveness, exotoxin production, serum resistance, and outer membrane vesicle secretion are potential weapons [16–19]. In the sections below, we will further address and discuss the tools behind the ability of this bacterium to evade and suppress the host immune response. The aim of the present review is to identify and describe virulence mechanisms of *A. actinomycetemcomitans*, which are associated with immune subversion, as well as bacterial pathogenicity.

2. Invasive Properties

Invasion of periodontal tissues by different bacterial species has been reported in human periodontitis for several decades [20–22]. The study by Saglie and co-workers [22] observed the prevalence and gingival localization of *A. actinomycetemcomitans* in periodontal lesions of young patients. Transmission electron microscopic examination showed microcolonies of small Gram-negative rods in the connective tissue, as well as single bacterial cells between collagen fibers and in areas of cell debris [20]. In addition to these intra-tissue bacterial cells, bacteria were also found within phagocytic cells, which had invaded the gingival connective tissue. More recent studies have demonstrated invasion of *A. actinomycetemcomitans* into epithelial cells in vitro [23–25]. Interestingly, some *A. actinomycetemcomitans* genotypes have been suggested to have different tissue invasive-properties [23]. If this difference in invasive properties interferes with the ability of *A. actinomycetemcomitans* to cause various periodontal or systemic diseases is not known.

A number of *A. actinomycetemcomitans* factors that likely contribute to host cell invasion have been elucidated. These include the *tad* (tight adherence) gene locus, which mediates adhesion and is required for virulence in a rat model for periodontal disease [26]. OmpA1 (also known as Omp29) is associated with the entry of *A. actinomycetemcomitans* into gingival epithelial cells by up-regulating F-actin rearrangement via the FAK signaling pathway [27], and Omp100 (also known as ApiA) promotes adhesion of *A. actinomycetemcomitans* cells, and their invasion of human gingival keratinocytes [28,29]. It has also been described that bacteria that express a cytolethal distending toxin, such as *A. actinomycetemcomitans,* can cause disruption of the epithelial barrier and promote tissue invasion [30]. A role of *A. actinomycetemcomitans* invasion in immune modulation is supported by in vitro evidence of a subsequent induction of pro-inflammatory cytokine production, and/or apoptosis, in epithelial cells and macrophage-like cells, respectively [31,32].

Severe extra-oral infections caused by *A. actinomycetemcomitans* include brain abscesses, meningitis, septicemia, urinary tract infections, osteomyelitis, and endocarditis [18,33–35]. Whether the systemic translocation through the epithelial barrier is due to an active invasive process, or a result of a passive leakage into the blood stream is not known [36,37]. Bacterial invasion of the periodontal tissues has been suggested as a relevant stage in the etiopathogenesis of periodontal disease, however, there is insufficient evidence to support or exclude this mechanism as a key step in periodontal disease [38,39]. Despite the lack of conclusive studies, the invasive properties of *A. actinomycetemcomitans* have the potential to help the bacterium to evade mechanical and chemical strategies immune responses, and mechanical or chemical eradication strategies [40] (Figure 1). If these properties of the bacterium contribute to systemic translocation and survival has not yet been studied. Evidently, major reasons for bacteremia caused by oral bacteria such as *A. actinomycetemcomitans* are gingival inflammation and mechanical manipulation [41].

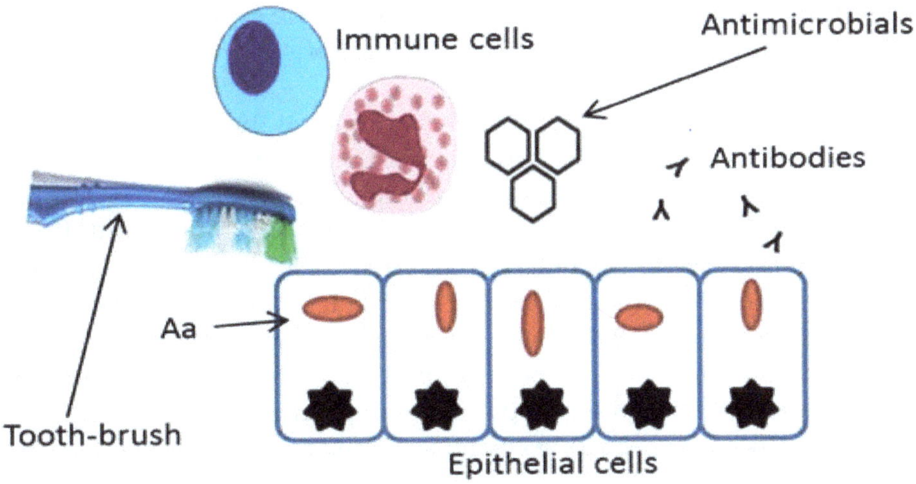

Figure 1. Invasion of *A. actinomycetemcomitans* into epithelial cells can protect the bacterial cells from mechanical removal, antibiotics, immune cell phagocytosis, and antibody binding.

3. Production of Exotoxins

A. actinomycetemcomitans is the only bacterium colonizing the oral cavity known to produce two exotoxins [42,43], leukotoxin (LtxA) that specifically induces killing of human leukocytes, and a cytolethal distending toxin (CDT), which is a genotoxin, causing growth arrest by affecting DNA in proliferating cells [16,44]. Both toxins are highly conserved and occur also in several other Gram-negative pathogens [45,46]. As a sign of the large genetic diversity of *A. actinomycetemcomitans*, there are strains, representing various genotypes, which produce highly different levels of these toxins [2,6,47]. All hitherto studied *A. actinomycetemcomitans* strains carry a complete *ltxCABD* gene locus, encoding for LtxA, activation and secretion [6]. Mutations, i.e., deletions and insertions in the *ltx* promoter region have been shown to influence leukotoxin production in *A. actinomycetemcomitans* [48–50]. The so called JP2 genotype, which harbors a 530-bp deletion in the *ltx* promoter region is well studied, and known to be strongly associated with disease risk in the individuals carrying it [5,6,51]. Its high LtxA production is considered to be an important factor for the enhanced pathogenicity of this genotype [52].

LtxA induces several pathogenic mechanisms in human leukocytes that can all be linked to the progression of periodontal disease [16]. A substantial humoral immune response against LtxA is initiated in all the infected individuals [53,54]. LtxA kills immune cells and protects the bacterium from phagocytic killing [55]. Neutrophils exposed to LtxA activate degranulation, concomitant with an extracellular release of proteolytic enzymes and metalloproteases, such as elastase and metallproteases [56,57]. LtxA can also affect human macrophages by activating the inflammasome complex, which results in the activation and secretion of pro-inflammatory enzymes (i.e., IL-1β and IL-18) [58]. In this context, an interesting observation was recently made that *A. actinomycetemcomitans* expresses an outer membrane lipoprotein, which binds host cytokines, including IL-1β [59]. The IL-1β binding protein was designated bacterial interleukin receptor I (BilRI) and has the ability to internalize IL-1β into the viable bacterial biofilm [60]. Taken together, the abilities of LtxA to cause a proteolytic environment that can degrade immunoproteins, internalize inflammatory proteins, and kill immune cells may all contribute to the survival of *A. actinomycetemcomitans* in the infected host.

The CDT is expressed by a majority of *A. actinomycetemcomitans* genotypes, even though some of them lack a complete gene operon for expression of an active holo-toxin [45]. In vitro and in vivo studies have shown that CDT affects cellular physiology involved in inflammation, immune response modulation, and causes tissue damage [61,62]. The holo-toxin consists of three subunits (CdtA, B, and C) and is transported to the nucleus of the mammalian target cells [63]. Cells exposed for CDT induce a growth arrest followed by apoptotic cell death [44,63]. In cultures of periodontal fibroblasts, CDT induces expression of cytokines and the osteoclast activating protein, receptor activator of nuclear factor kappa-B ligand (RANKL) [64,65]. The role of CDT in the pathogenesis of periodontitis is not entirely clear, and the literature contains studies that demonstrate an association, as well as those reporting no correlation [42,66,67].

Together LtxA and CDT can act as strong weapons against the immune response raised against *A. actinomycetemcomitans*. They can cause an imbalance in the host response by activating inflammation, killing immune cells, affecting antigen presenting cells, and inhibiting lymphocyte proliferation (Figure 2). The impact of these exotoxins in the pathogenesis of periodontal disease is apparent, whereas their role in systemic diseases is not known. However, LtxA-exposed neutrophils do release net-like structures and express patterns of citrullinated proteins that are similar to those observed in synovial fluid from inflamed joints [12,68]. Moreover, antibiotic treatment of a periodontitis patient, infected with the highly leukotoxic JP2 genotype of *A. actinomycetemcomitans*, and suffering from rheumatoid arthritis, was also cured of the joint pain after the treatment [69]. These observations indicate that *A. actinomycetemcomitans* is an interesting organism in the etiopathogenesis of rheumatoid arthritis.

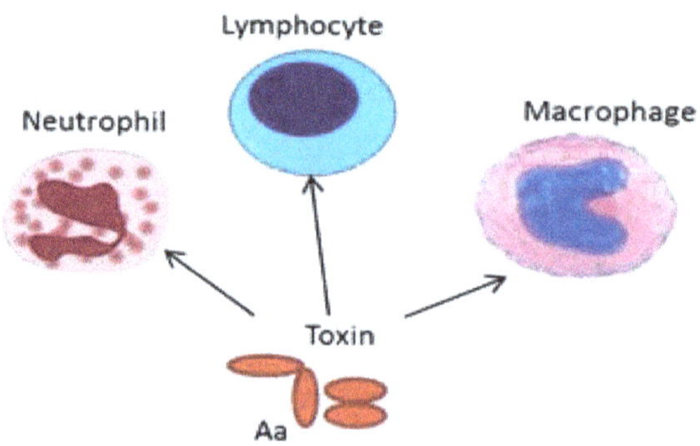

Figure 2. Expression of exotoxins can result in resistance of *A. actinomycetemcomitans* to phagocytosis and neutrophil degranulation. The cytolethal distending toxin (CDT) can cause inhibited proliferation of stimulated lymphocytes, and LtxA induces an inflammatory cell death in the antigen presenting cells, macrophages, and monocytes.

4. Serum Resistance

Serum resistance represents an important virulence factor of bacteria that enter into the bloodstream and cause infection, allowing the bacterial cells to evade the innate immune defense mechanisms present in serum, including the complement system and antimicrobial peptides [70–72]. The recognition of bacterial products mediating serum resistance, therefore, represents an approach to the vaccine and drug development [73,74]. Resistance to complement-mediated killing by human serum appears to be important for *A. actinomycetemcomitans* virulence, and is a common characteristic among strains of this species, although they typically do not form capsules [28,75]. The outer membrane protein, Omp100 (ApiA), was earlier demonstrated to be important for serum resistance in some serotype b and d strains and to physically interact with and trap the alternative complement pathway negative regulator, Factor H, in vitro [28,76] (Figure 3).

Evidently, Omps produced by *A. actinomycetemcomitans* strains are immuno-reactive in the human host [77]. As the presence of antibodies towards bacterial antigens such as Omps is a known trigger of classical complement activation [78], serum resistance of *A. actinomycetemcomitans* strains would be expected to also include mechanisms interacting with this activation. We recently presented evidence that the major outer membrane protein, OmpA1, is critical for serum survival in the *A. actinomycetemcomitans* serotype a model strain, D7SS [17]. Outer membrane integrity may be one mechanism behind OmpA-mediated serum resistance in Gram-negative bacteria [79]. Interestingly, serum resistant *ompA1* mutants were fortuitously obtained, which expressed increased levels of the paralogue, OmpA2. Thus, OmpA2 can apparently operate as a functional homologue to OmpA1 in *A. actinomycetemcomitans*, and both proteins seemingly act, at least partly by binding and trapping of C4-binding protein [17] (Figure 3), which is an inhibitor of classical and mannose-binding lectin (MBL) complement activation [80]. Further to these activation pathways, alternative complement activation is needed to fully eliminate serum-sensitive *ompA* mutant *A. actinomycetemcomitans* derivatives [17]. It is plausible that serum resistance in this species, similar to in *Acinetobacter baumanii* [81], is highly complex and relies on a large number of gene products, including host factors. For example, whether cleavage of the complement molecule C3 by elastase [82], which release is triggered by leukotoxin [57], may contribute to *A. actinomycetemcomitans* serum resistance is not known. Moreover, albeit *A. actinomycetemcomitans* strains are ubiquitously serum resistant, strains not expressing their immunodominant, serotype-specific polysaccharide (S-PA) antigen are occasionally isolated [83]. As speculated previously [83], the lack of S-PA expression may represent a mechanism to evade from antibody-based host responses, which could be advantageous in blood circulation. However, an inconsistency with this notion is that the absence of S-PA expression in *A. actinomycetemcomitans* appears to be scarce.

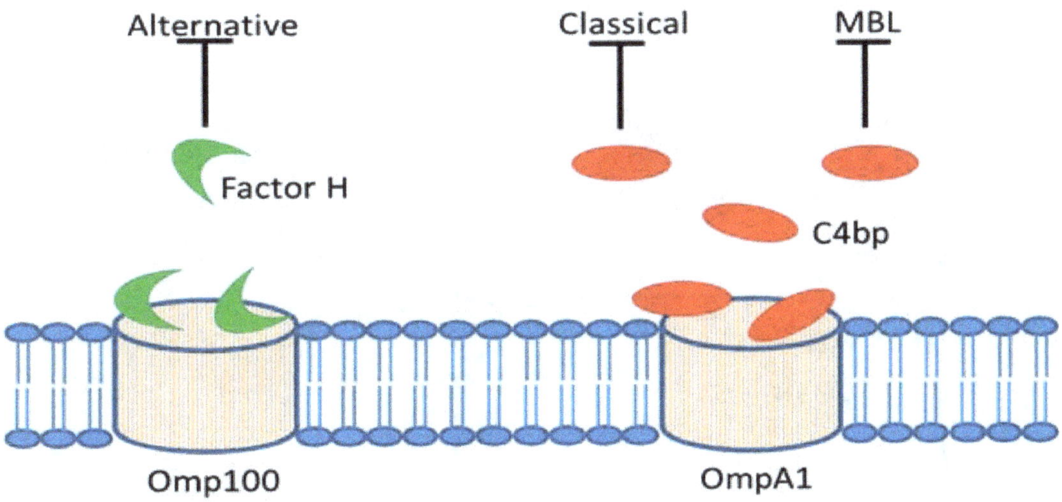

Figure 3. Serum resistance. In vitro evidence supports that *A. actinomycetemcomitans* outer membrane proteins, Omp100 and OmpA1, may allow trapping of soluble repressors of complement activation, i.e., Factor H and C4 binding protein (C4bp), respectively. This would result in downregulation of the alternative, classical, and mannose-binding lectin (MBL) pathway of complement activation.

5. Outer Membrane Vesicles

Outer Membrane Vesicles (OMVs) of Gram-negative bacteria are spherical membrane-enclosed nanostructures that are released from the outer membrane. They can operate as a fundamental mechanism for discharging proteins and additional bacterial components into the surrounding environment and to target host cells [84,85]. Evidence from in vitro experiments shows that *A. actinomycetemcomitans* OMVs can deliver an abundance of biologically active virulence factors to host cells, and which can modulate the immune response (Figure 4).

One such example is CDT, which is delivered into HeLa cells and human gingival fibroblasts via OMVs [86]. OMVs are also involved in the export of LtxA, peptidoglycan-associated lipoprotein (Pal), and the chaperonin GroEL to host cells [87–90]. Proteomics and Western blot analysis of *A. actinomycetemcomitans* OMVs has identified additional proteins that can contribute to evasion of the immune defense, including the IL1β-binding lipoprotein, BilRI, the outer membrane proteins Omp100, OmpA1, and OmpA2, and a Factor H-binding protein homologue [17,91,92]. A functional role in the interaction with complement by vesicles is supported by observations that *A. actinomycetemcomitans* OMVs in an OmpA1-dependent manner can bind to the classical and MBL complement inhibitor, C4-binding protein [17]. It has also been demonstrated that *A. actinomycetemcomitans* OMVs can carry small molecules, including lipopolysaccharide (LPS), which can interact with complement [93]. LPS may also play a role in the observed binding of *A. actinomycetemcomitans* OMVs to IL-8 [94]. Evidence that *A. actinomycetemcomitans* OMVs carry NOD1- and NOD2-active peptidoglycan, which can be internalized into non-phagocytic human cells including gingival fibroblasts [19], reveals a role of the vesicles as a trigger of innate immunity. Moreover, OMV-dependent release of microRNA-size small RNAs (msRNAs), may potentially represent a mechanism to transfer a novel class of bacterial signaling molecules into host cells [95]. It is not completely understood how *A. actinomycetemcomitans* OMVs may physically interact with and/or enter into human host cells to enhance bacterial evasion of the immune defense. The OMVs appear to enter into human cells via clathrin-mediated endocytosis [19,96], but can also fuse with host membranes in a process dependent on cholesterol [86]. Toxins exported via OMVs can function as adhesins in receptor-mediated endocytosis of the vesicles [97], albeit neither CDT nor leukotoxin are required *per se* for the OMV uptake into host cells [86,87]. Concomitantly, although LtxA has an apparent localization on the *A. actinomycetemcomitans* OMV surface, its receptor LFA-1 is not required for delivering the toxin into host cells [98].

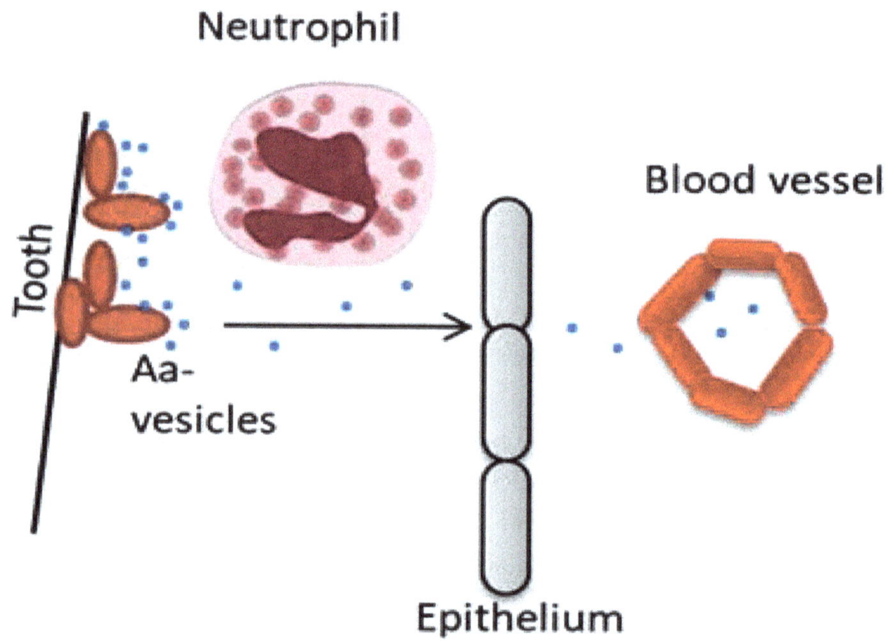

Figure 4. Release of outer membrane vesicles may serve as protection of *A. actinomycetemcomitans* from phagocytic- and serum killing, and also as a means to transport virulence factors to tissues that not are in close contact with the infecting bacteria.

6. Conclusions

We have summarized current knowledge regarding major attributes and strategies of *A. actinomycetemcomitans*, allowing this organism to evade the host response. Without doubt, the numerous virulence properties of *A. actinomycetemcomitans* can be linked to the pathogenesis of periodontal disease [99]. Utilization of these properties for systemic translocation of *A. actinomycetemcomitans* and its subsequent survival in this new environment has been excellently summarized and illustrated [1,100]. It is today hypothesized that the virulence characteristics of *A. actinomycetemcomitans* allow this organism to induce an immune subversion that tip the balance from homeostasis over to disease in oral and/or extra-oral sites [101]. Hence, in order to prohibit the negative systemic consequences that are associated with periodontitis, successful treatment in an early phase of the disease is fundamental. Development of specific diagnostic tools for assessment of periodontal pathogens and inflammatory components in the saliva of young individuals might make it possible to prevent the disease before its onset.

Author Contributions: Conceptualization, A.J., J.O. and, R.C.; writing—original draft preparation, A.J. and, J.O.; writing—review and editing, A.J., J.O., R.C., M.L., and C.H.Å.; funding acquisition, A.J., M.L. and, J.O.; supervision, C.H.Å., R.C., A.J. and, J.O.

References

1. Fine, D.H.; Patil, A.G.; Velusamy, S.K. *Aggregatibacter actinomycetemcomitans* (*Aa*) Under the Radar: Myths and Misunderstandings of *Aa* and Its Role in Aggressive Periodontitis. *Front. Immunol.* **2019**, *10*, 728. [CrossRef] [PubMed]
2. Henderson, B.; Ward, J.M.; Ready, D. *Aggregatibacter* (*Actinobacillus*) *actinomycetemcomitans*: A triple A* periodontopathogen? *Periodontol. 2000* **2010**, *54*, 78–105. [CrossRef] [PubMed]
3. Könönen, E.; Muller, H.P. Microbiology of aggressive periodontitis. *Periodontol. 2000* **2014**, *65*, 46–78. [CrossRef] [PubMed]
4. Höglund Åberg, C.; Kelk, P.; Johansson, A. *Aggregatibacter actinomycetemcomitans*: Virulence of its leukotoxin and association with aggressive periodontitis. *Virulence* **2015**, *6*, 188–195. [CrossRef] [PubMed]
5. Haubek, D.; Ennibi, O.K.; Poulsen, K.; Vaeth, M.; Poulsen, S.; Kilian, M. Risk of aggressive periodontitis in adolescent carriers of the JP2 clone of *Aggregatibacter* (*Actinobacillus*) *actinomycetemcomitans* in Morocco: A prospective longitudinal cohort study. *Lancet* **2008**, *371*, 237–242. [CrossRef]
6. Höglund Åberg, C.; Kwamin, F.; Claesson, R.; Dahlen, G.; Johansson, A.; Haubek, D. Progression of attachment loss is strongly associated with presence of the JP2 genotype of *Aggregatibacter actinomycetemcomitans*: A prospective cohort study of a young adolescent population. *J. Clin. Periodontol.* **2014**, *41*, 232–241. [CrossRef] [PubMed]
7. Kittichotirat, W.; Bumgarner, R.E.; Chen, C. Evolutionary Divergence of *Aggregatibacter actinomycetemcomitans*. *J. Dent. Res.* **2016**, *95*, 94–101. [CrossRef]
8. Paju, S.; Carlson, P.; Jousimies-Somer, H.; Asikainen, S. *Actinobacillus actinomycetemcomitans* and *Haemophilus aphrophilus* in systemic and nonoral infections in Finland. *APMIS* **2003**, *111*, 653–657. [CrossRef]
9. van Winkelhoff, A.J.; Slots, J. *Actinobacillus actinomycetemcomitans* and *Porphyromonas gingivalis* in nonoral infections. *Periodontol. 2000* **1999**, *20*, 122–135. [CrossRef]
10. Demmer, R.T.; Jacobs, D.R., Jr.; Singh, R.; Zuk, A.; Rosenbaum, M.; Papapanou, P.N.; Desvarieux, M. Periodontal Bacteria and Prediabetes Prevalence in ORIGINS: The Oral Infections, Glucose Intolerance, and Insulin Resistance Study. *J. Dent. Res.* **2015**, *94*, 201S–211S. [CrossRef]
11. Diaz-Zuniga, J.; Munoz, Y.; Melgar-Rodriguez, S.; More, J.; Bruna, B.; Lobos, P.; Monasterio, G.; Vernal, R.; Paula-Lima, A. Serotype b of *Aggregatibacter actinomycetemcomitans* triggers pro-inflammatory responses and amyloid beta secretion in hippocampal cells: A novel link between periodontitis and Alzheimer's disease? *J. Oral Microbiol.* **2019**, *11*, 1586423. [CrossRef] [PubMed]
12. Konig, M.F.; Abusleme, L.; Reinholdt, J.; Palmer, R.J.; Teles, R.P.; Sampson, K.; Rosen, A.; Nigrovic, P.A.; Sokolove, J.; Giles, J.T.; et al. *Aggregatibacter actinomycetemcomitans*-induced hypercitrullination links periodontal infection to autoimmunity in rheumatoid arthritis. *Sci. Transl. Med.* **2016**, *8*, 369ra176. [CrossRef] [PubMed]
13. Laugisch, O.; Johnen, A.; Maldonado, A.; Ehmke, B.; Burgin, W.; Olsen, I.; Potempa, J.; Sculean, A.; Duning, T.; Eick, S. Periodontal Pathogens and Associated Intrathecal Antibodies in Early Stages of Alzheimer's Disease. *J. Alzheimers Dis.* **2018**, *66*, 105–114. [CrossRef] [PubMed]
14. Liljestrand, J.M.; Paju, S.; Pietiainen, M.; Buhlin, K.; Persson, G.R.; Nieminen, M.S.; Sinisalo, J.; Mantyla, P.; Pussinen, P.J. Immunologic burden links periodontitis to acute coronary syndrome. *Atherosclerosis* **2018**, *268*, 177–184. [CrossRef] [PubMed]
15. Revest, M.; Egmann, G.; Cattoir, V.; Tattevin, P. HACEK endocarditis: State-of-the-art. *Expert Rev. Anti-Infect. Ther.* **2016**, *14*, 523–530. [CrossRef] [PubMed]
16. Johansson, A. *Aggregatibacter actinomycetemcomitans* leukotoxin: A powerful tool with capacity to cause imbalance in the host inflammatory response. *Toxins* **2011**, *3*, 242–259. [CrossRef] [PubMed]
17. Lindholm, M.; Min Aung, K.; Nyunt Wai, S.; Oscarsson, J. Role of OmpA1 and OmpA2 in *Aggregatibacter actinomycetemcomitans* and *Aggregatibacter aphrophilus* serum resistance. *J. Oral Microbiol.* **2019**, *11*, 1536192. [CrossRef] [PubMed]
18. Raja, M.; Ummer, F.; Dhivakar, C.P. *Aggregatibacter actinomycetemcomitans*—A tooth killer? *J. Clin. Diagn. Res.* **2014**, *8*, ZE13–ZE16. [CrossRef]
19. Thay, B.; Damm, A.; Kufer, T.A.; Wai, S.N.; Oscarsson, J. *Aggregatibacter actinomycetemcomitans* outer membrane vesicles are internalized in human host cells and trigger NOD1- and NOD2-dependent NF-kappaB activation. *Infect. Immun.* **2014**, *82*, 4034–4046. [CrossRef]

20. Christersson, L.A.; Albini, B.; Zambon, J.J.; Wikesjo, U.M.; Genco, R.J. Tissue localization of *Actinobacillus actinomycetemcomitans* in human periodontitis. I. Light, immunofluorescence and electron microscopic studies. *J. Periodontol.* **1987**, *58*, 529–539. [CrossRef]
21. Christersson, L.A.; Wikesjo, U.M.; Albini, B.; Zambon, J.J.; Genco, R.J. Tissue localization of *Actinobacillus actinomycetemcomitans* in human periodontitis. II. Correlation between immunofluorescence and culture techniques. *J. Periodontol.* **1987**, *58*, 540–545. [CrossRef] [PubMed]
22. Saglie, F.R.; Marfany, A.; Camargo, P. Intragingival occurrence of *Actinobacillus actinomycetemcomitans* and *Bacteroides gingivalis* in active destructive periodontal lesions. *J. Periodontol.* **1988**, *59*, 259–265. [CrossRef] [PubMed]
23. Lepine, G.; Caudry, S.; DiRienzo, J.M.; Ellen, R.P. Epithelial cell invasion by *Actinobacillus actinomycetemcomitans* strains from restriction fragment-length polymorphism groups associated with juvenile periodontitis or carrier status. *Oral Microbiol. Immunol.* **1998**, *13*, 341–347. [CrossRef] [PubMed]
24. Meyer, D.H.; Sreenivasan, P.K.; Fives-Taylor, P.M. Evidence for invasion of a human oral cell line by *Actinobacillus actinomycetemcomitans*. *Infect. Immun.* **1991**, *59*, 2719–2726. [PubMed]
25. Meyer, D.H.; Lippmann, J.E.; Fives-Taylor, P.M. Invasion of epithelial cells by *Actinobacillus actinomycetemcomitans*: A dynamic, multistep process. *Infect. Immun.* **1996**, *64*, 2988–2997.
26. Schreiner, H.C.; Sinatra, K.; Kaplan, J.B.; Furgang, D.; Kachlany, S.C.; Planet, P.J.; Perez, B.A.; Figurski, D.H.; Fine, D.H. Tight-adherence genes of *Actinobacillus actinomycetemcomitans* are required for virulence in a rat model. *Proc. Natl. Acad. Sci. USA* **2003**, *100*, 7295–7300. [CrossRef] [PubMed]
27. Kajiya, M.; Komatsuzawa, H.; Papantonakis, A.; Seki, M.; Makihira, S.; Ouhara, K.; Kusumoto, Y.; Murakami, S.; Taubman, M.A.; Kawai, T. *Aggregatibacter actinomycetemcomitans* Omp29 is associated with bacterial entry to gingival epithelial cells by F-actin rearrangement. *PLoS ONE* **2011**, *6*, e18287. [CrossRef]
28. Asakawa, R.; Komatsuzawa, H.; Kawai, T.; Yamada, S.; Goncalves, R.B.; Izumi, S.; Fujiwara, T.; Nakano, Y.; Suzuki, N.; Uchida, Y.; et al. Outer membrane protein 100, a versatile virulence factor of *Actinobacillus actinomycetemcomitans*. *Mol. Microbiol.* **2003**, *50*, 1125–1139. [CrossRef]
29. Yue, G.; Kaplan, J.B.; Furgang, D.; Mansfield, K.G.; Fine, D.H. A second *Aggregatibacter actinomycetemcomitans* autotransporter adhesin exhibits specificity for buccal epithelial cells in humans and Old World primates. *Infect. Immun.* **2007**, *75*, 4440–4448. [CrossRef]
30. DiRienzo, J.M. Breaking the Gingival Epithelial Barrier: Role of the *Aggregatibacter actinomycetemcomitans* Cytolethal Distending Toxin in Oral Infectious Disease. *Cells* **2014**, *3*, 476–499. [CrossRef]
31. Dickinson, B.C.; Moffatt, C.E.; Hagerty, D.; Whitmore, S.E.; Brown, T.A.; Graves, D.T.; Lamont, R.J. Interaction of oral bacteria with gingival epithelial cell multilayers. *Mol. Oral Microbiol.* **2011**, *26*, 210–220. [CrossRef] [PubMed]
32. Okinaga, T.; Ariyoshi, W.; Nishihara, T. *Aggregatibacter actinomycetemcomitans* Invasion Induces Interleukin-1beta Production Through Reactive Oxygen Species and Cathepsin B. *J. Interferon. Cytokine Res.* **2015**, *35*, 431–440. [CrossRef] [PubMed]
33. Rahamat-Langendoen, J.C.; van Vonderen, M.G.; Engstrom, L.J.; Manson, W.L.; van Winkelhoff, A.J.; Mooi-Kokenberg, E.A. Brain abscess associated with *Aggregatibacter actinomycetemcomitans*: Case report and review of literature. *J. Clin. Periodontol.* **2011**, *38*, 702–706. [CrossRef] [PubMed]
34. Stepanovic, S.; Tosic, T.; Savic, B.; Jovanovic, M.; K'Ouas, G.; Carlier, J.P. Brain abscess due to *Actinobacillus actinomycetemcomitans*. *APMIS* **2005**, *113*, 225–228. [CrossRef] [PubMed]
35. Tang, G.; Kitten, T.; Munro, C.L.; Wellman, G.C.; Mintz, K.P. EmaA, a potential virulence determinant of *Aggregatibacter actinomycetemcomitans* in infective endocarditis. *Infect. Immun.* **2008**, *76*, 2316–2324. [CrossRef]
36. Doran, K.S.; Banerjee, A.; Disson, O.; Lecuit, M. Concepts and mechanisms: Crossing host barriers. *Cold Spring Harb. Perspect. Med.* **2013**, *3*. [CrossRef] [PubMed]
37. Ribet, D.; Cossart, P. How bacterial pathogens colonize their hosts and invade deeper tissues. *Microbes Infect.* **2015**, *17*, 173–183. [CrossRef]
38. Ji, S.; Choi, Y.S.; Choi, Y. Bacterial invasion and persistence: Critical events in the pathogenesis of periodontitis? *J. Periodontal Res.* **2015**, *50*, 570–585. [CrossRef]

39. Mendes, L.; Azevedo, N.F.; Felino, A.; Pinto, M.G. Relationship between invasion of the periodontium by periodontal pathogens and periodontal disease: A systematic review. *Virulence* **2015**, *6*, 208–215. [CrossRef]
40. Eick, S.; Pfister, W. Efficacy of antibiotics against periodontopathogenic bacteria within epithelial cells: An in vitro study. *J. Periodontol.* **2004**, *75*, 1327–1334. [CrossRef]
41. Hirschfeld, J.; Kawai, T. Oral inflammation and bacteremia: Implications for chronic and acute systemic diseases involving major organs. *Cardiovasc. Hematol. Disord. Drug Targets* **2015**, *15*, 70–84. [CrossRef] [PubMed]
42. Höglund Åberg, C.; Antonoglou, G.; Haubek, D.; Kwamin, F.; Claesson, R.; Johansson, A. Cytolethal distending toxin in isolates of *Aggregatibacter actinomycetemcomitans* from Ghanaian adolescents and association with serotype and disease progression. *PLoS ONE* **2013**, *8*, e65781. [CrossRef]
43. Höglund Åberg, C.; Haubek, D.; Kwamin, F.; Johansson, A.; Claesson, R. Leukotoxic activity of *Aggregatibacter actinomycetemcomitans* and periodontal attachment loss. *PLoS ONE* **2014**, *9*, e104095. [CrossRef] [PubMed]
44. Belibasakis, G.N.; Mattsson, A.; Wang, Y.; Chen, C.; Johansson, A. Cell cycle arrest of human gingival fibroblasts and periodontal ligament cells by *Actinobacillus actinomycetemcomitans*: Involvement of the cytolethal distending toxin. *APMIS* **2004**, *112*, 674–685. [CrossRef] [PubMed]
45. Fais, T.; Delmas, J.; Serres, A.; Bonnet, R.; Dalmasso, G. Impact of CDT Toxin on Human Diseases. *Toxins* **2016**, *8*, 220. [CrossRef] [PubMed]
46. Linhartova, I.; Bumba, L.; Masin, J.; Basler, M.; Osicka, R.; Kamanova, J.; Prochazkova, K.; Adkins, I.; Hejnova-Holubova, J.; Sadilkova, L.; et al. RTX proteins: A highly diverse family secreted by a common mechanism. *FEMS Microbiol. Rev.* **2010**, *34*, 1076–1112. [CrossRef] [PubMed]
47. Johansson, A.; Claesson, R.; Hoglund Aberg, C.; Haubek, D.; Oscarsson, J. The cagE gene sequence as a diagnostic marker to identify JP2 and non-JP2 highly leukotoxic *Aggregatibacter actinomycetemcomitans* serotype b strains. *J. Periodontal. Res.* **2017**, *52*, 903–912. [CrossRef]
48. Brogan, J.M.; Lally, E.T.; Poulsen, K.; Kilian, M.; Demuth, D.R. Regulation of *Actinobacillus actinomycetemcomitans* leukotoxin expression: Analysis of the promoter regions of leukotoxic and minimally leukotoxic strains. *Infect. Immun.* **1994**, *62*, 501–508.
49. Claesson, R.; Gudmundson, J.; Höglund Åberg, C.; Haubek, D.; Johansson, A. Detection of a 640-bp deletion in the *Aggregatibacter actinomycetemcomitans* leukotoxin promoter region in isolates from an adolescent of Ethiopian origin. *J. Oral Microbiol.* **2015**, *7*, 26974. [CrossRef]
50. He, T.; Hayashi, J.; Yamamoto, M.; Ishikawa, I. Genotypic characterization of *Actinobacillus actinomycetemcomitans* isolated from periodontitis patients by arbitrarily primed polymerase chain reaction. *J. Periodontol.* **1998**, *69*, 69–75. [CrossRef]
51. Ennibi, O.K.; Claesson, R.; Akkaoui, S.; Reddahi, S.; Kwamin, F.; Haubek, D.; Johansson, A. High salivary levels of JP2 genotype of *Aggregatibacter actinomycetemcomitans* is associated with clinical attachment loss in Moroccan adolescents. *Clin. Exp. Dent. Res.* **2019**, *5*, 44–51. [CrossRef] [PubMed]
52. Haubek, D.; Johansson, A. Pathogenicity of the highly leukotoxic JP2 clone of *Aggregatibacter actinomycetemcomitans* and its geographic dissemination and role in aggressive periodontitis. *J. Oral Microbiol.* **2014**, *6*. [CrossRef]
53. Brage, M.; Holmlund, A.; Johansson, A. Humoral immune response to *Aggregatibacter actinomycetemcomitans* leukotoxin. *J. Periodontal. Res.* **2011**, *46*, 170–175. [CrossRef] [PubMed]
54. Johansson, A.; Buhlin, K.; Sorsa, T.; Pussinen, P.J. Systemic *Aggregatibacter actinomycetemcomitans* Leukotoxin-Neutralizing Antibodies in Periodontitis. *J. Periodontol.* **2017**, *88*, 122–129. [CrossRef] [PubMed]
55. Johansson, A.; Sandstrom, G.; Claesson, R.; Hanstrom, L.; Kalfas, S. Anaerobic neutrophil-dependent killing of *Actinobacillus actinomycetemcomitans* in relation to the bacterial leukotoxicity. *Eur. J. Oral Sci.* **2000**, *108*, 136–146. [CrossRef] [PubMed]
56. Claesson, R.; Johansson, A.; Belibasakis, G.; Hanstrom, L.; Kalfas, S. Release and activation of matrix metalloproteinase 8 from human neutrophils triggered by the leukotoxin of *Actinobacillus actinomycetemcomitans*. *J. Periodontal. Res.* **2002**, *37*, 353–359. [CrossRef] [PubMed]
57. Johansson, A.; Claesson, R.; Hänström, L.; Sandström, G.; Kalfas, S. Polymorphonuclear leukocyte degranulation induced by leukotoxin from *Actinobacillus actinomycetemcomitans*. *J. Periodontal. Res.* **2000**, *35*, 85–92. [CrossRef] [PubMed]

58. Kelk, P.; Abd, H.; Claesson, R.; Sandström, G.; Sjöstedt, A.; Johansson, A. Cellular and molecular response of human macrophages exposed to *Aggregatibacter actinomycetemcomitans* leukotoxin. *Cell Death Dis.* **2011**, *2*, e126. [CrossRef]
59. Ahlstrand, T.; Tuominen, H.; Beklen, A.; Torittu, A.; Oscarsson, J.; Sormunen, R.; Pollanen, M.T.; Permi, P.; Ihalin, R. A novel intrinsically disordered outer membrane lipoprotein of *Aggregatibacter actinomycetemcomitans* binds various cytokines and plays a role in biofilm response to interleukin-1beta and interleukin-8. *Virulence* **2017**, *8*, 115–134. [CrossRef]
60. Paino, A.; Ahlstrand, T.; Nuutila, J.; Navickaite, I.; Lahti, M.; Tuominen, H.; Valimaa, H.; Lamminmaki, U.; Pollanen, M.T.; Ihalin, R. Identification of a novel bacterial outer membrane interleukin-1Beta-binding protein from *Aggregatibacter actinomycetemcomitans*. *PLoS ONE* **2013**, *8*, e70509. [CrossRef]
61. Belibasakis, G.N.; Bostanci, N. Inflammatory and bone remodeling responses to the cytolethal distending toxins. *Cells* **2014**, *3*, 236–246. [CrossRef] [PubMed]
62. Kawamoto, D.; Ando-Suguimoto, E.S.; Bueno-Silva, B.; DiRienzo, J.M.; Mayer, M.P. Alteration of Homeostasis in Pre-osteoclasts Induced by *Aggregatibacter actinomycetemcomitans* CDT. *Front. Cell. Infect. Microbiol.* **2016**, *6*, 33. [CrossRef] [PubMed]
63. DiRienzo, J.M. Uptake and processing of the cytolethal distending toxin by mammalian cells. *Toxins* **2014**, *6*, 3098–3116. [CrossRef] [PubMed]
64. Belibasakis, G.N.; Johansson, A.; Wang, Y.; Chen, C.; Kalfas, S.; Lerner, U.H. The cytolethal distending toxin induces receptor activator of NF-kappaB ligand expression in human gingival fibroblasts and periodontal ligament cells. *Infect. Immun.* **2005**, *73*, 342–351. [CrossRef] [PubMed]
65. Belibasakis, G.N.; Johansson, A.; Wang, Y.; Chen, C.; Lagergard, T.; Kalfas, S.; Lerner, U.H. Cytokine responses of human gingival fibroblasts to *Actinobacillus actinomycetemcomitans* cytolethal distending toxin. *Cytokine* **2005**, *30*, 56–63. [CrossRef] [PubMed]
66. Ando, E.S.; De-Gennaro, L.A.; Faveri, M.; Feres, M.; DiRienzo, J.M.; Mayer, M.P. Immune response to cytolethal distending toxin of *Aggregatibacter actinomycetemcomitans* in periodontitis patients. *J. Periodontal. Res.* **2010**, *45*, 471–480. [PubMed]
67. Tan, K.S.; Song, K.P.; Ong, G. Cytolethal distending toxin of *Actinobacillus actinomycetemcomitans*. Occurrence and association with periodontal disease. *J. Periodontal. Res.* **2002**, *37*, 268–272. [CrossRef] [PubMed]
68. Hirschfeld, J.; Roberts, H.M.; Chapple, I.L.; Parcina, M.; Jepsen, S.; Johansson, A.; Claesson, R. Effects of *Aggregatibacter actinomycetemcomitans* leukotoxin on neutrophil migration and extracellular trap formation. *J. Oral Microbiol.* **2016**, *8*, 33070. [CrossRef] [PubMed]
69. Mukherjee, A.; Jantsch, V.; Khan, R.; Hartung, W.; Fischer, R.; Jantsch, J.; Ehrenstein, B.; Konig, M.F.; Andrade, F. Rheumatoid Arthritis-Associated Autoimmunity Due to *Aggregatibacter actinomycetemcomitans* and Its Resolution With Antibiotic Therapy. *Front. Immunol.* **2018**, *9*, 2352. [CrossRef] [PubMed]
70. Abreu, A.G.; Barbosa, A.S. How Escherichia coli Circumvent Complement-Mediated Killing. *Front. Immunol.* **2017**, *8*, 452. [CrossRef] [PubMed]
71. Berends, E.T.; Kuipers, A.; Ravesloot, M.M.; Urbanus, R.T.; Rooijakkers, S.H. Bacteria under stress by complement and coagulation. *FEMS Microbiol. Rev.* **2014**, *38*, 1146–1171. [CrossRef] [PubMed]
72. Hovingh, E.S.; van den Broek, B.; Jongerius, I. Hijacking Complement Regulatory Proteins for Bacterial Immune Evasion. *Front. Microbiol.* **2016**, *7*, 2004. [CrossRef] [PubMed]
73. Jongerius, I.; Schuijt, T.J.; Mooi, F.R.; Pinelli, E. Complement evasion by Bordetella pertussis: Implications for improving current vaccines. *J. Mol. Med.* **2015**, *93*, 395–402. [CrossRef] [PubMed]
74. Vila-Farres, X.; Parra-Millan, R.; Sanchez-Encinales, V.; Varese, M.; Ayerbe-Algaba, R.; Bayo, N.; Guardiola, S.; Pachon-Ibanez, M.E.; Kotev, M.; Garcia, J.; et al. Combating virulence of Gram-negative bacilli by OmpA inhibition. *Sci. Rep.* **2017**, *7*, 14683. [CrossRef] [PubMed]
75. Sundqvist, G.; Johansson, E. Bactericidal effect of pooled human serum on *Bacteroides melaninogenicus*, *Bacteroides asaccharolyticus* and *Actinobacillus actinomycetemcomitans*. *Scand. J. Dent. Res.* **1982**, *90*, 29–36. [CrossRef] [PubMed]
76. Ramsey, M.M.; Whiteley, M. Polymicrobial interactions stimulate resistance to host innate immunity through metabolite perception. *Proc. Natl. Acad. Sci. USA* **2009**, *106*, 1578–1583. [CrossRef] [PubMed]
77. Komatsuzawa, H.; Asakawa, R.; Kawai, T.; Ochiai, K.; Fujiwara, T.; Taubman, M.A.; Ohara, M.; Kurihara, H.; Sugai, M. Identification of six major outer membrane proteins from *Actinobacillus actinomycetemcomitans*. *Gene* **2002**, *288*, 195–201. [CrossRef]

78. Aung, K.M.; Sjostrom, A.E.; von Pawel-Rammingen, U.; Riesbeck, K.; Uhlin, B.E.; Wai, S.N. Naturally Occurring IgG Antibodies Provide Innate Protection against Vibrio cholerae Bacteremia by Recognition of the Outer Membrane Protein U. *J. Innate. Immun.* **2016**, *8*, 269–283. [CrossRef] [PubMed]
79. Confer, A.W.; Ayalew, S. The OmpA family of proteins: Roles in bacterial pathogenesis and immunity. *Vet. Microbiol.* **2013**, *163*, 207–222. [CrossRef]
80. Suankratay, C.; Mold, C.; Zhang, Y.; Lint, T.F.; Gewurz, H. Mechanism of complement-dependent haemolysis via the lectin pathway: Role of the complement regulatory proteins. *Clin. Exp. Immunol.* **1999**, *117*, 442–448. [CrossRef]
81. Sanchez-Larrayoz, A.F.; Elhosseiny, N.M.; Chevrette, M.G.; Fu, Y.; Giunta, P.; Spallanzani, R.G.; Ravi, K.; Pier, G.B.; Lory, S.; Maira-Litran, T. Complexity of Complement Resistance Factors Expressed by Acinetobacter baumannii Needed for Survival in Human Serum. *J. Immunol.* **2017**, *199*, 2803–2814. [CrossRef] [PubMed]
82. Claesson, R.; Kanasi, E.; Johansson, A.; Kalfas, S. A new cleavage site for elastase within the complement component 3. *APMIS* **2010**, *118*, 765–768. [CrossRef] [PubMed]
83. Kanasi, E.; Dogan, B.; Karched, M.; Thay, B.; Oscarsson, J.; Asikainen, S. Lack of serotype antigen in *A. actinomycetemcomitans*. *J. Dent. Res.* **2010**, *89*, 292–296. [CrossRef] [PubMed]
84. Deatherage, B.L.; Cookson, B.T. Membrane vesicle release in bacteria, eukaryotes, and archaea: A conserved yet underappreciated aspect of microbial life. *Infect. Immun.* **2012**, *80*, 1948–1957. [CrossRef] [PubMed]
85. Jan, A.T. Outer Membrane Vesicles (OMVs) of Gram-negative Bacteria: A Perspective Update. *Front. Microbiol.* **2017**, *8*, 1053. [CrossRef] [PubMed]
86. Rompikuntal, P.K.; Thay, B.; Khan, M.K.; Alanko, J.; Penttinen, A.M.; Asikainen, S.; Wai, S.N.; Oscarsson, J. Perinuclear localization of internalized outer membrane vesicles carrying active cytolethal distending toxin from *Aggregatibacter actinomycetemcomitans*. *Infect. Immun.* **2012**, *80*, 31–42. [CrossRef] [PubMed]
87. Demuth, D.R.; James, D.; Kowashi, Y.; Kato, S. Interaction of *Actinobacillus actinomycetemcomitans* outer membrane vesicles with HL60 cells does not require leukotoxin. *Cell Microbiol.* **2003**, *5*, 111–121. [CrossRef] [PubMed]
88. Goulhen, F.; Hafezi, A.; Uitto, V.J.; Hinode, D.; Nakamura, R.; Grenier, D.; Mayrand, D. Subcellular localization and cytotoxic activity of the GroEL-like protein isolated from *Actinobacillus actinomycetemcomitans*. *Infect. Immun.* **1998**, *66*, 5307–5313. [PubMed]
89. Karched, M.; Ihalin, R.; Eneslätt, K.; Zhong, D.; Oscarsson, J.; Wai, S.N.; Chen, C.; Asikainen, S.E. Vesicle-independent extracellular release of a proinflammatory outer membrane lipoprotein in free-soluble form. *BMC Microbiol.* **2008**, *8*, 18. [CrossRef] [PubMed]
90. Kato, S.; Kowashi, Y.; Demuth, D.R. Outer membrane-like vesicles secreted by *Actinobacillus actinomycetemcomitans* are enriched in leukotoxin. *Microb. Pathog.* **2002**, *32*, 1–13. [CrossRef] [PubMed]
91. Kieselbach, T.; Zijnge, V.; Granstrom, E.; Oscarsson, J. Proteomics of *Aggregatibacter actinomycetemcomitans* Outer Membrane Vesicles. *PLoS ONE* **2015**, *10*, e0138591. [CrossRef] [PubMed]
92. Kieselbach, T.; Oscarsson, J. Dataset of the proteome of purified outer membrane vesicles from the human pathogen *Aggregatibacter actinomycetemcomintans*. *Data Brief* **2017**, *10*, 426–431. [CrossRef] [PubMed]
93. Iino, Y.; Hopps, R.M. The bone-resorbing activities in tissue culture of lipopolysaccharides from the bacteria *Actinobacillus actinomycetemcomitans*, *Bacteroides gingivalis* and *Capnocytophaga ochracea* isolated from human mouths. *Arch. Oral Biol.* **1984**, *29*, 59–63. [CrossRef]
94. Ahlstrand, T.; Kovesjoki, L.; Maula, T.; Oscarsson, J.; Ihalin, R. *Aggregatibacter actinomycetemcomitans* LPS binds human interleukin-8. *J. Oral Microbiol.* **2019**, *11*, 1549931. [CrossRef]
95. Choi, J.W.; Kim, S.C.; Hong, S.H.; Lee, H.J. Secretable Small RNAs via Outer Membrane Vesicles in Periodontal Pathogens. *J. Dent. Res.* **2017**, *96*, 458–466. [CrossRef] [PubMed]
96. O'Donoghue, E.J.; Krachler, A.M. Mechanisms of outer membrane vesicle entry into host cells. *Cell Microbiol.* **2016**, *18*, 1508–1517. [CrossRef] [PubMed]
97. Kesty, N.C.; Mason, K.M.; Reedy, M.; Miller, S.E.; Kuehn, M.J. Enterotoxigenic Escherichia coli vesicles target toxin delivery into mammalian cells. *EMBO J.* **2004**, *23*, 4538–4549. [CrossRef] [PubMed]
98. Nice, J.B.; Balashova, N.V.; Kachlany, S.C.; Koufos, E.; Krueger, E.; Lally, E.T.; Brown, A.C. *Aggregatibacter actinomycetemcomitans* Leukotoxin Is Delivered to Host Cells in an LFA-1-Indepdendent Manner When Associated with Outer Membrane Vesicles. *Toxins* **2018**, *10*, 414. [CrossRef] [PubMed]

99. Gholizadeh, P.; Pormohammad, A.; Eslami, H.; Shokouhi, B.; Fakhrzadeh, V.; Kafil, H.S. Oral pathogenesis of *Aggregatibacter actinomycetemcomitans*. *Microb. Pathog.* **2017**, *113*, 303–311. [CrossRef]
100. Hajishengallis, G. Periodontitis: From microbial immune subversion to systemic inflammation. *Nat. Rev. Immunol.* **2015**, *15*, 30–44. [CrossRef]
101. Johansson, A.; Dahlén, G. Bacterial virulence factors that contribute to periodontal pathogenesis. In *Pathogenesis of Periodontal Diseases*; Bostanci, N., Belibasakis, G., Eds.; Springer Nature: Cham, Switzerland, 2018; pp. 31–49. [CrossRef]

Permissions

All chapters in this book were first published by MDPI; hereby published with permission under the Creative Commons Attribution License or equivalent. Every chapter published in this book has been scrutinized by our experts. Their significance has been extensively debated. The topics covered herein carry significant findings which will fuel the growth of the discipline. They may even be implemented as practical applications or may be referred to as a beginning point for another development.

The contributors of this book come from diverse backgrounds, making this book a truly international effort. This book will bring forth new frontiers with its revolutionizing research information and detailed analysis of the nascent developments around the world.

We would like to thank all the contributing authors for lending their expertise to make the book truly unique. They have played a crucial role in the development of this book. Without their invaluable contributions this book wouldn't have been possible. They have made vital efforts to compile up to date information on the varied aspects of this subject to make this book a valuable addition to the collection of many professionals and students.

This book was conceptualized with the vision of imparting up-to-date information and advanced data in this field. To ensure the same, a matchless editorial board was set up. Every individual on the board went through rigorous rounds of assessment to prove their worth. After which they invested a large part of their time researching and compiling the most relevant data for our readers.

The editorial board has been involved in producing this book since its inception. They have spent rigorous hours researching and exploring the diverse topics which have resulted in the successful publishing of this book. They have passed on their knowledge of decades through this book. To expedite this challenging task, the publisher supported the team at every step. A small team of assistant editors was also appointed to further simplify the editing procedure and attain best results for the readers.

Apart from the editorial board, the designing team has also invested a significant amount of their time in understanding the subject and creating the most relevant covers. They scrutinized every image to scout for the most suitable representation of the subject and create an appropriate cover for the book.

The publishing team has been an ardent support to the editorial, designing and production team. Their endless efforts to recruit the best for this project, has resulted in the accomplishment of this book. They are a veteran in the field of academics and their pool of knowledge is as vast as their experience in printing. Their expertise and guidance has proved useful at every step. Their uncompromising quality standards have made this book an exceptional effort. Their encouragement from time to time has been an inspiration for everyone.

The publisher and the editorial board hope that this book will prove to be a valuable piece of knowledge for researchers, students, practitioners and scholars across the globe.

List of Contributors

Se-Yeon Kim and Ji-Soo Kim
Department of Preventive and Community Dentistry, School of Dentistry, Pusan National University, 49 Busandaehak-ro, Yangsan 50612, Korea

Min-Ji Byon and Jin-Bom Kim
Department of Preventive and Community Dentistry, School of Dentistry, Pusan National University, 49 Busandaehak-ro, Yangsan 50612, Korea
BK21 FOUR Project, School of Dentistry, Pusan National University, Yangsan 50612, Korea

Hyun Kyung Kang
Department of Dental Hygiene, Silla University, Baekyang-daero, 700, Sasang-gu, Busan 46958, Korea

Jonas Conrad, Christof Dörfer and Mohamed Mekhemar
Clinic for Conservative Dentistry and Periodontology, School of Dental Medicine, Christian-Albrecht's University, 24105 Kiel, Germany

Jan Retelsdorf
Department of General, Faculty of Education, Intercultural and International Comparative Education University of Hamburg, 20146 Hamburg, Germany

Sameh Attia
Department of Cranio Maxillofacial Surgery, Justus-Liebig University, 35392 Giessen, Germany

Sudhir L. Munasur, Eunice B. Turawa and Alfred Musekiwa
Division of Epidemiology and Biostatistics, Department of Global Health, Faculty of Medicine and Health Sciences, Stellenbosch University, Cape Town 7530, South Africa

Usuf M.E. Chikte
Division of Health Systems and Public Health, Department of Global Health, Faculty of Medicine and Health Sciences, Stellenbosch University, Cape Town 7530, South Africa

Joonas Liukkonen and Ulvi K. Gürsoy
Institute of Dentistry, University of Turku, 20100 Turku, Finland

Eija Könönen
Institute of Dentistry, University of Turku, 20100 Turku, Finland
Oral Health Care, Welfare Division, 20100 Turku, Finland

Timo Sorsa and Kåre Buhlin
Oral and Maxillofacial Diseases, University of Helsinki and Helsinki University Hospital, 00100 Helsinki, Finland
Department of Periodontology, Institute of Odontology, Karolinska Institutet, 12343 Huddinge, Sweden

G. Rutger Persson
Departments of Periodontics and Oral Medicine, University of Washington, Seattle, WA 98101, USA
Department of Periodontology, University of Bern, 3001 Bern, Switzerland

Päivi Mäntylä
Oral and Maxillofacial Diseases, University of Helsinki and Helsinki University Hospital, 00100 Helsinki, Finland
Institute of Dentistry, University of Eastern Finland, 70100 Kuopio, Finland
Oral and Maxillofacial Diseases, Kuopio University Hospital, 70100 Kuopio, Finland

Juha Sinisalo
HUCH Heart and Lung Center, Helsinki University Central Hospital, 00100 Helsinki, Finland

Pirkko J. Pussinen
Institute of Dentistry, University of Turku, 20100 Turku, Finland
Oral and Maxillofacial Diseases, University of Helsinki and Helsinki University Hospital, 00100 Helsinki, Finland

Barbora Konečná and L'ubomíra Tóthová
Institute of Molecular Biomedicine, Faculty of Medicine, Comenius University in Bratislava, 811 08 Bratislava, Slovakia

Alexandra Gaál Kovalčíková
Department of Pediatrics, National Institute of Children's Diseases and Faculty of Medicine, Comenius University in Bratislava, 831 01 Bratislava, Slovakia

Alexandra Pančíková
School of Biological Sciences, University of Edinburgh, Edinburgh EH9 3FF, UK

Bohuslav Novák
Department of Stomatology and Maxillofacial Surgery, Faculty of Medicine, Comenius University, 811 08 Bratislava, Slovakia

Eva Koval'ová
Department of Maxillofacial Surgery and Dental Hygiene of J.A. Reiman Hospital in Prešov, 080 01 Prešov, Slovakia

Peter Celec
Institute of Molecular Biomedicine, Faculty of Medicine, Comenius University in Bratislava, 811 08 Bratislava, Slovakia
Institute of Pathophysiology, Faculty of Medicine, Comenius University in Bratislava, 811 08 Bratislava, Slovakia
Department of Molecular Biology, Faculty of Natural Sciences, Comenius University in Bratislava, 841 04 Bratislava, Slovakia

Nobuhisa Furuse
Department of Periodontology, Nihon University School of Dentistry at Matsudo, Matsudo, Chiba 271-8587, Japan

Hideki Takai and Yorimasa Ogata
Department of Periodontology, Nihon University School of Dentistry at Matsudo, Matsudo, Chiba 271-8587, Japan
Research Institute of Oral Science, Nihon University School of Dentistry at Matsudo, Matsudo, Chiba 271-8587, Japan

Milla Pietiäinen, John M. Liljestrand, Susanna Paju, Aino Salminen, Leo Tjäderhane and Pirkko J. Pussinen
Oral and Maxillofacial Diseases, University of Helsinki and Helsinki University Hospital, FI-00014 Helsinki, Finland

Pratikshya Pradhan-Palikhe
Oral and Maxillofacial Diseases, University of Helsinki and Helsinki University Hospital, 00100 Helsinki, Finland

Ramin Akhi and Sohvi Hörkkö
Medical Microbiology and Immunology, Research Unit of Biomedicine, University of Oulu, FI-90014 Oulu, Finland
Medical Research Center, Oulu University Hospital and University of Oulu, FI-90014 Oulu, Finland
Nordlab, Oulu University Hospital, FI-90220 Oulu, Finland

Kåre Buhlin
Oral and Maxillofacial Diseases, University of Helsinki and Helsinki University Hospital, FI-00014 Helsinki, Finland
Division of Periodontology, Department of Dental Medicine, Karolinska Institutet, S-141 04 Huddinge, Sweden

Päivi Mäntylä
Institute of Dentistry, University of Eastern Finland, FI-70211 Kuopio, Finland
Kuopio University Hospital, Oral and Maxillofacial Diseases, FI-70029 Kuopio, Finland

Juha Sinisalo
HUCH Heart and Lung Center, Helsinki University Hospital, FI-00029 Helsinki, Finland

Yuko Yamamoto
Department of Dental Hygiene, Kanagawa Dental University, Junior College, 82 Inaoka, Yokosuka 2388580, Kanagawa, Japan

Toshiya Morozumi, Takahisa Hirata and Masato Minabe
Division of Periodontology, Department of Oral Interdisciplinary Medicine, Graduate School of Dentistry, Kanagawa Dental University, 82 Inaoka, Yokosuka 2388580, Kanagawa, Japan

Toru Takahashi
Department of Health and Nutrition, Faculty of Human Health, Kanazawa Gakuin University, 10 Sue-machi, Kanazawa 9201392, Ishikawa, Japan

Shinya Fuchida
Department of Disaster Medicine and Dental Sociology, Graduate School of Dentistry, Kanagawa Dental University, 82 Inaoka, Yokosuka 2388580, Kanagawa, Japan

Masami Toyoda and Shigeru Nakajima
Nakajima Internal Medicine Clinic, 1-17 Yonegahamadori, Yokosuka 2380011, Kanagawa, Japan

Gunnar Dahlen, Amina Basic and Johan Bylund
Department of Oral Microbiology and Immunology, Institute of Odontology, Sahlgrenska Academy, University of Gothenburg, SE-40530 Gothenburg, Sweden

Yoshiaki Nomura and Nobuhiro Hanada
Department of Translational Research, Tsurumi University School of Dental Medicine, Yokohama 230-8501, Japan

Mitsuo Fukuda
Department of Periodontology, School of Dentistry, Aichi Gakuin University, Nagoya 464-8650, Japan

Erika Kakuta
Department of Oral Microbiology, Tsurumi University School of Dental Medicine, Yokohama 230-8501, Japan

Hiroaki Kobayashi
Department of Periodontology, Graduate School of Medical and Dental Sciences, Tokyo Medical and Dental University, Tokyo 113-8510, Japan

Toshiaki Nakamura and Kazuyuki Noguchi
Department of Periodontology, Kagoshima University Graduate School of Medical and Dental Sciences, Kagoshima 890-8544, Japan

Yohei Nakayama
Department of Periodontology, Nihon University School of Dentistry at Matsudo, Matsudo 271-8587, Japan

Fusanori Nishimura
Section of Periodontology, Division of Oral Rehabilitation, Faculty of Dental Science, Kyushu University, Fukuoka 819-0395, Japan

Yukihiro Numabe and Satoshi Sekino
Department of Periodontology, School of Life Dentistry at Tokyo, The Nippon Dental University, Tokyo 102-8159, Japan

Atsushi Saito
Department of Periodontology, Tokyo Dental College, Tokyo 101-0061, Japan

Soh Sato
Department of Periodontology, School of life Dentistry at Niigata, The Nippon Dental University, Niigata 951-8580, Japan

Naoyuki Sugano
Department of Periodontology, Nihon University School of Dentistry, Tokyo 101-8310, Japan

Tsutomu Sugaya
Division of Periodontology and Endodontology, Department of Oral Health Science, Hokkaido University Graduate School of Dental Medicine, Sapporo 060-8586, Japan

Fumihiko Suzuki
Division of Dental Anesthesiology, Department of Oral Surgery, Ohu University School of Dentistry, Koriyama 963-8611, Japan

Keiso Takahashi
Division of Periodontics, Department of Conservative Dentistry, Ohu University School of Dentistry, Koriyama 963-8611, Japan

Shogo Takashiba
Department of Pathophysiology-Periodontal Science, Okayama University Graduate School of Medicine, Dentistry and Pharmaceutical Sciences, Okayama 700-8525, Japan

Makoto Umeda
Department of Periodontology, Osaka Dental University, Hirakata 573-1121, Japan

Hiromasa Yoshie
Division of Periodontology, Department of Oral Biological Science, Niigata University Graduate School of Medical and Dental Sciences, Niigata 951-8514, Japan

Atsutoshi Yoshimura
Department of Periodontology and Endodontology, Nagasaki University Graduate School of Biomedical Sciences, Nagasaki 852-8588, Japan

Taneaki Nakagawa
Department of Dentistry and Oral Surgery, School of Medicine, Keio University, Tokyo 60-8582, Japan

Nagihan Bostanci and Georgios N. Belibasakis
Division of Oral Diseases, Department of Dental Medicine, Karolinska Institutet, 14104 Huddinge, Sweden
Center of Dental Medicine, University of Zürich, 8032 Zürich, Switzerland

Toshiharu Abe and George Hajishengallis
Department of Basic and Translational Sciences, School of Dental Medicine, University of Pennsylvania, Philadelphia, PA 19104, USA

Shuichi Sato
Department of Periodontology, Nihon University School of Dentistry, Chiyoda-ku, Tokyo 101-8310, Japan

Norihisa Watanabe and Sho Yokoe
Department of Periodontology, Nihon University School of Dentistry, Chiyoda-ku, Tokyo 101-8310, Japan
Department of Microbiology, Nihon University School of Dentistry, 1-8-13 Kanda-Surugadai, Chiyoda-ku, Tokyo 101-8310, Japan

Kenichi Imai
Department of Microbiology, Nihon University School of Dentistry, 1-8-13 Kanda-Surugadai, Chiyoda-ku, Tokyo 101-8310, Japan

Eija Könönen
Department of Periodontology, Institute of Dentistry, University of Turku, 20520 Turku, Finland
Oral Health Care,Welfare Division, City of Turku, 20101 Turku, Finland

Mervi Gursoy and Ulvi Kahraman Gursoy
Department of Periodontology, Institute of Dentistry, University of Turku, 20520 Turku, Finland

Eduardo Gómez-Bañuelos, Amarshi Mukherjee, Erika Darrah and Felipe Andrade
Division of Rheumatology, The Johns Hopkins University School of Medicine, Baltimore, MD 21224, USA

Yuhei Takayanagi, Takeshi Kikuchi, Hisashi Goto, Kousuke Okada, Iichiro Okabe, Yosuke Kamiya, Yuki Suzuki, Noritaka Sawada, Teppei Okabe, Shun Kondo, Tasuku Ohno, Jun-Ichiro Hayashi and Akio Mitani
Department of Periodontology, School of Dentistry, Aichi Gakuin University, 2-11 Suemoridori, Chikusaku, Nagoya, Aichi 464-8651, Japan

Yoshiaki Hasegawa and Yoshikazu Naiki
Department of Microbiology, School of Dentistry, Aichi Gakuin University, 1-100 Kusumoto-cho, Chikusaku, Nagoya, Aichi 464-8651, Japan

Melissa M. Grant
School of Dentistry, Institute of Clinical Sciences, University of Birmingham and Birmingham Community Healthcare Foundation Trust, Birmingham B5 7EG, UK

Daniel Jönsson
Swedish Dental Service of Skåne, 222 37 Lund, Sweden
Department of Periodontology, Faculty of Odontology, Malmö University, 214 21 Malmö, Sweden

Jan Oscarsson, Rolf Claesson and Mark Lindholm
Department of Odontology, Oral Microbiology, Umeå University, S-90187 Umeå, Sweden

Carola Höglund Åberg and Anders Johansson
Department of Odontology, Molecular Periodontology, Umeå University, S-901 87 Umeå, Sweden

Index

www.ingramcontent.com/pod-product-compliance
Lightning Source LLC
LaVergne TN
LVHW060523210926
848485LV00005B/1133